Magnetic Resonance Scanning and Epilepsy

NATO ASI Series

Advanced Science Institutes Series

A series presenting the results of activities sponsored by the NATO Science Committee, which aims at the dissemination of advanced scientific and technological knowledge, with a view to strengthening links between scientific communities.

The series is published by an international board of publishers in conjunction with the NATO Scientific Affairs Division

A	Life Sciences	Plenum Publishing Corporation
B	Physics	New York and London
C	Mathematical and Physical Sciences	Kluwer Academic Publishers
D	Behavioral and Social Sciences	Dordrecht, Boston, and London
E	Applied Sciences	
F	Computer and Systems Sciences	Springer-Verlag
G	Ecological Sciences	Berlin, Heidelberg, New York, London,
H	Cell Biology	Paris, Tokyo, Hong Kong, and Barcelona
I	Global Environmental Change	

Recent Volumes in this Series

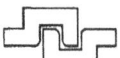

Series A: Life Sciences

Magnetic Resonance Scanning and Epilepsy

Edited by

S. D. Shorvon and D. R. Fish

Institute of Neurology and National Society for Epilepsy
London, United Kingdom

F. Andermann

Montreal Neurological Institute
Montreal, Quebec, Canada

G. M. Bydder

Hammersmith Hospital
London, United Kingdom

and

H. Stefan

University of Erlangen
Erlangen, Germany

Springer Science+Business Media, LLC

Proceedings of a NATO Advanced Research Workshop on
Advanced Magnetic Resonance and Epilepsy,
held October 1–3, 1992,
in Chalfont St. Peter, Buckinghamshire, United Kingdom

NATO-PCO-DATA BASE

The electronic index to the NATO ASI Series provides full bibliographical references (with keywords and/or abstracts) to more than 30,000 contributions from international scientists published in all sections of the NATO ASI Series. Access to the NATO-PCO-DATA BASE is possible in two ways:

—via online FILE 128 (NATO-PCO-DATA BASE) hosted by ESRIN, Via Galileo Galilei, I-00044 Frascati, Italy

—via CD-ROM "NATO Science and Technology Disk" with user-friendly retrieval software in English, French, and German (©WTV GmbH and DATAWARE Technologies, Inc. 1989). The CD-ROM also contains the AGARD Aerospace Database.

The CD-ROM can be ordered through any member of the Board of Publishers or through NATO-PCO, Overijse, Belgium.

Library of Congress Cataloging-in-Publication Data

Magnetic resonance scanning and epilepsy / edited by S.D. Shorvon ...
[et al.].
     p.   cm. -- (NATO ASI series. Series A, Life sciences ; v.
264)
     "Proceedings of a NATO Advanced Research Workshop on Advanced
Magnetic Resonance and Epilepsy, held October 1-3, 1992, in Chalfont
St. Peter, Buckinghamshire, United Kingdom"--T.p. verso.
   Includes bibliographical references and index.
   ISBN 978-0-306-44735-8   ISBN 978-1-4615-2546-2 (eBook)
   DOI 10.1007/978-1-4615-2546-2
   1. Epilepsy--Magnetic resonance imaging--Congresses.   I. Shorvon,
S. D. (Simon D.) II. North Atlantic Treaty Organization.
Scientific Affairs Division. III. NAT) Advanced Research Workshop
on Advanced Magnetic Resonance and Epilepsy (1992 : Buckinghamshire,
England) IV. Series.
   [DNLM: 1. Epilepsy--diagnosis. 2. Magnetic Resonance Imaging.
WL 385 M196 1994]
RC372.A2M34   1994
616.8'5307548--dc20
DNLM/DLC
for Library of Congress   94-33185
                                                             CIP

ISBN 978-0-306-44735-8

© 1994 Springer Springer Science+Business Media New York
Originally published by Plenum Press, New York in 1994

PREFACE

It was only in 1980 that the first recognisable magnetic resonance images of the human brain were published, by Moore and Holland from Nottingham University in England. There then followed a number of clinical trials of brain imaging, the most notable from the Hammersmith Hospital in London using a system designed by EMI, the original manufacturers of the first CT machines. A true revolution in medicine has ensued; in only a few years there are thousands of scanning units, and magnetic resonance imaging (MRI) has assumed a central importance in medical investigation. It is an extraordinary fact that within a few years of development, the esoteric physics of nuclear spin, angular momentum, and magnetic vector precession were harnessed to provide exquisite images of living anatomy; modern science has no greater tribute.

That indisputable king of neurology and the oldest of recorded conditions, epilepsy, has not been untouched by the new technology; indeed, it is our view that the introduction of MRI has been as important to epilepsy as was that of electroencephalography (EEG) in the late 1930s. Now, for the first time, the structural and aetiological basis of the condition is susceptible to thorough investigation, and MRI can provide structural detail to parallel the functional detail of EEG. MRI has the same potential as had EEG over 50 years ago, to provide a new level of understanding of the basic mechanisms, the clinical features and the treatment of epilepsy.

It was against this background that the present volume was conceived. The time seemed right for a review of the current position of MRI and MRS in epilepsy, a summary of current research, and an indication of the likely direction of future research. No single alternative text exists on this topic, and as research crosses the conventional boundaries of disciplines, much original work is not easily accessible to the general reader. The volume contains contributions from neurologists, neurophysiologists, radiologists, physicists and neurosurgeons, from Europe, North America and Australia; we see this drawing together of experience from widely differing backgrounds as an important feature of the work. We have organised the book into sections, each dealing with specific clinical issues, and have throughout attempted closely to apply the subject to the important clinical questions (of diagnosis, treatment, outcome, prevention) as well as the basic issues of pathophysiology and pathogenesis. We hope that the book will be of interest to medical specialists in different disciplines (neurologists, radiologists, neurophysiologists, neurosurgeons, psychiatrists) as well as to physicists working in the field of epilepsy.

Our grateful thanks are extended to the Scientific Division of NATO who saw the importance of the topic, and kindly sponsored the work, and to Ms Carolyn Cowey for her invaluable assistance in preparing this manuscript.

Simon Shorvon, for the editors

CONTENTS

Section 1

Introduction

MAGNETIC RESONANCE IMAGING IN EPILEPSY

The Central Clinical Research Questions

S.D. Shorvon

Institute of Neurology and
National Hospitals for Neurology and Neurosurgery
Queen Square
London, WC1N 3BG

National Society for Epilepsy
Chalfont St. Peter
Bucks, SL9 0RJ
United Kingdom

INTRODUCTION

The advent of magnetic resonance imaging (MRI) seems likely to have as great an impact on clinical epilepsy as did that of electroencephalography (EEG) in the late 1930s. Although the initial reactions to MRI in the imaging of epilepsy were dismissive, after only a few years of further experience its clinical importance became established. The technique was viewed in its initial phase of development simply as a superior alternative to computed tomography (CT). As experience has grown, however, the flexibility of MRI and its potential to provide clinical information well beyond routine imaging are now being recognised. There seems no doubt that clinical practice in epilepsy will be changed, sometimes radically, as MRI is more fully exploited in both the investigation and the treatment.

The purpose of this introductory chapter is to point to those clinical research questions which seem, to the author at least, to be those that will be most appropriately addressed over the next five years or so. This is inevitably a personal view, coloured by and biased towards my own experience of MRI research, but will I hope form a framework for approaching the wider issues of MRI research in epilepsy. Clinical research in MRI only will be considered, and not the equally exciting physics research questions, MR spectroscopy or experimental epilepsy research which are discussed in later chapters.

Clinical MRI research in epilepsy should be essentially goal-directed, and applied to one or more of the following five issues:

Magnetic Resonance Scanning and Epilepsy, Edited by S.D. Shorvon et al.,
Plenum Press, New York, 1994

    i. Detection and diagnosis.
    ii. Pathophysiology and pathogenesis.
    iii. Treatment (surgical and medical).
    iv. Prognosis and outcome.
    v. Prevention.

The more directly these questions are addressed, the more useful the research is. The tendency to explore unfocused questions (the MRI equivalent of computer games) should be strongly resisted. The research undertaken should be feasible and practicable, in terms of both time and scrutiny of resources, and be susceptible to audit and clinical cost-effectiveness. In this chapter, a general overview is taken; many questions are posed and no attempt is made to set these in order of priority, although this too should be a concern of any research programmes.

THE AETIOLOGICAL BASIS OF EPILEPSY

The first task allotted to MRI on its introduction into clinical practice was to determine aetiology, this being an obvious choice. Initial research papers were concerned with a comparison of the ability of MRI and CT to detect cerebral tumours and other structural cerebral lesions; the superiority of MRI in this regard soon became apparent. MRI epilepsy research then largely turned its attention to mesial temporal sclerosis (MTS), and more recently has been widened to consider other aetiological factors.

Mesial Temporal Sclerosis

The pathology of this condition is associated with (and probably the cause of) many cases of focal epilepsy. Except when very severe, it was undetectable in vivo prior to MRI. Because of the insensitivity of imaging with CT (or other imaging modalities), diagnosis previously had to be largely inferred from EEG, which as a functional measure is unsuited at a fundamental level to structural diagnosis. MRI has already demonstrated its effectiveness in the detection of MTS, using both anatomical and signal intensity measures, and the routine features of MTS on images are now largely defined. The following research questions should now be addressed, many of which have important implications for surgical therapy.

    i. What are the most sensitive and specific MRI signs of MTS? Most emphasis has been placed on anatomical and volumetric imaging: is this more or less reliable (sensitive and specific) than measures of signal intensity? In this regard, it will be especially important to relate the imaging features to pathological findings, using "blind" investigators. The extent to which false positives occur, the importance of concordance with other investigations (e.g. EEG), the degree to which these measures can be detected by eye without recourse to objective measurement, and the reliability of the MRI methods need to be established.

    ii. Can bilateral MTS be reliably determined? Most studies to date have used side to side comparisons, a potentially insensitive and unreliable method if pathology is bilateral. Attempts to quantify volumes in absolute rather than relative terms have not so far proved fruitful, although early work on quantitation of signal intensity has shown promise.

    iii. What are the electroclinical correlations of MTS? Prior to MRI, the full range of clinical correlations of MTS could not be determined. Clinicopathological correlation has previously been carried out only on epilepsy surgery material, a highly biased sample. Furthermore, atrophy confined to localised regions of the amygdalohippocampal structures is now detectable, and early work suggests that the electroclinical correlations of anterior, posterior or diffuse sclerosis may differ as may those of bilateral MTS.

iv. Are there different types of MTS which can be defined by MRI?   It has been suggested that there are several pathological subtypes of MTS, perhaps with differing causations. The MRI features of these subtypes may differ, and correlation of imaging and pathological findings will be necessary to determine the reliability of MRI in detecting pathological differences.

v. What are the causative mechanisms of MTS?   Over the past 30 years, there has been an inconclusive debate about whether or not MTS is a congenital or an acquired lesion (secondary to a febrile convulsion, ongoing seizure activity or status epilepticus). Serial MRI scanning following febrile seizures, in the early years of epilepsy or after status epilepticus, will help resolve this question. The presence of extrahippocampal abnormalities (e.g. dysplastic cortex, abnormal gyration, loss of white/grey matter boundary definition, ectopic neurons) in cases of MTS also needs further evaluation, as evidence of a congenital causation, and as a factor influencing surgical outcome.

Foreign Tissue Lesions

The first application of MRI to epilepsy was to detect cerebral tumours and other foreign tissue lesions, and the superiority of MRI over all other imaging methods is no longer in doubt. The avoidance of bony artefact, the increased tissue contrast and the ability to image in any plane are important advantages of MRI over CT. The detection of lesions depends on both anatomical and image intensity imaging, and detection can be maximised by manipulating imaging methods. The ability to change hardware and software parameters adds a further dimension to MRI research: the use of volumetric 1.5 T acquisition of thin (< 5 mm) T1-weighted contiguous image slices, for instance, allows reformatting in any plane and images of excellent anatomical detail.

Cerebral Tumours

Using conventional sequences, both benign and malignant cerebral tumours are diagnosed reliably. The small indolent gliomas in the temporal lobe are well shown, a particular advantage over CT which often misses these lesions. Research questions include the following.

i. Can the anatomical extent of the tumour be clearly determined?   The accuracy of MRI in determining the extent of tumour tissue is still uncertain. A difficult problem concerns the differentiation of tumour from surrounding oedema and tissue reaction. The use of differing MRI sequences may help in this regard.

ii. Can the pathological nature of the tumour or its degree of malignancy be reliably determined by MRI?   The tissue characteristics of the lesion or the spectroscopic patterns may assist in differentiating the types of tumour and also in grading malignancy.

iii. What proportion of tumours goes undetected by MRI and for what reasons? A few cerebral tumours may be missed by anatomical imaging or by signal intensity measures. It is not known how often this occurs, and whether or not this is due to the inherent imaging characteristics of some types of pathology.

Cerebral Haemorrhage and Infarction

Stroke accounts for many cases of late-onset epilepsy. Vascular pathology is well demonstrated by MRI, but the imaging correlates of vascular epilepsy are not well defined.

i. To what extent do vascular changes cause late-onset epilepsy in patients without a history of overt stroke?   CT studies showed subclinical vascular changes in patients with late-onset epilepsy without stroke. The use of MRI should allow accurate assessment of the extent of such changes, and the characteristics of the vascular disease. This might assist early detection and prevention.

ii. What are the anatomical features of stroke which result in epilepsy?   The site, size and nature of the cerebral damage in stroke vary. The characterisation of those aspects which result in epilepsy would help elucidate the pathogenesis of epilepsy in stroke, and might assist in treatment or prevention.

Arteriovenous Malformations and Other Vascular Lesions

As with tumours, using appropriate sequences, MRI will detect vascular lesions with greater sensitivity than CT. Indeed, it is now clear that the importance of these vascular lesions underlying focal epilepsy was underestimated prior to MRI. MRI has proved particularly useful in demonstrating small arteriovenous malformations especially in the temporal lobe and cavernous haemangiomas (cavernomas), both of which were often invisible on CT or angiography. Important research questions include the following.

i. What is the natural history of these vascular lesions?   It is not clear to what extent some types of vascular lesions grow in size, what the risks of bleeding are, or the extent to which new cavernous haemangiomas develop during adult life. Answers to these questions are important for making rational decisions about surgery or prognosis.

ii. What aspects predispose to epilepsy?   A particular issue concerns the significance of haemosiderin at the edges of the vascular lesions (often a sign of previous haemorrhage or leakage of blood).

iii. Are venous haemangiomas pathological?   It is unclear to what extent venous haemangiomas cause epilepsy or whether they other pathological states, or are simply normal variants. A study of their occurrence and electroclinical correlates should help resolve this question.

Congenital Anomalies

Only the largest structural congenital anomalies were detectable by CT or other pre-MRI imaging methods. With appropriate sequencing and reformatting, MRI, can however, detect even subtle anatomical variation in the cerebral cortex and pathological white matter states. Some congenital metabolic disorders alter chemistry in a way that can be detected by MR spectroscopy. The sensitivity of MRI in the detection and characterisation of the congenital abnormalities underlying epilepsy is only just being recognised. It seems likely that many apparently "idiopathic" or "cryptogenic" epilepsies do in fact have a congenital structural basis. Important research questions include the following.

i. What are the electroclinical features of the various types of congenital structural anomaly? Although the features of the gross lesions are more or less understood from previous pathological studies (e.g. corpus callosal agenesis, hemimegencephaly, agyria etc.), less severe anomalies have been largely undetectable and this has prevented systematic study. The cortical dysplasias and other neuronal migration disorders are examples of pathologies likely to be of particular importance in cryptogenic epilepsy. The optimal modes of detecting dysplasia have not yet been determined, and scanning methods are improving. With new imaging techniques, it is probable that a range of new congenital syndromes will be revealed.

ii. What are the frequency and range of types of congenital structural anomalies underlying epilepsy? The application of MRI to large numbers of patients with epilepsy and to unselected patient populations will for the first time provide an accurate estimate of the range and frequency of the differing structural lesions (including mesial temporal sclerosis dysplasias and migrational disorders) underlying epilepsy.

iii. What are the features of congenital metabolic disorders? The same questions arise with regard to the congenital metabolic disorders without gross structural change. MRI can detect white matter signal intensity changes in many such conditions, as well as anatomical abnormalities. MR spectroscopy also has the potential to detect diagnostic biochemical changes and to provide a method for monitoring progress or treatment. These are areas in which only preliminary research has so far been undertaken.

iv. Will imaging in utero permit early investigation of congenital anomalies? MRI in utero will detect congenital anomalies and can potentially also be used to monitor fetal development. This technique could provide data of theoretical and practical importance, which could allow: the early detection of fetal malformation or congenital metabolic disorders, the study of fetal development, the identification of aetiological agents, and ultimately prevention.

Atrophies and Other Cerebral-destructive Aetiologies

Cerebral damage can be caused by trauma, infection, perinatal injury and ischaemia. These result in atrophy, neuronal loss and gliosis—pathological changes that are well visualised by MRI, causing both volume and signal intensity changes. Very little specific MRI epilepsy research has so far been carried out on these pathologies, other than to define their usual imaging features. This is partly because surgical therapy is generally disappointing, because the epileptogenic zones associated with these lesions are often wide or diffuse.

THE CLASSIFICATION OF EPILEPSY

Since the advent of EEG, the classifications of epilepsy have been dominated by clinical and electrographic correlation. The structural or aetiological bases of epilepsy have been largely ignored, not least because, before the advent of MRI, there was no sensitive method of investigation. Epilepsy has both structural and functional features, and there is now a need to reevaluate clinical classification, in its broadest sense, in the light of the structural/aetiological basis of epilepsy. Quite where this will lead is unclear. It may improve treatment by providing more specific clinical categorisation, allow more accurate prognostication and lead to prevention.

THE STRUCTURAL BASIS OF EPILEPSY

MRI provides an unrivalled method for visualising brain structure. Anatomical detail is exquisitely demonstrated, and to a certain extent tissue can be characterised by signal intensity measures and spectroscopy. Modern techniques such as the volumetric acquisition of thin contiguous T1-weighted slices, two-dimensional and three-dimensional reformatting, and surface rendering have all enhanced the ability of MRI to display anatomy; because epilepsy is essentially a disease of grey matter, the anatomical information provided about the cerebral cortex (both archicortex and neocortex) has proved especially valuable.

i. What are the limits of normal anatomical variation? The identification of anatomical abnormalities in epilepsy depends on a knowledge of normal variation. A databank of normal volumetric and morphometric data is required for (1) the cerebral neocortex, (2) the hippocampus and amygdala, and (3) other deep nuclei. The normal variation in the size, shape and position of gyri and sulci needs to be established. Quantitative measures (for instance, of signal intensity) of cortex and white matter are also required. These measures should be age matched, and the extent of side to side variation should also be assessed. These data already exist in part, but definitive databanks are lacking. From the anatomical point of view, the importance of thin and contiguous imaging slices must be emphasised to avoid partial volume effects and to maximise the accuracy of volumetric or surface area measures. Some anatomical structures of interest in epilepsy may have complex shapes with edges that are difficult to differentiate (e.g. the border of the amygdala and hippocampus, the posterior fornices); these sources of potential inaccuracy should be recognised and arbitrary boundaries agreed.

ii. To what extent is anatomy altered in idiopathic epilepsy? There are indications that deviations from normal gyral and sulcal patterns may occur in patients with apparently idiopathic epilepsy, perhaps on the basis of subtle developmental changes. Disorders of the process of neuronal migration range from microdysgenesis seen only at the microscopic level to gross cerebral disruption. Using new MRI analytical techniques, it is possible that even the subtle forms of cerebral anomaly will be detected. The extent to which such changes underlie epilepsy, the type of epilepsy, and the clinical and investigatory correlations are quite unknown.

iii. In what situations and to what extent does epilepsy result in cerebral damage? The clinical importance of acquired cerebral damage in epilepsy is unknown, but a number of issues arise:

(a) It has been suggested that severe seizures (e.g. early childhood convulsions, convulsive status epilepticus, seizures with anoxia) may result directly in cerebral damage, but firm evidence is lacking.

(b) Drug treatment has been implicated in cerebral atrophy and in various psychometric disturbances. MRI has also already been used to assess the intramyelinic vacuolation due to vigabatrin therapy.

(c) Kindling and secondary epileptogenesis are phenomena which are readily observable in experimental models of epilepsy, but which are of unknown significance in humans.

(d) In a proportion of patients with epilepsy, intellectual decline occurs, often of memory or other specific functions, and sometimes this is progressive. The physiological and anatomical basis of this decline is uncertain.

Serial MRI scanning with quantitative measurement provide, for the first time, the potential for visualising and measuring these changes in a clinical setting. Potential measurements include those of signal intensity and volumetric anatomical measures (e.g. of atrophy). The relation of scanning changes to clinical parameters will help elucidate the mechanisms of cerebral damage, and possibly their prevention.

iv. Can MRI help define the anatomical basis of epileptogenesis?   The functional process of human epileptogenesis is complex. On the assumption that these functional changes have structural correlates, MRI might have a role in elucidating underlying mechanisms. Research issues include:

(a) Studies of the anatomical changes underlying generalised epilepsy. Widely differing anatomical changes have been proposed, including cortical microdysgenesis, deep thalamic pacemaker changes or widespread cortical biochemical abnormalities. MRI studies using volumetric or signal intensity measures or MR spectroscopy may provide a method of investigating these possibilities.

(b) The anatomical basis of focal epileptogenesis is also ill-understood. The minimum extent of neuronal aggregates and the neuronal systems necessary to sustain focal epilepsy are not known; they may be susceptible to MRI investigation.

(c) Methods for defining the extent of the epileptogenic zone would be invaluable in planning surgical resection. Signal intensity, volumetric quantitation and functional imaging may be useful in defining epileptogenic areas.

(d) Seizures spread along well-defined pathways, and these pathways may be identifiable, at least in part, using functional imaging techniques, diffusion or flow scanning.

iv. What degree of inaccuracy occurs in MRI anatomical measures?   This is an important question for the use of MRI in epilepsy surgery, where accuracy in resection and in depth electrode placement is crucial. The MR image is subject to deformation and distortion, which depends upon the characteristics of the magnetic field, the sequences used, and other hard and software considerations. Brain structures also move during the respiratory cycle, and errors are introduced due to imaging parameters (e.g. partial volume effects). Research is needed to quantify and develop methods of imaging to minimise these errors. The ability to carry out postoperative MRI allows the accuracy of surgical method to be gauged, but not any inherent or internal inaccuracies due to MRI methodology.

THE SURGICAL TREATMENT OF EPILEPSY

Any investigatory method which can define cerebral structural changes is of course potentially useful surgically, and MRI has indeed already had a major impact in epilepsy surgery. Current research is focusing on the use of MRI for defining indications for surgery/improving outcome, and refining surgical technique.

Temporal Lobectomy for Mesial Temporal Sclerosis

MRI is now indispensable in the investigation of temporal lobe epilepsy. As outlined above, volumetric studies can demonstrate small degrees of atrophy and define the exact position of the atrophy within the hippocampus, and quantitative studies may be able to detect bilateral changes. Questions which arise include the following.

i. Is the surgical outcome of temporal lobectomy related to the pattern of atrophy/signal change on MRI?   The outcome of surgical resection of mesial temporal structures can now be related to such factors as: the overall extent (volume) of the hippocampal resection (which can be measured by postoperative MRI), the completeness of resection of atrophic areas, the severity of the MRI changes, and unilateral resection in cases where quantitative MRI measures suggest bilateral disease. These are potentially important prognostic factors which require evaluation.

ii. Is the surgical outcome of temporal lobectomy influenced more by MRI or EEG findings, in cases where data are discordant? Not infrequently, patients with temporal lobe epilepsy are encountered in whom MRI atrophy is demonstrated with discordant EEG (or psychometric or clinical) data. The relative importance of the EEG (functional) and MRI (structural) data is of great interest from both clinical and theoretical points of view.

iii. Does outcome differ in the selective temporal lobe operations and the standard temporal lobectomy? This question is best considered in relation to the pre- and post-operative MRI findings, to ensure standard comparisons. A large multicentre clinical trial will be necessary satisfactorily to address this issue.

Resective Surgery For Foreign Tissue Lesions

MRI can define lesions preoperatively and the extent of resection post-operatively with a precision that is not possible with previous imaging methods. Thus, questions of surgical indication and outcome can be clearly related to anatomical and structural issues.

i. How is the surgical outcome for resective surgery related to the degree of resection? It will be important to relate surgical outcome to such issues as: the completeness of lesional resection, the extent of resection of the epileptogenic zone, and the nature of the pathology. For vascular lesions, it is not clear whether resection of surrounding haemosiderin-stained tissue influences outcome.

Other Surgical Therapy

Issues related to the extent and nature of resection have to date dominated clinical surgical research in MRI. Other areas of research include:

(a) The display by MRI of pre-operative and post-operative anatomical detail for corpus callosal section, multiple subpial transections and invasive EEG electrode placement should greatly improve the accuracy of the procedures and post-operative surgical assessment.

(b) The study of the pathways of seizure spread may allow surgical intervention which aims to interrupt pathways rather than to resect seizure foci. Stereotactic lesioning, focused radiotherapy and the stereotactic infusion of anticonvulsant compounds are all potential methods of interest. This is an exciting area of future surgical research which is currently in its infancy.

(c) If MRI methods for the identification of the extent or even the severity of the epileptogenic zone were found to be reliable, this would also have a great impact on the surgical approaches to neocortical epilepsy.

Surgical Technique

The surgical techniques employed in epilepsy surgery have been modified since the introduction of MRI in a number of ways.

(a)   As indicated above, the ability to measure pre- and post-operative resection volumes and the ability to assess the accuracy of resection are important research tools.

(b)   The detailed display of anatomy and aetiology by MRI has also allowed novel stereotactic surgical methods. MRI stereotaxy is now used in tailored resections, in biopsy and in EEG depth electrode placement. Research in this field is likely to concentrate upon: an assessment of the limits of accuracy of MRI stereotaxy (compared to CT stereotaxy); the potential for frameless stereotaxy, a technique which has not as yet been refined sufficiently for clinical practice; the development of new stereotactic methods for electrode implantation; the application of stereotactic surgical methods currently used in tumour surgery to resective epilepsy surgery.

(c)   MRI imaging data can now be coregistered with data from other modalities (including CT, angiography, positron emission tomography (PET), single photon emission computerised tomography (SPECT), EEG). These coregistered data can be displayed using two or three-dimensional techniques, for surgical purposes. The surgical value of coregistered data requires assessment; although this is clear, for instance, in the use of coregistered angiographic data to guide electrode placement, no specific advantage has yet accrued from coregistered PET or SPECT data. The coregistration of EEG data, particularly from invasive EEG, is a method of potential value for defining the extent of the epileptogenic zone or the pathways of seizure spread. The use of MR angiography may supersede that of conventional contrast angiograms, a development which will render redundant the coregistration of MRI and contrast angiographic data.

(d)   Peroperative MRI will be possible in the future, allowing the surgeon to monitor the anatomical aspects of the operation during its course, improving surgical precision.

CORRELATION OF MRI FINDINGS WITH DATA FROM OTHER INVESTIGATIONS

Correlation of the findings from MRI and those of CT, EEG, magnetic electroencephalogram (MEG), PET, SPECT and other imaging modalities is now possible. This can be enhanced by computerised on-screen co-registration, by two- or three-dimensional display, or by quantitative statistical methods. How useful such correlative studies will be depends on the research questions being addressed, and there is a danger of producing redundant (often highly visual) information. Furthermore, because the anatomical and structural detail of MRI is superior to other modalities, co-registration to improve anatomical information is not required The co-registration of functional (whether this be based on neurophysiological (EEG, MEG) or blood flow/metabolism (SPECT, PET) data) and structural data carries promise in epilepsy which has functional and structural elements; however ictal rather than inter-ictal functional data are likely to yield more interesting research data. Where this will take epilepsy research, and which questions will be addressed by such developments are as yet unclear.

The correlation of MRI and psychometric data is another area of great interest, with potential for elucidating the structural basis of psychometric function. In epilepsy this will be important:

(a) as part of pre-surgical assessment;
(b) in understanding the effects of childhood epilepsy on the development of brain function;
(c) in monitoring the effects of ongoing epilepsy on established brain function.

NEW DEVELOPMENTS IN MRI TECHNIQUE

The clinical questions posed above require a range of imaging approaches. A great advantage of MRI is its flexibility, and the physics-based capability to vary both image acquisition and post-processing parameters. The application of the appropriate technique requires an understanding of the advantages and limitations of each method, and thus inevitably, a grasp of basic physics as well as clinical and anatomical issues is required. The following gives those technical developments that we most likely (in the author's view at least) to be of value in clinical imaging research in epilepsy.

New Imaging Parameters

There is considerable scope for the use of novel imaging parameters to address specific problems in epilepsy, examples include (1) the use of long T2-weighted sequences such as FLAIR for demonstrating subtle cortical changes, and multiecho decay; (2) magnetisation transfer contrast scanning, an alternative to measuring T2 decay, which may be useful to quantify the density of abnormal tissue, and for demonstrating tissue breakdown or gliosis; and (3) the use of diffusion-weighted scanning, another method of great promise in its application to epilepsy, which, by measuring spatial restriction in flow, can potentially identify seizure pathways.

Echo Planar Imaging

This imaging method allows very fast image acquisition, and is likely to be of benefit especially in functional imaging and in serial imaging studies. This method is now possible on 1.5 T machines. Image quality currently is suboptimum, but has the potential for improvement.

Three Dimensional Analysis

This post-processing technology is now available, and is likely to be of great assistance in anatomical imaging, especially of the cerebral cortex. Methods to make quantitative measures from three-dimensional data, and to assess the accuracy of volumetric assessments are required.

Other Post-processing Methods

The mathematical manipulation of digitally acquired MRI images can provide another level of MRI analysis. Fractal analysis of the grey-white matter junction has already been shown to be of value in clinical imaging, and other post-processing methods may be of similar potential benefit, including image analysis using mathematical morphology, shape analysis, textural analysis and tissue characterisation.

Functional MRI Imaging

Functional imaging of bolus injections of gadolinium or non-invasive cerebral blood volume, and changes in blood oxygenation and flow are now possible. These can be carried out on conventional MRI machines, but are easier and more sensitive on high field or echoplanar scanners. Superimposition of the functional image onto conventional anatomical images provides data of great potential interest in epilepsy.

Chemical Shift Imaging and Spectroscopy

Proton and phosphorus spectroscopy have provided information of limited value in clinical epilepsy to date. Chemical shift imaging may provide more useful clinical information, and other spectroscopic techniques also show promise, including carbon-13, fluorine-19 and carbon-23 imaging. The spectra from gamma-aminobutyric acid (GABA) and glutamate are now possible to identify, and serial biochemical measures to identify drug effects are a promising area of future research. Labelling of biochemical compounds or drugs may also allow their regional quantitation in brain.

THE ANATOMICAL BASES OF THE EPILEPSIES AND MRI

Implications for MRI

D.R. Fish

Institute of Neurology and
The National Hospitals for Neurology and Neurosurgery
Queen Square
London, WC1N 3BG
United Kingdom

INTRODUCTION

An understanding of the anatomical bases of the epilepsies is crucially important in order to evaluate the immense impact that MR offers in this domain. Historically, and with good pragmatic justification, the epilepsies have been divided into primary generalised and partial (with or without secondary generalisation).

Until recently the primary generalised epilepsies were not recognised to be associated with discrete pathological abnormalities. They are characterised by epileptic discharges that usually appear bilaterally, synchronously and with an anterior predominance. Different schools of thought attributed this pattern to either an undisclosed central generator (such as the thalamus) or a widespread primary cortical event. Although their neurophysiological basis remains uncertain, it has now become apparent that at least some patients with primary generalised epilepsy may harbour widespread subtle cortical dysplastic abnormalities (see Chapter 23). For the most part these are only apparent on detailed microscopic analysis of post-mortem human tissue, and therefore would not normally be expected to be detectable with current in vivo MR techniques. However, although in its infancy, more detailed methods of post-processing MRI may yet offer the opportunity to detect subtle variations in gyral architecture associated with such underlying changes (see Chapter 7).

At the present time the main impact of MRI is likely to be in pre-surgical evaluation or classification of partial epilepsies, and the remainder of this chapter will address the anatomical basis of this type of seizure disorder.

Magnetic Resonance Scanning and Epilepsy, Edited by S.D. Shorvon et al.,
Plenum Press, New York, 1994

Definitions

The "epileptogenic zone" is usually considered as a hypothetical brain region corresponding to the minimum amount of tissue that needs to be resected in order to render the patient seizure free. It is useful to consider it in terms of three major components (see Figure 1):

(1) The epileptic lesion—this is the pathological abnormality (e.g. a foreign tissue lesion or hippocampal sclerosis) responsible for the patient developing epilepsy.

(2) The cerebral regions responsible for the various electro-clinical findings. These can be subdivided into:

    (a) the epileptic pacemaker—the brain region from which the ictal electrographic onset is generated.

    (b) the symptomogenic zone—the brain region which becomes active during the seizure to produce the typical features of the habitual clinical attack.

    (c) the irritative zone—the brain region responsible for the generation of the inter-ictal spike field.

(3) The functional deficit—the area of brain with associated functional impairments such as those defined by neuropsychometry or cerebral perfusion studies.

These three zones are often overlapping or adjacent, but at times there are marked incongruities. It remains uncertain how much contribution each of these three regions makes to the minimum neuronal aggregate that needs to be resected to render the patient seizure free. However, historical series provide an important insight into their relative contributions, placing particular emphasis on removal of the pathological lesion.

The modern era of epilepsy surgery began more than 100 years ago. At that time case selection was dependent upon clinical signs: either fixed neurological deficits or focal ictal phenomena such as unilateral jerking. In consequence many of the earlier cases had abnormalities in or around the primary motor cortex. The advent of the EEG some 50 years later was a major step forward, allowing a new dimension of localisation. However, the logic of the epileptologist remained confined to the prediction of pathology (both type and location) from the electroclinical features or functional characteristics. Most of the lesions were too small or subtle to be visualised by CT or even early MRI. The former had an estimated pick-up rate in pre-surgical candidates of the order of 5–10% and the latter of approximately 30% depending upon methodologies and patient populations.

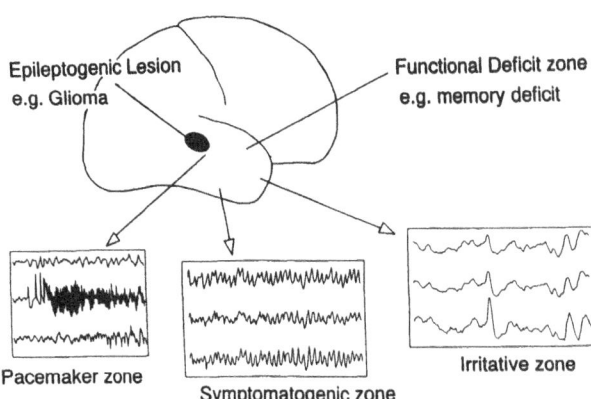

Epileptogenic Lesion
e.g. Glioma

Functional Deficit zone
e.g. memory deficit

Pacemaker zone

Symptomatogenic zone

Irritative zone

Figure 1. Schematic representation of the different areas which may be used to describe the epileptogenic abnormalities.

Review of the surgical series with post-operative follow-up reveals that pathology has two important influences on outcome; these relate to the nature of the pathology and the extent of its resection (see Cascino et al., 1993 for review).

In broad terms the most favourable lesional pathologies are low-grade gliomas and dysembryoplastic neuroepithelial tumours. These have proved difficult to distinguish pathologically in some earlier series. Kirkpatrick et al. (1993) reported that 78% of 36 temporal lobe cases with such indolent tumours were seizure free following resection. Similarly, Daumas-Duport et al. (1988) reported 75% of 39 patients with dysembryoplastic neuroepithelial tumours (DNT) were seizure free at long-term follow-up. In both these papers there was a suggestion that a good outcome could be seen with a microscopically incomplete resection, although presumably the main bulk of the tumour was usually removed. The outcome from vascular lesions is more variable, presumably reflecting their pathological and anatomical diversity. In a mixed series of such cases, Yeh et al. (1990) reported that 78% of 27 such patients became seizure free following surgery. Clinical experience suggests that small single cavernomas have a more favourable outcome than large or more complex vascular anomalies. The outcome of surgery for gross cortical dysplasia appears to be less favourable. In a large recent series from Montreal, Palmini et al. (1991), reported that only 2 of 24 (8%) were seizure free following surgery, although a much larger proportion had some reduction in seizure frequency. Failure to demonstrate a major effect of pathological lesion type on outcome in some other series may have reflected the histological categorisations used, failure to take account of the extent of their removal or limited numbers of cases in each pathological category (e.g. Awad et al., 1991). However, reviewing the early series of Rasmussen (1975), it is still noticeable that slightly higher seizure-free rates were observed in patients with small nodular lesions or vascular lesions (56%), than with astrocytomas or other relatively low-grade tumours (43%), whereas more malignant lesions such as glioblastomas had an inferior outcome (10% seizure free).

In patients with hippocampal sclerosis the prognosis for post-operative seizure control is generally good (Falconer et al., 1964; Davidson and Falconer, 1975; Engel et al., 1975, Jensen and Klinken, 1976; Babb and Brown, 1987) with some of the variability perhaps related to differing definitions; however, overall it is probably slightly less favourable than that of small indolent tumours. For example, seizure-free rates of 14 of 24 (Davidson and Falconer, 1975), and 16 of 19 (Duncan and Sagar, 1987) have been reported.

Although the outcome of epilepsy surgery appears to depend at least in part on the precise nature of the underlying pathology, it is clear that the finding of "normal" pathology in the resected specimen usually carries a poor prognosis for both the behavioural and the seizure outcome. For example, Green and Scheetz (1964) reported that 26 of 34 patients with hippocampal sclerosis became independent following temporal lobectomy, whereas only 1 of 14 with normal pathology did so. Davidson and Falconer (1975) reported significant behavioural improvement or normalisation in 17 of 24 children with hippocampal sclerosis, but this did not occur in any of the 7 children with normal pathology. Similarly, in patients with normal or non-specific pathology in the resected tissue, seizure-free rates of, for example, 1 of 7 (Davidson and Falconer, 1975), 1 of 7 (Duncan and Sagar, 1987) and 1 of 7 (Adler et al., 1991) have been reported. Review of 118 children with medically intractable frontal or temporal lobe epilepsy who underwent surgery at the Montreal Neurological Institute confirmed the prognostic importance of establishing the aetiology, and of identifying pathological abnormalities that should be detected by MRI in this age group (Fish et al., 1993). Of course, caution should be exercised in considering some series in which pathological tissue may have been removed without histological examination (e.g. use of suction/piecemeal resection), if detailed analysis of the tissue was not provided (e.g. cell counts in hippocampal specimens), or if the proportion of seizure-free cases was not described.

The second major contribution of pathology relates to the extent of its resection. Awad et al. (1991) reported the outcome of surgery in 47 patients with lesions undergoing epilepsy surgery. Removal of the lesion was classified as complete (18 patients), partial (23 patients) or none (6 patients). Extent of the lesion resection correlated with post-operative seizure outcome ($P < 0.003$ two-level outcome, $P < 0.002$ three-level outcome): 16 of 18 with a complete removal, 9 of 23 with a partial removal and 2 of 6 with no removal of the lesion became seizure free. The results of lesional epilepsy surgery have been encouraging (Cascino et al., 1990), with seizure-free rates of up to 83% reported (Boon et al., 1991).

The importance of removal of the pathology remains clear even when the EEG abnormalities are incongruent with the pathological lesion (e.g. Awad et al., 1991; Clarke et al., 1992; Williamson et al., 1992). For example, Fish et al. (1991) reported disappointing results in 20 patients with complex partial seizures and surgically inaccessible lesions in whom the EEG-defined areas of abnormality were resected (anterior temporal lobectomy for posterior lesions). None remained seizure free at follow-up of more than 2 years, 5 had > 95% seizure reduction, 5 had 50–95% seizure reduction, but 50% showed no improvement. Conversely, the following year Clarke et al. (1992) reported a favourable outcome in 20 similar patients from the same institution with incongruent EEG and imaging findings in whom the surgery was directed at the pathological lesion: 6 remained seizure free at follow-up of more than 2 years, 13 > 95% reduction in seizures (or seizure free at less than 2 years follow-up), and only one was not improved. Similarly, Williamson et al. (1992) reported excellent results in 10 patients with parietal lesions treated by lesionectomy, in whom the EEG findings were largely unhelpful or discordant.

The ability of MRI to detect the underlying pathological epileptic lesion is of crucial importance to our understanding of the mechanisms of epilepsy and the planning of rational surgical treatment. In our experience detection rates have been high using a volumetric SPGR sequence with the ability to reconstruct 1.5 mm contiguous slices throughout the whole brain, in addition to routine scanning protocols (see Table 1).Eighty-four of the abnormalities were demonstrated on volumetric imaging; one patient had multiple lesions demonstrated on gadolinium enhanced and heavily T2-weighted MRI, one being a cavernoma.

Obviously the exact proportion of cases in each category will depend upon the patient population. However, it is apparent that the main improvement in detection has come with the recognition of the two common, but often subtle, pathologies, i.e. hippocampal sclerosis and cortical dysplasia.

PROBABLE DEVELOPMENT OVER THE NEXT FIVE YEARS

Future MR work in this domain is likely to concentrate on enhancing the following:

(1) The pick-up rate of lesions (are there really no pathological abnormalities in 15% of cases, or do these represent subtle cortical dysgeneses/gliosis or atrophies?).
(2) The nature and precise extent of pathologies (including dual or multiple lesions).
(3) The characteristics of secondary changes (e.g. hippocampal atrophy in neocortical lesions).

This will require continued improvements in the anatomical resolution of MRI. In addition it remains of fundamental importance to consider why structural lesions cause seizures, and whether the mechanisms differ between pathologies. High-resolution MRI may allow a more rational classification of the partial epilepsies by pathology as well as the conventional use of the electroclinical features. In patients being evaluated for surgery, MRI will radically change the agenda. It will be necessary to determine, for each MRI and clinically defined category, which tests add information that alters the decision-making process or the surgical outcome.

Table 1. The Principal MRI Findings in 100 Adults with Chronic Partial Epilepsy (94 CT Negative)

Presumed Pathology	Number of Cases (n = 100)
Hippocampal sclerosis	38
Cortical dysgeneses	17
Small vascular lesion	11
DNT	7
Large arteriovenous malfunction	6
Post-traumatic	3
Glioma	2
Porencephalic cyst	1
Total abnormal	85
Normals	15

Clearly in some (e.g. parietal lesions, indolent tumours), MRI will be of dominant importance, whereas in others (e.g. dual pathologies) functional techniques will remain crucial. MR spectroscopy or other functional techniques may be more fruitful in terms of considering the mechanisms responsible for the lesions causing epileptic activity.

REFERENCES

Adler, J., Erba, G., Winston, K.R., Welch, K., and Lombroso, C.T., 1991, Result of extratemporal partial epilepsy that began in childhood, Arch Neurol 48: 133–140.

Awad, I.A., Rosenfeld, J., Ahl, H., Hahn, J.F. and Luders, H., 1991, Intractable epilepsy and structural lesions in the brain: mapping, resection strategies and seizure outcome, Epilepsia 32: 179–186.

Babb, T.L., and Brown, W.J., 1987, Pathological findings in epilepsy, in: "Surgical Treatment of the Epilepsies", J. Engel, Jr, ed., Raven Press, New York.

Boon, P.A., Williamson, P.D., Fried, I., Spencer, D.D., Novelly, R.A., Spencer, S.S., and Mattson, R.H., 1991, Intracranial, intraaxial space occupying lesions in patients with intractable partial seizures: an anatomico-clinical, neuropsychological and surgical correlation, Epilepsia 32: 467–476.

Cascino, G.D., Boon, P.A.J.M., and Fish, D.R. (1993) Surgically remedial lesional syndromes, in: "Surgical Treatment of the Epilepsies", second edition, J. Engel, Jr, ed., Raven Press, New York, pp. 77–87.

Cascino, G.D., Kelly, P.J., Hirschorn, K.A., Marsh, W.R., and Sharbrough, F.W., 1990, Stereotactic lesion resection in partial epilepsy, Mayo Clin Proc 65: 1053–1060.

Clarke, Olivier, A., Fish, D.R., and Andermann, F., 1992, Surgical treatment of eplilespy: the problem of focus/lesion incongruence, Epilepsia 33(Suppl 3): 99.

Daumas-Duport, C., Scheithauser, B.W., Chodkiewicz, J.P., Laws, E.R., and Vedrenne, C., 1988, Dysembryoplastic neuroepithelial tumour: a surgically curable tumour of young patients with intractable partial seizures, Neurosurgery 23: 545–556.

Davidson, S., and Falconer, M.A., 1975, Outcome of surgery in 40 children with temporal lobe epilepsy, Lancet 1260–1263.

Duncan, J.D., and Sagar, H.J., 1987, Seizure characteristics, pathology, and outcome after temporal lobectomy, Neurology 37: 405–409.

Falconer, M.A., Serafetinides, E.A., and Corsellis, J.A.N., 1964, Etiology and pathogenesis of temporal lobe epilepsy, Arch Neurol 10: 233–248.

Fish, D.R., Andermann, F., and Olivier, A., 1991, Complex partial seizures and posterior temporal or extratemporal lesions: surgical strategies, Neurology 41: 1781–1784.

20   D.R. Fish

Fish, D.R., Smith, S.J.M., Quesney, L.F., Andermann, F., and Rasmussen, T., 1993, Epilepsy surgery in children with medically intractable temporal or frontal lobe epilepsy: highlights and results of 40 years experience, Epilepsia. 34: 244–247

Green, J.R., and Scheetz, D.G., 1964, Surgery of epileptogenic lesions of the temporal lobe, Arch Neurol. 10: 135–148.

Jensen, I., and Klinken, L., 1976, Temporal lobe epilepsy and neuropathology: histological findings in resected temporal lobes correlated to surgical results and clinical aspects, Acta Neurol Scand. 54: 391–414.

Kirkpatrick, P.J., Honavar, M., Janota, I., and Polkey, C.E., 1993, Control of temporal lobe epilepsy following en bloc resection of low-grade tumors. Neurosurgery 78: 19–25.

Palmini, A., Andermann, F., Olivier, A., Tampieri, D., and Robitaille, Y., 1991, Focal neuronal migration disorders and intractable epilepsy, Ann Neurol. 30: 750–757

Rasmussen, T., 1975, Surgery of epilepsy associated with brain tumours, in: "Advances in Neurology: Neurosurgical Management of the Epilepsies," vol. 8, D.P. Purpura, J.K. Penry, R.D. Walter, eds, Raven Press, New York.

Williamson, P.D., Boon, P.A., Thadani, V.M., Darce, T.M., Spencer, D.D., Spencer, S.S., Novelly, R.A., and Mattson, R.H., 1992, Parietal lobe epilepsy: diagnostic considerations and results of surgery, Ann Neurol. 31: 193–201

Yeh, H., Kashiwaga, S., Tew, J.M., and Berger, T.S., 1990, Surgical management of epilepsy associated with cerebral arteriovenous malformations, J Neurosurg. 72: 216–223.

BRAIN STRUCTURE IN EPILEPSY

The Crucial Role of MRI

F. Andermann

Montreal Neurological Hospital and Institute
3801 University Street
Montreal, Quebec
Canada H3A 2B4

INTRODUCTION

The relationship between cerebral localization and partial epilepsy has been recognized for a long time. The stimulation experiments of Fritsch and Hitzig which illustrated cortical localization (Fritsch and Hitzig, 1870) were carried out just before the development of modern surgical treatment. The earliest patients operated by Victor Horsley had lesions involving eloquent areas of the brain, usually the central region (Horsley, 1886). Early in the history of surgical treatment for intractable epilepsy, epileptogenic lesions were demonstrated radiologically. The hemangioma calcificans described by Penfield and Ward (1948) was a good example of such imaging-clinical correlation. However, recognizable lesions were few and virtually limited to those containing calcifications.

Radiographic studies of the skull produced valuable lateralizing information in patients with intractable epilepsy who were considered for surgical resection. Signs such as flattening or thickening of the vault, elevation of the petrous ridge, enlargement of the sinuses and smallness of the middle fossa were greatly stressed from the 1940s on. This work was spear-headed by Arthur Childe (Childe and Penfield, 1937) and Donald McRae (1974, 1948).

Pneumoencephalography often provided only indirect evidence of intracerebral lesions. When it represented the most effective method for demonstrating focal abnormalities, many epileptogenic lesions were missed. It was common to find unsuspected small tumours or other lesions in electrically defined epileptogenic areas resected at surgery. This was the experience of the groups of Theodore Rasmussen (Leblanc and Rasmussen, 1974) and Murray Falconer (Cavanagh, 1958; Falconer and Kennedy, 1962). Up to 30% of patients operated for intractable epilepsy at the Montreal Neurological Institute were found to have relatively inert lesions of this type. Because the potential benefits of surgical treatment of epilepsy were not widely recognized, many patients with intractable seizures and small focal lesions were advised that they should continue with the ineffective medical treatment and be followed with periodic

Magnetic Resonance Scanning and Epilepsy, Edited by S.D. Shorvon et al.,
Plenum Press, New York, 1994

examinations. This was considered preferable to having their epileptogenic lesions investigated further and giving consideration to removal of the lesion. There was considerable uncertainty and debate about the best approach to epilepsy related to small tumours and to other focal lesions. Electroencephalography and corticography were the only guides to resection. It was generally considered inadvisable to rely on resection of a lesion alone, no matter where it was localized or how it correlated with the clinical pattern. The main emphasis was placed on mapping the epileptogenic area and removing it if possible, leaving the lesion unless it was superimposed on the area of electrical discharge.

The advent of CT was a major milestone in the recognition of epileptogenic lesions. It led to a veritable explosion of information with recognition of innumerable cavernous angiomas, small neoplastic lesions and gangliogliomas situated in more or less close proximity to electrographically identified epileptogenic areas (Adams et al., 1974). The significance of these structural lesions was not then recognized. Many patients with posterior temporal or temporo-occipital lesions were found to have major electrographic abnormalities in anterior and inferomesial temporal areas. When resection of these electrographically active areas did not lead to good surgical result, attention turned to the role of the structural abnormalities themselves. The work of Fish et al. (1991) was a logical extension of the work of Falconer who had stressed the importance of resecting the lesion in order to achieve a good surgical result (Falconer et al., 1962).

CT scanning was found to have a major blind spot in the evaluation of abnormalities in the temporal region. Attempts to study this area with coronal cuts and with better orientation of slices (Adams et al., 1974) led to some improvement, but temporal "foreign tissue" lesions at times still eluded pre-operative detection.

Though the early results of magnetic resonance imaging were disappointing it soon became clear that mesial temporal structures could be visualized by MRI and that good comparison between these investigations and anatomical studies was possible (Berkovic et al., 1986a,b; Kuzniecky et al., 1987). In selected groups of patients known to harbour mesial temporal sclerosis, such as individuals with a history of prolonged febrile convulsions, both the small size of mesial temporal structures and an abnormal signal were recognized. Despite initial scepticism these findings were gradually accepted (Berkovic et al., 1991). There followed attempts at quantitating these changes using semi-automated volumetric studies with renewed emphasis on recognizing the anatomy and limits of the amygdala, hippocampus and other structures within the temporal lobe (Press et al., 1989; Jack, 1989; Squire et al., 1990). These studies are ongoing and have greatly facilitated the assessment of patients with temporal lobe epilepsy (Jack et al., 1990, 1992; Cook et al., 1992; Lencz et al., 1992; Watson et al., 1992; Cendes et al., 1993a,b). When unequivocal asymmetries are found, the pre-operative investigation is greatly facilitated and the correlation of imaging, electrographic and neuropsychological findings permits an accurate prognosis in a great majority of patients with temporal lobe epilepsy. In many individuals these determinations render invasive recording, once considered essential in all candidates for surgery, unnecessary. Sometimes there is conflicting evidence between the small size of the hippocampus and amygdala and surface EEG findings which may suggest contralateral onset of seizures. Such patients are fortunately few, as are those with bilateral smallness of mesial temporal structures. Depth electrode studies have confirmed that the clinically important side is the one with maximal structural shrinkage; thus, in such patients the ambiguity generated by surface EEG is usually corrected by the volumetric studies (Cendes et al. in prep.).

Patients who have seizures originating independently in mesial temporal structures of both hemispheres are presently studied with a view to assessing side predominance, which could allow the consideration of restricted resection such as cortico-amygdalectomy (Kim et al., 1992). Some patients who have memory deficits and would not previously have been surgical candidates may have a chance to benefit from surgical treatment along these lines. The question of progressive atrophy versus initial damage leading to sclerosis of mesial temporal structures may also be assessed by MRI volumetric studies. Linear regression analysis suggests that duration of epilepsy, number of seizures or the presence of generalized seizures do not correlate with the degree of atrophy of mesial temporal structures. Thus, any ongoing and progressive changes relating to these parameters should be a minor factor if present at all in mesial temporal sclerosis (Cendes et al., 1993b).

A current thrust of investigation involves the management of small stereotactically accessible lesions. Unlike what was expected earlier, resections of such lesions have been shown to be effective in leading to improvement in the seizure tendency in most, although not all patients (Adams et al., 1974; Cascino et al., 1990). Further studies of the relationship of such small lesions to the electrographically defined epileptogenic area should lead to clarification and to planning of effective surgical strategies for the control of the epilepsy associated with them.

CT scanning began to demonstrate architectonic abnormalities such as abnormally wide gyri, bands of what appeared to be excessively thick and featureless grey matter, subcortical heterotopias or periventricular structural irregularities (Andermann et al., 1987). Pathological studies of epileptogenic tissue removed from these areas or consisting of spiking cortex resected from the proximity of these abnormalities showed the pathological changes of focal cortical dysplasia or of the forme fruste of tuberous sclerosis (Perot et al., 1966).

Focal cortical dysplasia was described by David Taylor, working with Murray Falconer and his group at the Maudsley Hospital (Taylor et al., 1971). The abnormal tissue could at that time not be visualized during life and the disorganized brain structure was first recognized by the pathologists Corsellis and Bruton (Taylor et al., 1971). The dysplastic areas in these early patients were fairly restricted. At that time only few patients were surgically treated for their intractable epilepsy and only rarely was cortical dysplasia discussed in the literature (Mathieson, 1975), until the advent of modern imaging. A clinically similar unsuspected finding was the forme fruste of tuberous sclerosis as defined by Rasmussen, Mathieson and their group (Mathieson, 1975). In these patients the pathological changes are similar except for the presence of clusters of subpial giant astrocytes which render these lesions pathologically indistinguishable from those found in patients with typical tuberous sclerosis. There are, however, crucial differences from a clinical point of view. These patients do not have the dermatological, cardiac, bony and other abnormalities found in tuberous sclerosis, the forme fruste is genetically quite different in that these patients are always sporadic, and there have been no patients with the dominant inheritance characteristic of many patients with the classical form. Thus the distinction between focal cortical dysplasia and the forme fruste of tuberous sclerosis is a purely pathological one, and comparison of the clinical history and findings in these patients shows that they cannot be distinguished a priori.

The pathological examples of neuronal migration disorders were initially derived from patients with severe abnormalities who died early, and thus these developmental disorders were not considered to be compatible with prolonged survival (Matell, 1893; Bielschowsky, 1923).

The advent of MRI has permitted identification of a number of anatomoclinical syndromes of neuronal or neuroblast migration disorders which until then had depended largely on demonstration at autopsy.

In our experience the largest number of patients with neuronal migration defects who present with intractable epilepsy have a focal unilateral dysplastic lesion (Palmini et al., 1991a). Pachygyria may be associated with an abnormal subcortical signal or heterotopic grey matter may be present below the cortex, and any part of the hemisphere may be involved. In most of these patients the associated epilepsy is intractable and a surgical approach was required in 26 of 30 patients we have studied. The success of surgery depended on the extent of removal of the visibly abnormal area more than on the extent of electroencephalographically or cortico-graphically abnormal tissue resected (Palmini et al., 1991b). Lesions involving the peri-sylvian region tend to lead to anterior and inferomesial temporal epileptic discharges and resection of these structures may lead to some improvement but not to cessation of seizures (Andermann et al., 1987). Maximal improvement, although very exceptionally complete cessation of seizures, was achieved when the major portion of the lesion was resected (Palmini et al., 1991b). The results were the same in patients who had a pathological diagnosis of focal cortical dysplasia and in those whose pathological diagnosis was that of the forme fruste of tuberous sclerosis (Palmini et al., 1991a,b).

In many patients with neuronal migration defects, the abnormality is much more wide-spread across the hemisphere than the changes visible by CT or even by MRI would lead one to expect. It is probably for this reason that seizures only exceptionally cease entirely following surgical treatment, although the improvement following surgery in the great majority of these patients is well worthwhile.

The whole hemisphere may be abnormal and enlarged, with pachygyria, overall enlarge-ment of the ventricle and gliotic changes. This disorder or hemimegalencephaly may be associated with congenital dermatological abnormalities such as the linear naevus syndrome of Jadassohn or the achromic nevus of Ito (Vigevano et al., 1989; Andermann and Palmini, 1991). The mechanism of these prenatal neuroectodermal abnormalities has not been clarified to date. In these children it is sometimes not clear whether the other hemisphere is involved as well, although to a lesser degree. Are electrographic abnormalities involving the more normal appearing side transmitted or due to secondary epileptogenesis or are they related to a neuronal migration defect involving that side as well? When a maximal hemiparesis is present functional hemispherectomy remains the treatment of choice of the intractable epilepsy associated with this abnormality (Tinuper et al., 1988; Vigevano et al., 1989).

Megalencephaly may be associated with visible architectonic changes in the area of maximal epileptic abnormality, but in some patients with megalencephaly and seizures no architectonic changes can be demonstrated by current MRI techniques. Arrest of migration of neuroblasts from the periventricular germinal layer towards the cortex may result in band or linear heterotopia, also described as the double cortex syndrome (Marchal et al., 1989; Livingston and Aicardi, 1990; Palmini et al., 1991c). The thickness of the band of arrested cells separated from the cortex by a narrow zone of white matter is quite variable, and there is still much discussion as to whether this type of heterotopia is always generalized or whether it may predominate or exist only in certain regions. In some of the patients the non-migrating cells may remain arrested in the periventricular region, and in some patients the heterotopic band is intermediate between the subcortical region and the periventricular area. There is thus a geographical spectrum of generalized migration disorders (Palmini et al., 1993). The patients have seizures of different types but usually secondary generalized patterns predominate. Some focalization may be present but this is usually not sufficient to consider a resection. The degree of mental change varies from low average intelligence to moderate retardation. Patients with a Lennox–Gastaut syndrome have, as expected, the worst outcome in intellectual development. In patients with the double cortex syndrome, the cortex itself may appear relatively normal or show varying degrees of pachygyria. Recognition of this abnormality is dependent on high-quality MRI because CT and preliminary MRI studies have caused us to miss or misinterpret the nature of the abnormality (Palmini et al., 1991c).

Nodular periventricular heterotopia is probably related to persistence of non-migrating islands of cells in the germinal layer. These can later be demonstrated in the periventricular region with striking predominance in the posterior portion of the hemisphere and sometimes extension into temporal areas (Dubeau et al., 1993). The lesions, usually bilateral, are commonly, but not always, associated with intractable epilepsy and in some of these patients electrographic abnormalities tend to predominate over anterior and inferomesial temporal regions. Resection of those areas, however, should not be expected to bring about complete cessation of seizures. Generalized epileptic disorders are not, in our limited experience, associated with nodular periventricular heterotopia and the intelligence of the patients is often normal. Exceptionally these lesions may not be associated with intractable epilepsy (Dubeau and Andermann, personal observations).

Bilateral peri-sylvian polymicrogyria (Kuzniecky et al., 1989) is commonly associated with a degree of mental retardation. Dysarthria, ranging all the way to almost complete anarthria and mild pyramidal changes are the rule. The CT changes are in some ways more striking than abnormalities demonstrated by MRI and have led us to misinterpret the lesions as representing macrogyria. Pathological studies have unequivocally demonstrated micropolygyria in these areas, and the time of onset and nature of the aetiological abnormalities are probably different from those leading to focal or generalized migration disorders (Becker and Dixon, 1989; Shevell et al., 1992). A characteristic peri-oral seizure pattern has been described in patients with this malformation and secondary generalized epilepsy or bilateral independent epileptogenic areas are common (Ambrosetto and Tassinari, 1990; Andermann et al., 1990). Resective surgery has not been possible but callosotomy has provided useful palliation in patients with a secondary generalized epileptic process and drop attacks (Kuzniecky et al., 1990). The relationship of this malformation to schizencephaly remains unclear (Leblanc et al., 1993).

Not all neuronal migration defects are visible by current MRI technology. In several patients, intractable focal status epilepticus led to repeated MR studies which did not show a structural abnormality but cortical dysplasia was clearly demonstrated in material removed at the time of surgery (Desbiens et al., 1991). Such patients and children with less severe, but still at times intractable, partial epilepsy without other explanation or cause are quite likely to harbour neuronal migration defects. Improved imaging techniques should enable recognition pre-operatively of yet other groups of more subtle neuronal migration defects, and allow improvement in selection criteria and in results of surgical treatment.

Functional MRI will hopefully lead to identification of language and other essential areas by non-invasive means. It should provide insight into shifts of function both within one hemisphere and contralaterally and thus into plasticity of the brain. Magnetic resonance imaging is currently revolutionizing our approaches to the investigation, diagnosis and treatment of patients with intractable epilepsy. It is generating an excitement which is comparable to that aroused by the introduction and development of EEG half a century ago.

REFERENCES

Adams, C.B.T., Anslow, P., Molyneux, A., and Oxbury, J., 1974, Radiological Detection of Surgically Treatable Pathology, in: "Handbook of Clinical Neurology," Vol. 15, P.K. Vinken and G.W. Bruyn, eds, North-Holland Publishing, Amsterdam.

Ambrosetto, G., and Tassinari, C.A., 1990, Sleep-related focal motor seizures in bilateral central macrogyria [Letter], Ann Neurol. 28:840–841.

Andermann, F., Olivier, A., Melanson, D., and Robitaille, Y., 1987, Epilepsy due to focal cortical dysplasia with macrogyria and the forme fruste of tuberous sclerosis: a study of 15 patients, in: "Advances in Epileptology," vol. 16, P. Wolfe, M. Dam, D. Janz, and F.E. Dreifuss, eds, Raven Press, New York.

Andermann, F., Kuzniecky, R., Tampieri, D., and Palmini A., 1990, Sleep-related focal motor seizures in bilateral central macrogyria [Letter], Ann Neurol. 28: 841–842.

Andermann, F., and Palmini, A.L., 1991, Neuronal migration disorders, tuberous sclerosis, and Sturge-Weber syndrome, in: "Epilepsy Surgery," H. Luders, ed., Raven Press, New York.

Becker, P.S., Dixon, A.M., and Troncoso, J.C., 1989, Bilateral opercular polymicrogyria, Ann Neurol. 25:90–92.

Berkovic, S.F., Ethier, R., Olivier, A., et al., 1986a, Magnetic resonance imaging of the hippocampus: I. normal anatomy, Epilepsia 27:611–612.

Berkovic, S.F., Ethier, R., Robitaille, Y., et al., 1986b, Magnetic resonance imaging of the hippocampus: II. mesial temporal sclerosis, Epilepsia 27:612.

Berkovic, S.F., Andermann, F., Olivier, A., Ethier, R., Melanson, D., Robitaille, Y., Kuzniecky, R., Peters, T., and Feindel, W., 1991, Hippocampal sclerosis in temporal lobe epilepsy demonstrated by magnetic resonance imaging, Ann Neurol. 29:175–182.

Bielschowsky, M., 1923, Uber die Oberflächengestaltung des Grosshirnmantels bei Pachygyrie, Mikrogyrie und bei normaler Hirnentwicklung, J Psychol Neurol. 30: 29–76.

Cascino, G.D., Kelly, P., Hirschorn, K.A., Marsh, W.R., and Sharbrough, F.W., 1990, Stereotactic resection of intra-axial cerebral lesions in partial epilepsy, Mayo Clin Proc. 65:1053–1060.

Cavanagh, JB., 1958, On certain small tumours encountered in the temporal lobe, Brain 81:389–405.

Cendes, F., Andermann, F., Gloor, P., et al., 1993a, MRI volumetric measurements of amygdala and hippocampus in temporal lobe epilepsy, Neurology 43:719–725.

Cendes, F., Andermann, F., Gloor, P., et al., 1993b, Atrophy of mesial structures in patients with temporal lobe epilepsy: cause or consequence of repeated seizures?, Ann Neurol. 34:795–801.

Cendes, F., Dubeau, F., Andermann, F., et al., in prep., Depth EEG investigation in patients with mesial temporal atrophy and bitemporal EEG abnormalities.

Childe, A., and Penfield, W., 1937, Anatomic and pneumographic studies of the temporal horn with a further note on the pneumographic analysis of the cerebral ventricles, Arch Neurol Psychiat (Chic.) 37:1021–1034.

Cook, M.J., Fish, D.R., Shorvon, S.D., Straughan, K., and Stevens, J.M., 1992, Hippocampal volumetric and morphometric studies in frontal and temporal lobe epilepsy, Brain 115:1001–1015.

Desbiens, R., Berkovic, S.F., Andermann, F., et al., 1991, Prolonged life-threatening focal status epilepticus due to cortical dysplasia not visible by MRI (abst), Epilepsia 32:89.

Dubeau, F., Lee, N., Tampieri, D., Andermann, E., Leblanc, R., Villemure, J-G., and Andermann, F., 1993, Periventricular nodular heteropia (PNH) genetic aspects and strategies for surgical treatment of intractable seizures, AAN, Scientific program Abst. Neurology suppl.

Falconer, M.A., and Kennedy, W.A., 1962, Epilepsy due to small focal temporal lesions with bilateral independent spike-discharge foci: A study of seven cases relieved by operation, Brain 85:521–534.

Falconer, M.A., Driver, M.V., and Serafetinides, E.A., 1962, Temporal lobe epilepsy due to distant lesions: two cases relieved by operation, Brain 85:521–534.

Fish, D., Andermann, F., and Olivier, A., 1991, Complex partial seizures and small posterior temporal or extratemporal structural lesions: Surgical management, Neurology 41:1781–1784.

Fritsch, G., and Hitzig, E., 1870, Ueber die elektrische Erregbarkeit des Grosshirns, Arch Anat Physiol. 37:300–332.

Horsley, Sir V., 1886, Brain surgery, BMJ. 2:670–675.

Jack, C.R. Jr, Twomey, C.K., Zinsmeister, A.R., et al., 1989, Anterior temporal lobes and hippocampal formations: normative volumetric measurements from MR images in young adults, Radiology 172:549–554.

Jack, C.R., Sharbrough, F.W., Twomey, C.K., et al., 1990, Temporal lobe seizures: lateralization with MR volume measurements of the hippocampal formation, Radiology 175:423–429.

Jack, C.R., Sharbrough, F.W., Cascino, G., et al., 1992, Magnetic resonance image-based hippocampal volumetry: correlation with outcome after temporal lobectomy, Ann Neurol. 31:138–146.

Kim, H-I., Olivier, A., Jones-Gotman, M., and Andermann, F., 1992, Corticoamygdalectomy in memory impaired patients, Stereotactic Funct Neurosurg. 58:162–167.

Kuzniecky, R., de la Sayette, V., Ethier, R., et al., 1987, Magnetic resonance imaging in temporal lobe epilepsy: pathological correlation, Ann Neurol. 22:341–347.

Kuzniecky, R., Andermann, F., Tampieri, D., Melanson, D., Olivier, A., and Leppik, I., 1989, Bilateral central macrogyria: epilepsy, pseudobulbar palsy, and mental retardation—a recognizable neuronal migration disorder, Ann Neurol. 25:547–554.

Kuzniecky, R., Andermann, F., Fusco, L., Melanson, D., Olivier, A., Faught, E., Morawetz, R., Palmini, A., and Tampieri, D., 1990, Corpus callosotomy in the management of the congenital bilateral peri-sylvian syndrome, Epilepsia 31:639.

Leblanc, F.E., and Rasmussen T., 1974, Cerebral seizures and brain tumors, in: "Handbook of Clinical Neurology," Vol. 15, P.K. Vinken and G.W. Bruyn, eds, North-Holland Publishing, Amsterdam.

Leblanc, R., Tampieri, D., Robitaille, Y., Feindel, W., Olivier, A., Andermann, F., and Silverberg, D., 1993, Surgical treatment of intractable epilepsy associated with schizencephaly, Neurology, in press.

Lencz, T., McCarty, G., Bronen, R.A., et al., 1992, Quantitative magnetic resonance imaging in temporal lobe epilepsy: Relationship to neuropathology and neuropsychological function, Ann Neurol. 31:629–637.

Livingston, J.H., and Aicardi, J., 1990, Unusual MRI appearance of diffuse subcortical heterotopia or "double cortex" in two children, J Neurol Neurosurg Psych. 53:617–620.

Marchal, G., Andermann, F., Tampieri, D., Robitaille, Y., Melanson, D., Sinclair, B., Olivier, A., Silver, K., and Langevin, P., 1989, Generalized cortical dysplasia manifested by diffusely thick cerebral cortex, Arch Neurol. 46:430–434.

Matell, M., 1893, Ein Fall von Heterotopie der grauen Substanz in den beiden Hemispheren des Großhirns, Arch Psychiatr Nervenkr. 25:124–136.

Mathieson, G., 1975, Pathology of temporal lobe foci, in: "Advances in Neurology," Vol. 11: Complex Partial Seizures and Their Treatment, J.K. Penry and D.P. Daly, eds, Raven Press, New York.

McRae, D.L., 1948, Focal epilepsy: correlation of the pathological and radiological findings, Radiology 50:439–457.

McRae, D.L., 1974, Radiology in epilepsy, in: "Handbook of Clinical Neurology," Vol. 15, P.J. Vinken and G.W. Bruyn, eds, North-Holland Publishing, Amsterdam.

Palmini, A., Andermann, F., Olivier, A., Tampieri, D., Robitaille, Y., Andermann, E. and Wright, G., 1991a, Focal neuronal migration disorders and intractable partial epilepsy: A study of 30 Patients, Ann Neurol. 30:741–749.

Palmini, A., Andermann, F., Olivier, A., Tampieri, D., and Robitaille, Y., 1991b, Focal neuronal migration disorders and intractable partial epilepsy: results of surgical treatment, Ann Neurol. 30:750–757.

Palmini, A., Andermann, F., Aicardi, J., Dulac, O., Chaves, F., Ponsot, G., Brian, R., Goutieres, F., Livingston, J., Tampieri, D., and Robitaille, Y., 1991c, Diffuse cortical dysplasia or the "double-cortex" syndrome. The clinical and epileptic spectrum in 10 children, Neurology 41:1656–1662.

Palmini, A., Andermann, F., de Grissac, H., Tampieri, D., Robitaille, Y., Desbiens, R., and Andermann, E., 1993, Stages and patterns of centrifugal arrest in diffuse neuronal migration disorders, Dev Med Child Neurol. 35:331–339.

Penfield, W.P., and Ward, A., 1948, Calcifying epileptogenic lesions; hemangioma calcificans. Report of a case, Arch Neurol Psych. 60:20–36.

Perot, P., Weir, B., and Rasmussen, T., 1966, Tuberous sclerosis: surgical therapy for seizures, Arch Neurol. 15:498–506.

Press, G.A., Amaral, D.G., and Squire, L.R., 1989, Hippocampal abnormalities in amnesic patients revealed by high-resolution magnetic resonance imaging, Nature 341:54–57.

Shevell, M.I., Carmant, L., and Meagher-Villemure, K., 1992, Developmental bilateral peri-sylvian dysplasia Pediatr Neurol. 8:299–302.

Squire, L.R., Amaral, D.G., and Press, G.A., 1990, Magnetic resonance imaging of the hippocampal formation and mammillary nuclei distinguish medial temporal lobe and diencephalic amnesia, J Neurosci. 10:3106–3117.

Taylor, D.C., Falconer, M.A., Bruton, C.J., and Corsellis, J.A.N., 1971, Focal dysplasia of the cerebral cortex in epilepsy. J Neurol Neurosurg Psych. 34:369–387.

Tinuper, P., Andermann, F., Villemure, J-G., Rasmussen, T.B., and Quesney, L.F., 1988, Functional hemispherectomy for treatment of epilepsy associated with hemiplegia: rationale, indications, results and comparison with callosotomy, Ann Neurol. 24:27–34.

Vigevano, F., Bertini, E., Boldrini, R., Bosman, C., Claps, D., di Capua, M., di Rocco, C., and Rossi, G.F., 1989, Hemimegalencephaly and intractable epilepsy: benefits of hemispherectomy, Epilepsia 30: 833–843.

Watson, C., Andermann, F., Gloor, P., et al., 1992, Anatomical basis of amygdaloid and hippocampal volume measurements by magnetic resonance imaging, Neurology 42: 1743–1750.16.

4

MR SPECTROSCOPY IN EPILEPSY

H. Stefan

University of Erlangen-Nuremberg
Department of Neurology
Erlangen
Germany

In the pathogenesis of epilepsies genetic and acquired factors are involved. The elementary electrophysiological phenomenon is the so-called intracellular paroxysmal depolarisation shift (PDS). Spontaneous chronic recurrence of paroxysmal epileptiform activity indicates an epileptogenic process. This epileptogenic process is correlated to biochemical changes in metabolism. The activity on CNS circuits is influenced by dominant excitatory (e.g. glutamate, aspartate, quisqualate) or dominant inhibitory (e.g. gamma-aminobutyric acid (GABA), GABA agonist) transmitters and neuromodulators. The excitation (paroxysmal depolarisation) is mediated by glutamate receptors. Ion-bound receptors are, for example, of the N-methyl-D-aspartate, Ampa or kainate types. The release of glutamate and the depolarisation of the neuron are closely linked. The result of glutamate release and the binding to the N-methyl-D-aspartate receptor causes an increase of calcium into the neuron. This energy consuming process may be accompanied by an increase of inorganic phosphate and energy depletion with decrease of ATP and phosphocreatine. In addition to the intracellular neuronal release of glutamate, or in the case of inhibition of GABA and reaction with the GABA-receptor complex, metabolic pathways obviously involve glia cells. The uptake of GABA and glutamate in the glial cell is influenced by different enzymes and pharmacological mechanisms. Tetrahydroisoxacolopyridinol PHPD decreases GABA uptake into the glial cell. Glutamine synthetase decreases uptake of glutamate into the glial cell. Anti-epileptic drugs such as valproate acid or vigabatrin enhance the concentration of GABA in the neurotransmitter pool. Lamotrigine may lead to a decrease of glutamate in the region of the focus. The concentration of glutamate GABA-aspartate and taurine was found to be decreased in the focus centre (van Gelder et al., 1972), whereas Perry and Hansen (1981) found an increase of GABA and glutamate in the focus centre.

MR spectroscopy allows a monitoring of cerebral metabolites: by phosphorus-31 (^{31}P) MR spectroscopy, phosphomonoesters (PME), phosphodiesters (PDE), inorganic phosphate (Pi), phosphocreatine (PCr) and adenosine triphosphate (ATP) can be detected. The chemical shift of the Pi resonance allows a determination of the PH value. By proton (^{1}H) MR spectroscopy, choline (Cho), creatine (Cr) and N-acetylaspartate (NAA) can be evaluated.

Using techniques with short echo times, additional cerebral metabolites such as glutamate (Glu), inositols (Ino) and glucose (Glc) may be evaluated.

Differences in the concentration of excitatory amino acids and other compounds involving high-energy phosphate metabolism such as ATP, creatine and phosphocreatine, as well as the cerebral blood flow (CBF), cerebral metabolic glucose rate (CMRGlc) or cerebral metabolic oxygen consumption (CMRO$_2$) and the local lactate production as well as the intracellular pH may depend on several factors. One of the important factors contributing to the changes of metabolism is the change from inter-ictal to ictal epileptic activity. For cerebral metabolism during seizure activity, local lactate production is increased, CBF, CMRGlc and CMRO$_2$ are often increased, whereas increased cerebral energy utilisation leads to a decrease of the ratio PCr/PE and a decrease of ATP. In addition to these metabolic changes, the concentration of NAA seems to reflect a neuronal concentration because NAA is located primarily in neurons. Pressure of choline, a precursor for membrane constituents (phosphatidylcholine) and the transmitter acetylcholine, might reflect a membrane disturbance. In addition the question arises of whether a non-invasive differentiation of tumoral or gliotic tissue can be obtained measuring the ratio of Cho/NAA. If MR spectroscopy would allow the detection of regional metabolic changes in comparison to non-epileptic brain tissue, it could have the potential for an additional non-invasive diagnostic test for focus localisation. The advantage of MR spectroscopy could result from this technique mainly being used during the inter-ictal state. For recording of the concentration of excitatory amino acids, short relaxation times have to be used. Even using those special techniques the question of the reference (using an internal standard?) does not have an ideal solution. The combination of phospho-spectroscopy and proton spectroscopy could provide valuable information concerning: (1) the phosphocreatine/inorganic phosphate rate, (2) pH value concerning the functional metabolic changes in the focus, and (3) reflecting the morphological lesion (a reduction of neurons during gliosis) by means of decreased NAA. The spatial resolution obtained by phospho-spectroscopy is low compared to proton spectroscopy. Different methods are currently being investigated, e.g. single-voxel spectroscopy which demonstrates one spectrum of one region or chemical shift imaging (allowing spatial mapping of cerebral metabolites to larger areas, e.g. reaching from the lateral temporal neocortex to mesial parts).

The question arises of whether the sensitivity of MR spectroscopy is large enough for identification individual of pathological concentration of products of brain metabolism resulting focal epileptic activity. For the detection of metabolic pathways the carbon-12 spectroscopy is of great interest. A limiting factor is the sensitivity but this is less for spectroscopy than for PET. It is therefore questionable whether the labelling of NMDA-antagonists by means of carbon-13 could help us to show the receptor density by means of spectroscopy. This is still an interesting topic for further developments in spectroscopy. In the following chapters experiences with phosphorus, proton and carbon-13 spectroscopy are reported. This also includes the necessary comparison to other clinical techniques such as EEG for focus localisation, SPECT etc. Though MR spectroscopy at the moment is far from clinical routine application, the results indicate that the scientific evaluation should now be intensified with special emphasis on the clinical evaluation.

Section 2

MR Imaging in Patients with Temporal Lobe Epilepsy

5

MESIAL TEMPORAL LOBE STRUCTURES

Anatomy

P. Gloor

Montreal Neurological Hospital and Institute
3801 University Street
Montreal, Quebec
Canada H3A 2B4

INTRODUCTION

To properly evaluate magnetic resonance imaging (MRI) scans of the mesial temporal region, its specific human morphology (Duvernoy, 1988) should be well understood.

CURRENT RESEARCH

I have dissected temporal lobes of normal human brains and studied this region in coronal, sagittal and horizontal, serial Nissl and myelin-stained histological sections at the Yakovlev Collection in the Armed Forces Institute of Pathology in Washington D.C.

The mesial temporal region of primates is anatomically complex, because a series of flexions and rotations which have occurred in primate phylogeny have profoundly affected the original topographical relationships between amygdala, hippocampus and entorhinal cortex. The rostral hippocampus has undergone a medial, and in its terminal segment an upward, flexion which caused it to emerge on the brain surface forming the posterior one-third of the uncal surface (Figures 1 and 2).This led to the formation of the uncal notch or cleft which separates the hippocampus proper forming its roof from part of the subiculum, and the presubicular part of the parahippocampal gyrus in its floor (Figure 2). The amygdala has been rotated upwards such that its posterior part now lies dorsally on top of the rostral hippocampus (Figure 3). The amygdala underwent an additional rotation around its vertical axis. Both rotations carried the entorhinal cortex forward, thus wrapping much of it around the amygdala to form the gyrus ambiens which covers the anterior two-thirds of the mesial surface of the uncus (Figures 1 and 3). Below the uncal notch the entorhinal cortex forms the rostral extension of the parahippocampal gyrus, but it extends only for a short distance behind the posterior border of the uncus along this gyrus. The entorhinal cortex is bordered laterally by the perirhinal cortex which extends from the mesial temporal pole to about halfway along the posterior extent

Magnetic Resonance Scanning and Epilepsy, Edited by S.D. Shorvon et al.,
Plenum Press, New York, 1994

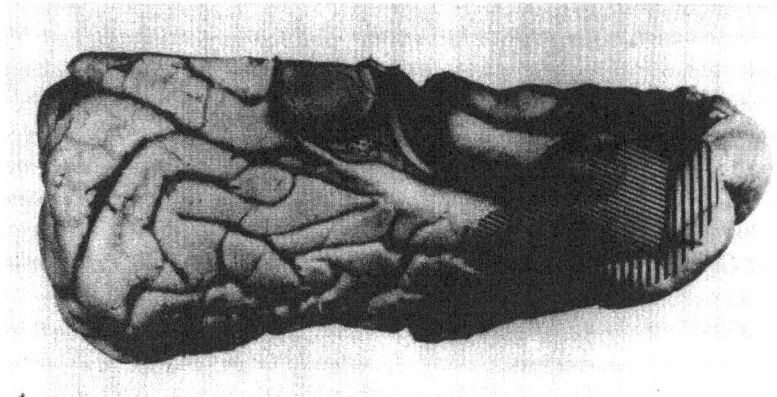

Figure 1. Subdivisions of the mesial temporal region. Stippled: hippocampus; cross-hatched: entorhinal cortex; vertically striped: perirhinal cortex. The small elevation on the top of the uncus left blank and located dorsal to the dorsal border of the entorhinal cortex is the part of the amygdala that rises to the brain surface.

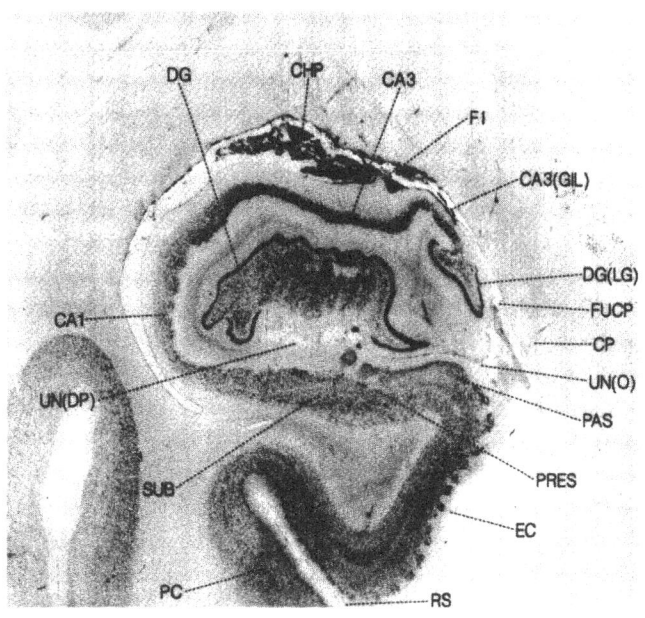

Figure 2. Coronal section through the posterior uncus. Note that the hippocampus forms the mesial surface of the uncus at this level as well as the roof of the uncal notch (specimen from the Yakovlev Collection, Armed Forces Institute of Pathology, Washington DC). Abbreviations in this and subsequent figures: A: amygdala; AAA: anterior amygdaloid area; ASA: amygdalostriatal area; CA1, CA3: hippocampal fields; CA3(GIL): hippocampal field CA3 forming part of the mesial surface of the uncus (gyrus intralimbicus); CAT: cortico-amygdaloid transition area (periamygdaloid cortex); CHP: choroid plexus within the temporal horn of the lateral ventricle; CP: cerebral peduncle; DG: dentate gyrus; DG(LG): dentate gyrus forming part of the mesial surface of the uncus (limbus Giacomini); EC: entorhinal cortex; EN: endopiriform nucleus; ES: endorhinal sulcus; FAH: zone of fusion between amygdala and hippocampus across obliterated ventricular cleft; FI: fimbria; FUCP: fissure between uncus and cerebral peduncle; GSL: gyrus semilunaris; HIP: hippocampus; IN: insula; OT: optic tract; PAS: parasubiculum; PC: perirhinal cortex; PPC: prepiriform (olfactory) cortex; PU: putamen; RS: rhinal sulcus; SF: sylvian fissure; SSA: sulcus semiannularis; SUB: subiculum; TN: tentorial notch; UD: uncal diverticulum of temporal horn of lateral ventricle; UN(DP): deep part of uncal notch; UN(O): opening of uncal notch on mesia l surface of uncus; UVC: unfused ventricular cleft between amygdala and hippocampus; VCL: ventral claustrum.

of the parahippocampal gyrus. Some aspects of mesial temporal anatomy raise difficulties in interpreting MRI data.

Anterior Limit of the Amygdala

Even histologically the rostral limit of the amygdala is difficult to define. The anterior amygdaloid area merges here with the ventral claustrum and the endopiriform nucleus. In coronal histological sections and in coronal MRI scans the first appearance of the endorhinal sulcus identifies fairly accurately the rostral extremity of the amygdala (Figure 4).

Differentiation of the Components of the Uncus

In histological sections these are easy to distinguish, but not on MRI scans. One must recall that the caudal third of the uncus dorsal to the uncal notch, including its mesial surface, is entirely hippocampal. More rostrally the roof of the temporal horn of the lateral ventricle is formed by the posterior portion of the amygdala which increases in bulk as one moves forward, whereas the size of the hippocampus on the ventricular floor decreases. Mesially amygdala and hippocampus are, however, fused to various degrees across an obliterated section of the temporal horn (Figure 3). Once the ventricle disappears, most of the uncus except for its medial surface covered by entorhinal cortex consists of amygdala. Its cortical nucleus emerges on the surface of the brain and forms a bump on the dorsal surface of the uncus, the gyrus semilunaris, bordered mesially by the sulcus semiannularis. Cortical nucleus and periamygdaloid cortex should be regarded as synonymous terms for practical purposes. Some boundaries of the amygdala which are easy to establish histologically are difficult to draw in MRI scans: (i) the boundary between amygdala and hippocampus where they are fused together; (ii) the dorsal

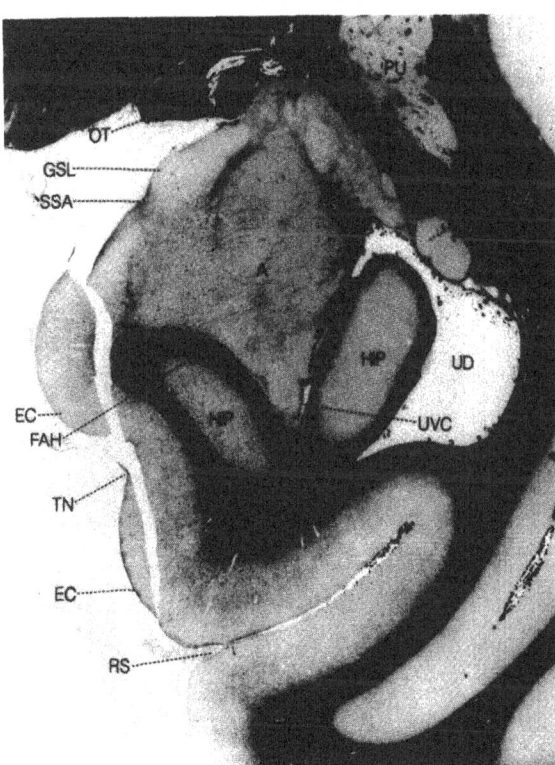

Figure 3. Coronal section through the mid-uncus. The amygdala lies on top of the rostral hippocampus and medially is partially fused with it. (Specimen from the Yakovlev Collection, Armed Forces Institute of Pathology, Washington, D.C.). For key to abbreviations, see legend of Figure 2.

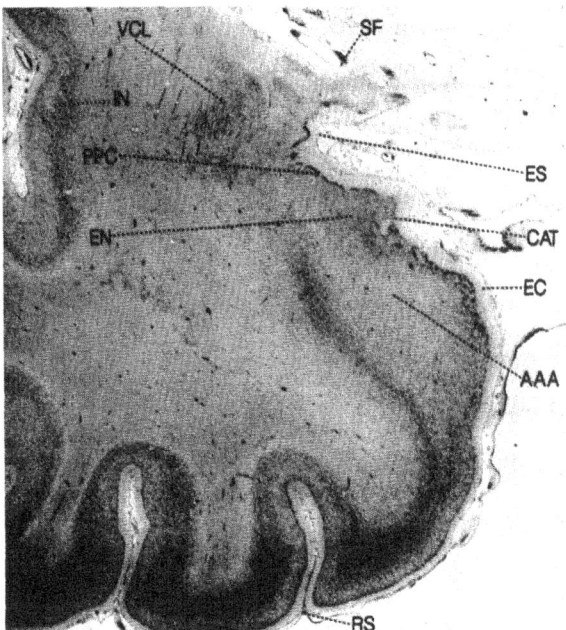

Figure 4. Coronal section through the rostral extremity of the amygdala at the level of the first appearance of the endorhinal sulcus. (Specimen from the Yakovlev Collection, Armed Forces Institute of Pathology, Washington DC). For key to abbreviations, see legend of Figure 2.

boundary separating the amygdala from the base of the lentiform nucleus; and (iii) the boundary between the entorhinal cortex and the amygdala on the medial aspect of the uncus. Watson et al. (1992) described how these boundaries can be drawn in MRI scans.

Posterior Limit of Hippocampus

As the hippocampus approaches the undersurface of the splenium of the corpus callosum, the posterior pillars of the fornix separate from it, whereas the hippocampus rapidly diminishes in size as it continues further posteriorly before fading into the indusium griseum of the corpus callosum. Caudal to the level of its separation from the pillars of the fornix, the hippocampus cannot be reliably identified in MRI scans.

POSSIBLE FUTURE DEVELOPMENTS

One boundary that is presently impossible to draw in MRI scans is the posterior limit of the entorhinal cortex. I found it difficult to establish it, even histologically, in the human brain. If a reliable landmark for the caudal limit of the entorhinal cortex could be defined in the human brain, it would become possible to estimate from MRI scans how much entorhinal cortex had been removed in temporal lobectomies or amygdalo-hippocampectomies. These data would be useful for assessing the relationships between deficits in post-operative memory function and the extent of removal of various key mesial temporal lobe structures.

REFERENCES

Duvernoy, H.M., 1988, "The Human Hippocampus. An Atlas of Applied Anatomy", J.F. Bergmann, ed.,Verlag, Munich.

Watson, C., Andermann, F., Gloor, P., Jones-Gotman, M., Peters, T., Evans, A., Olivier, A., Melanson, D., and Leroux, G., 1992, Anatomic basis of amygdaloid and hippocampal volume measurement by magnetic resonance imaging, Neurology 42.

MAGNETIC RESONANCE IMAGING OF HIPPOCAMPAL SCLEROSIS

Reliability of Visual Diagnosis and Implications for Surgical Treatment

S.F. Berkovic,[1] A.M. McIntosh,[1] R.M. Kalnins,[2] and P.F. Bladin[1]

[1] Department of Neurology
[2] Department of Anatomical Pathology
Austin Hospital
Heidelberg (Melbourne)
Victoria 3084
Australia

INTRODUCTION

Hippocampal sclerosis (HS) is found in approximately 65% of patients with refractory temporal lobe epilepsy undergoing temporal lobectomy. Prior to the development of magnetic resonance imaging (MRI) there was no reliable method to detect this lesion pre-operatively. The early literature on MRI in epilepsy regarding the detection of this abnormality was confusing and contradictory (Laster et al., 1985; McLachlan et al., 1985; Jabbari et al., 1986; Lesser et al., 1986; Sperling et al., 1986; Schörner et al., 1987; Heinz et al., 1988). Areas of high signal in T2-weighted images were frequently reported. These high signals were not always of diagnostic significance, in some cases being due to artefact or non-specific enlargement of the temporal horn. The early enthusiasm for the value of MRI in non-lesional cases of temporal lobe epilepsy waned in many centres, and it was widely regarded that it was not possible to detect HS by visual inspection of MRI scans (Sperling et al., 1987).

Recently, careful volumetric studies of the hippocampus showed unilateral hippocampal atrophy in a considerable proportion of cases (Ashtari et al., 1991; Cook et al., 1992; Jack et al., 1992) and in some studies, this has been shown to be correlated with the pathological finding of HS (Bronen et al., 1991; Cascino et al., 1991). Although the value of volumetric assessment has been widely endorsed, the possibility of accurate diagnosis of HS by visual inspection of MRI has received insufficient attention. This can be performed with great reliability, providing the scans are performed in the appropriate fashion, and are interpreted by an informed reader.

Magnetic Resonance Scanning and Epilepsy, Edited by S.D. Shorvon et al.,
Plenum Press, New York, 1994

DIAGNOSIS OF HIPPOCAMPAL SCLEROSIS BY VISUAL INSPECTION

Using a 0.5 T magnet in Montreal we identified hippocampal sclerosis in spin echo images using visual criteria of a reduction in cross-sectional area of the hippocampus (analogous to current volumetric techniques), in association with a high signal seen on T2-weighted images (Berkovic et al., 1986a,b,c). In view of the shape and orientation of the hippocampus, we realised that the conventional orbitomeatal plane was inappropriate, and that examination of the hippocampus was improved by using an axial plane parallel to the base of the temporal lobe and coronal planes at 90° to this (Berkovic et al., 1986b). Moreover, for correct diagnosis the increased T2 signal must be localised to the hippocampus and proper interpretation is only possible by comparing the high T2 signal area to an anatomically defined abnormality on the T1-weighted scans (Berkovic et al., 1986c). The early Montreal experience showed that the side of the MRI abnormality correlated with the side of the electrical focus, and with the presence of pathological abnormality in the surgical specimens (Kuzniecky et al., 1987). However, adequate pathological material from the hippocampus itself was not obtained, so the view that one could recognise HS was not widely accepted, and indeed full publication of our observations was delayed (Berkovic et al., 1991).

Subsequently, in studies from Melbourne, we compared pre-operative "blind" MRI diagnoses, using a 0.3 T magnet, in 41 surgical cases with adequate hippocampal specimens of which 27 had HS and 14 were normal. The sensitivity for detection of HS was 93% and the specificity was 86% (Jackson et al., 1990). We have since studied a further 73 cases with hippocampal specimens and no major foreign tissue lesion, including 59 cases of pathologically proven hippocampal sclerosis. All 59 cases were recognised on pre-operative MRI by blinded observers. False-positive diagnosis of HS was made on five cases, all of which on review showed quite subtle abnormalities in hippocampal size or shape with little or no change in T2 signal. In four cases the lateralisation was correct. Of these, two showed microdysgenesis of the mesial structures on pathology. There was no definite abnormality in the other two, but in one of these cases the whole hemisphere was atrophic and the hippocampal volume loss presumably reflected this. In the fifth case, EEG and other data pointed to the temporal lobe contralateral to the subtle hippocampal abnormality. Temporal lobectomy was performed on the side of the EEG abnormality and the pathology was normal. The overall sensitivity and specificity for visual diagnosis of HS in the Melbourne series of 114 cases were 98% and 75% respectively. It should be emphasised, however, that of the seven false positives in the whole series, there was strong evidence that the seizures originated from the designated hippocampus in six, even though there was no pathological evidence of hippocampal sclerosis.

The high sensitivity and specificity of visual diagnosis of HS in the Melbourne series were based on two radiological signs using spin echo images; hippocampal atrophy on first echo images and increased hippocampal signal on second echo (more T2-weighted) images. More recently, Jackson et al. (1992), using inversion recovery sequences, described two more features of HS. The abnormal hippocampus has reduced signal intensity on T1-weighted images, and the normally visible internal layering of the hippocampus is absent, which equates with the pathological abnormality of destruction of the pyramidal cell layer. These four hippocampal MRI signs of HS (Table 1) each have a sensitivity of approximately 80% in properly performed and interpreted studies (Jackson et al., 1992).

In addition to these specific signs of HS, other abnormalities may be present in extra-hippocampal regions of the temporal lobe. In some cases the whole temporal lobe may be atrophied; the cortex may show thinning and loss of T1 signal and there may be dilatation of the temporal horn. Recently, abnormalities of the grey–white matter junction have been described in cases of HS (see Meiners et al., Chapter 14). The sensitivity and specificity of these extra-hippocampal features for diagnosis of HS are not known.

Table 1. Signs of hippocampal sclerosis on MRI

Hippocampal abnormalities	Extra-hippocampal abnormalities
• Hippocampal atrophy	• Temporal lobe atrophy
• Increased T2 signal	• Thinning and loss of T1 signal in temporal neocortex
• Loss of T1 signal (inversion recovery sequences)	• Loss of grey–white distinction in the temporal lobe
• Loss of internal layering of hippocampus (inversion recovery sequences)	

It appears that visual diagnosis of hippocampal sclerosis has the sensitivity and specificity very similar to that of volumetric techniques although extensive comparisons have yet to be made. Our own experience, with a large pathological sample, confirms this even though our scans were performed on a low field strength magnet. Although the value of volumetrics is beyond doubt, and is especially useful for correlating a quantitative measure of atrophy with other variables, it is labour intensive and requires special techniques, whereas visual interpretation can be done by the informed clinician at the bedside or in the outpatient clinic.

SIGNIFICANCE OF ABNORMALITIES ON VISUAL INSPECTION

It has been known for many years, and particularly emphasised in early studies by Falconer (1974), that the finding of an abnormality in the surgical specimen was a good prognostic sign for seizure control whereas the normal specimen was more often associated with surgical failure. Visual inspection of the pre-operative MRI allows accurate prediction of the pathological abnormalities and we sought to determine if this was related to post-operative seizure control.

Table 2 shows the seizure outcome in a series of 135 patients with temporal lobe epilepsy followed for at least 24 months following unilateral temporal lobectomy classified according to the pre-operative MRI.

Twenty patients had foreign tissue lesions, and of these only four failed to become seizure free post-operatively. Three of these had large lesions extending outside the area of the temporal lobe resection. The fourth patient had occasional seizures despite the apparent complete removal of a grade 2 astrocytoma.

Eighty-five patients had hippocampal sclerosis, and of these 36 (58%) became seizure free. Thirty per cent were improved and the majority of these had only rare seizures. In many cases post-operative MRI scans suggested that there was hippocampal sclerosis extending posterior to the resection line; however, this was also present in patients who were seizure free. Other follow-up studies (Olivier et al., 1988; Wyler et al., 1989) suggest that improvement in surgical failures is most often achieved by increasing the mesial resection. Some 12% of patients had no significant improvement, despite the relatively favourable diagnosis of hippocampal sclerosis. The reasons for these failures are still being explored.

Amongst the patients with normal hippocampus only 29% became seizure free and 33% were not improved. This supports the volumetric findings of Jack et al. (1992),

Table 2. Pre-operative MRI versus Outcome in Temporal Lobe Epilepsy (n = 135 cases)

Pathology	Seizure free (%)
Foreign tissue (n = 20)	80
Hippocampal sclerosis (n = 85)	58
Normal (n = 24)	29
Other (n = 6)	33

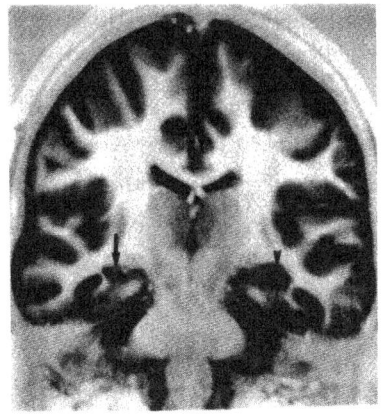

Figure 1. Inversion recovery MRI at 1.5 T showing unilateral right hippocampal atrophy (long arrow) with a normal left hippocampus (between arrow heads). The abnormal side also shows a loss of T1 signal and of internal detail of hippocampal structure. (From Jackson et al. (1992), with permission of authors and publisher.)

who observed that patients with normal hippocampal volumes had a poorer outcome than those with hippocampal atrophy.

CONCLUSIONS

(1) Careful visual inspection of MRI is very sensitive in the detection of hippocampal sclerosis. The specificity is also high, but other rarer abnormalities such as hippocampal microdysgenesis can also cause hippocampal atrophy.

(2) Pre-operative MRI in patients with well-localised temporal lobe foci provides useful prognostic data regarding the chances of post-operative improvement.

REFERENCES

Ashtari, M., Barr, W.B., Schaul, N., and Bogerts, B., 1991, Three dimensional fast low-angle shot imaging and computerised volume measurement of the hippocampus in patients with chronic epilepsy of the temporal lobe, ANJR 12: 941–947.

Berkovic, S.F., Ethier, R., Feindel, W., et al., 1986a, Magnetic resonance imaging in the evaluation of intractable temporal lobe epilepsy, Proceedings of the Society for Magnetic Resonance in Medicine, 587–588.

Berkovic, S.F., Ethier, R., Olivier, A., et al., 1986b, Magnetic resonance imaging of the hippocampus: I. normal anatomy, Epilepsia 27: 611–612.

Berkovic, S.F., Ethier, R., Robitaille, Y., et al., 1986c, Magnetic resonance imaging of the hippocampus: II. mesial temporal sclerosis, Epilepsia 27: 612.

Berkovic, S.F., Andermann, F., Ethier, R., et al., 1991, Hippocampal sclerosis in temporal lobe epilepsy demonstrated by magnetic resonance imaging, Ann Neurol. 29: 175–182.

Bronen, R.A., Cheung, G., Charles, J.T., et al., 1991, Imaging findings in hippocampal sclerosis: correlation with pathology, AJNR 12: 933–940.

Cascino, G.D., Jack, C.R., Parisi, J.E., et al., 1991, MRI-based volume studies in temporal lobe epilepsy: pathological correlations, Ann Neurol. 30: 31–36

Cook, M.J., Fish, D.R., Shorvon, S.D., Straughan, K., and Stevens, J.M., 1992, Hippocampal volumetric studies in frontal and temporal lobe epilepsy, Brain 115: 1001–1015.

Falconer, M.A., 1974, Mesial temporal (Ammon's horn) sclerosis as a common cause of epilepsy: aetiology, treatment and prevention, Lancet 2: 767–770.

Heinz, E.R., Heinz, T.R., Radtke, R. et al., 1988, Efficacy of MRI vs CT in epilepsy, ANJR 9: 1123–1128.

Jabbari, B., Gunderson, C.H., Wippold, F., et al., 1986, Magnetic resonance imaging in partial complex epilepsy, Arch Neurol. 43: 869–872.

Jack, C.R., Sharbrough, F.W., Cascino, G.D., Hirschorn, K.R., O'Brien, P.C., and Marsh, W.R., 1992, Magnetic resonance image-based hippocampal volumetry: correlation with outcome after temporal lobectomy, Ann Neurol. 31: 138–146.

Jackson, G.D., Berkovic, S.F., Tress, B.M., Kalnins, R.M., Fabinyi, G., and Bladin, P.F., 1990, Hippocampal sclerosis can be reliably detected by magnetic resonance imaging, Neurology 40: 1869–1875.

Jackson, G.D., Berkovic, S.F., Duncan, J.S., and Connelly, A., 1992, Optimising the diagnosis of hippocampal sclerosis using magnetic resonance imaging, ANJR.

Kuzniecky, R., de la Sayette, V., Ethier, R., et al., 1987, Magnetic resonance imaging in temporal lobe epilepsy: pathological correlations, Ann Neurol. 22: 341–347.

Laster, D.W., Penry, J.K., Moody, D.M., et al., 1985, Chronic seizure disorders: contribution of MR imaging when CT is normal, ANJR 6: 177–180.

Lesser, R., Modic, M.T., Weinstein, M.A., et al., 1986, Magnetic resonance imaging in patients with intractable focal seizures, Arch Neurol. 43: 367–371.

McLachlan, R.S., Nicholson, R.L., Black, S., Carr, T., and Blume, W.T., 1985, Nuclear magnetic resonance, a new approach to the investigation of refractory temporal lobe epilepsy, Epilepsia 26: 555–562.

Olivier, A., Tanaka, T., and Andermann, F., 1988, Reoperations in temporal lobe epilepsy, Epilepsia 29: 678.

Schörner, W., Meencke, W.J., and Felix, R., 1987, Temporal-lobe epilepsy: comparison of CT and MR imaging, ANJR 8: 773–781.

Sperling, M.R., Sutherling, W.W., and Nuwer, M.R., 1987, New techniques for evaluating patients for epilepsy surgery, in: "Surgical Treatment of the Epilepsies," J.Engel, Jr, ed., Raven Press, New York.

Sperling, M.R., Wilson, C., Engel, J.Jr, et al., 1986, Magnetic resonance imaging in intractable partial epilepsy: correlative studies, Ann Neurol. 20: 57–62.

Wyler, A.R., Herman, B.P., and Richey, E.T. 1989, Results of reoperation for failed epilepsy surgery, J Neurosurg. 71:815–819.

VOLUMETRIC MRI STUDIES OF THE HIPPOCAMPUS

M.J. Cook,[1] S.L. Free,[2] D.R. Fish,[1] S.D. Shorvon,[1] K. Straughan,[2] and J.M. Stevens[3]

[1] Institute of Neurology
Queen Square
London WC1N 3BG
[2] Imperial College
London
[3] St. Mary's Hospital
London
United Kingdom

INTRODUCTION

Volumetric MRI permits acquisition of fine, contiguous slices with excellent tissue contrast, and is ideal for detailed morphometric studies of the hippocampus.

Volumetric studies have shown that hippocampal volume loss occurs in patients with typical temporal lobe epilepsy (Jack et al., 1990; Ashtari et al., 1991; Cook et al., 1992). Several centres have shown correlation of this volume loss with histologically proven mesial temporal sclerosis (MTS), and a relationship between degree of cell loss in MTS and the degree of atrophy (Bronen et al., 1991; Cascino et al., 1991).

CURRENT RESEARCH

We have not seen hippocampal volume loss with extratemporal lesions, and this may provide a useful means of discrimination when clinical phenomenology is atypical (Cook et al., 1992). Large extratemporal lesions may cause distortion of the mesial temporal structures, but volumes are preserved. Definition of the distribution of volume loss by simple morphometry reveals focal anterior hippocampal atrophy to be the most commonly encountered pattern (Figure 1). Diffuse volume loss is associated with frequent secondarily generalised seizures. Isolated posterior volume loss is relatively uncommon. The relationship between the distribution of volume loss and post-operative seizure control is not yet known.

Quantification of volume loss in this way may allow more precise correlation between the distribution of atrophy and clinical features, as well as detecting minor degrees of

Magnetic Scanning Resonance and Epilepsy, Edited by S.D. Shorvon et al.,
Plenum Press, New York, 1993

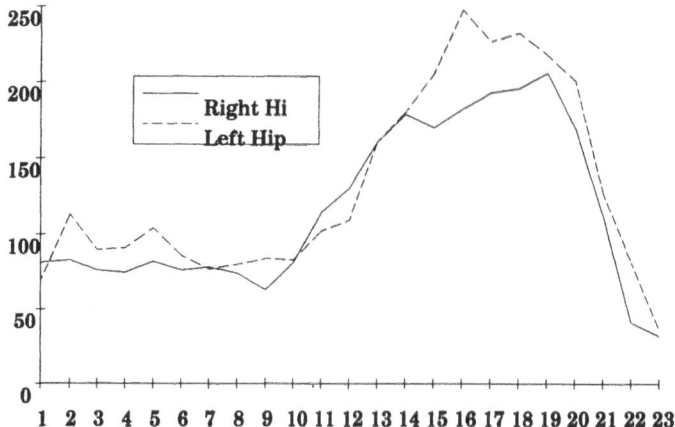

Figure 1. Typical anterior right hippocampal volume loss shown in this graph of hippocampal surface area vs slice number, representing approx. 10% total volume loss. Posterior hippocampus lower slice numbers, slice 23 most anterior hippocampus. Y-axis surface area, X-axis slice number.

asymmetry not seen on visual inspection of the images. Volume loss is often focal and mild (< 10%) in patients with temporal lobe epilepsy, necessitating fine (1–3 mm), contiguous slices if high sensitivity is expected (Cook et al., 1992). More obvious atrophy may be seen without detailed morphometry being performed, but valuable information regarding the degree and distribution of the atrophy may be lost. In addition, it is particularly difficult to estimate volumes by a reliable visual method if patients are tilted or obliquely placed when imaged. Inter- and intra-observer variation of volume measures is low, provided strict anatomical definitions are adhered to.

Image processing facilities are required to perform morphometry, though these are now widely available. Essentially, all methods rely on comparison of the two hippocampi, and so evidence of bilaterality may be concealed. Preservation of normal volume contours and absolute hippocampal volumes may allow this occurrence to be detected.

DISCUSSION

Volumetric techniques allow the limits and degree of hippocampal volume loss to be assessed. Normal hippocampal volumes in the presence of neocortical lesions may allow distinction of these groups. Morphometry may permit definition of high risk surgical groups, and aid in surgical planning. Post-operative studies reveal valuable prognostic information, relating extent of resection to seizure control (Nayel et al., 1991). Standardisation of these measures should allow multicentre collaborative studies of this type.

PROBABLE DEVELOPMENT OVER THE NEXT FIVE YEARS

These techniques are likely to become a regular part of pre- and post-operative assessment in partial epilepsy. Automation has proved difficult, largely due to the inhomogeneity of the structure, but more sophisticated image processing techniques may make this possible.

REFERENCES

Ashtari, M., Barr, W.B., Schaul, N., and Bogerts, B., 1991, Three dimensional fast low angle shot imaging and computerized volume measurements of the hippocampus in patients with chronic epilepsy of the temporal lobe, AJNR 12: 941–947.

Bronen, R.A., Cheung, G., Charles, J.T., Kim, J.H., Spencer, D.D., Spencer, S.S., Sze, G., and McCarthy, G., 1991, Imaging findings in hippocampal sclerosis: Correlation with pathology, H.J.N.I.L. 12: 933–940.

Cascino, G.D., Jack, C.R., Parisi, J.E., Sharbrough, F.W., Hirschorn, K.A., Meyer, F.B., Marsh, W.R., and O'Brien, P.C., 1991, Magnetic resonance imaging-based volume studies in temporal lobe epilepsy: pathological correlations, Ann Neurol. 30: 31–36.

Cook, M.J., Fish, D.R., Shorvon, S.D., Straughan, K., and Stevens, J.M., 1992, Hippocampal volumetric and morphometric studies in temporal and frontal lobe epilepsy, Brain 115: 1001–1015.

Jack, C.R. Jr., Sharbrough, F.W., Twomey, C.K., Cascino, G.D., Hirschorn, K.A., Marsh, W.R., Zinsmeister, A.R., and Scheithauer, B., 1990, Temporal lobe seizures: lateralisation with MR volume measurements of the hippocampal formation, Radiology 175: 423–429.

Nayel, M.H., Awad, I.A., and Luders, H., 1991, Extent of mesiobasal resection determines outcome after temporal lobectomy for intractable complex partial seizures, Neurosurgery 29: 55–60.

8

ADVANCES IN MORPHOMETRIC AND VOLUMETRIC ANALYSIS IN TEMPORAL LOBE EPILEPSY

C. Watson,[1] F. Andermann,[2] P. Gloor,[2] F. Cendes,[2] M. Jones-Gotman,[2]
T. Peters,[2] A. Evans,[2] A. Olivier,[2] D. Melanson,[2] G. Leroux,[2] and
B. Williamson[1]

[1] School of Medicine
University of California, Davis and
Sacramento Comprehensive Epilepsy Program and
Sutter Neuroscience Center Epilepsy Program
Sacramento, California

[2] Department of Neurology and Neurosurgery
McGill University and
Montreal Neurological Institute and Hospital
Montreal, Quebec, Canada

INTRODUCTION

Recently, quantitative MRI-based volumetric studies have been used in the investigation of patients with unilateral temporal lobe epilepsy (Jack et al., 1990, 1992; Cascino et al., 1991; Ashtari et al., 1991; Cook et al., 1992; Lencz et al., 1992). As each centre uses a different method in obtaining its results, it is difficult to compare them directly. To date, attention has been focused on hippocampal volume measurements. Because the amygdala also plays an important role in the pathophysiology of temporal lobe epilepsy, it seems reasonable to include volumetric analysis of this structure as well (Gloor et al., 1982; Feindel and Rasmussen, 1991; Feindel et al., 1991; Gloor, 1992).

CURRENT RESEARCH

To obviate many of these discrepancies, we developed a protocol for measuring approximately 90–95 % of the hippocampus. Because of the importance of distinguishing hippocampal from amygdaloid contributions to temporal lobe epilepsy, we also developed a protocol to measure the volume of the amygdala (Watson et al., 1991, 1992).

Magnetic Resonance Scanning and Epilepsy, Edited by S.D. Shorvon et al.,
Plenum Press, New York, 1994

Anatomical Guidelines

Anatomical guidelines for outlining the amygdala and hippocampus were established using multiple sources, including personal histological and whole brain sections belonging to the authors or studied at the Yakovlev Collection (Armed Forces Institute of Pathology, Washington DC), neuroanatomical atlases, and frequent correlation with cadaver brain specimens and special dissections.

Amygdaloid Volume

The anterior end of the amygdala was arbitrarily and consistently measured on the MRI section at the level of the closure of the lateral sulcus to form the endorhinal sulcus. Although we recognise that this procedure potentially excluded part of the anterior amygdaloid area, we thought that this region was too difficult to visualise reliably on MRI scan and might well consist of other structures such as the anterior-inferior extent of the claustrum and the endopyriform nucleus. The medial border of the amygdala is covered by part of the entorhinal cortex which forms the surface of the ambient gyrus in this region. The entorhinal cortex inferior to the tentorial indentation was excluded from the amygdaloid measurement. If the tentorial indentation was poorly defined or not visible in the anterior amygdaloid region, the line of demarcation between the amygdala and the adjacent entorhinal cortex that occupies the ambient gyrus was defined by a line drawn in direct continuation with the inferior and medial border of the amygdala within the substance of the temporal lobe. By proceeding in this manner a small amount of the superior extent of the entorhinal cortex will be included in the amygdaloid volume, as is the case when the tentorial indentation is used as the landmark. The inferior and lateral borders of the amygdala were formed by the inferior horn of the lateral ventricle or white matter (Figure 1).

To define the superior border of the amygdala, we drew a straight line laterally from the endorhinal sulcus to the fundus of the inferior portion of the circular sulcus of the insula. More posteriorly, the optic tract was utilised as a guide to the lateral extension of the crural cistern into the transverse cerebral fissure. This located the medial aspect of the posterior amygdala and was used as the point of departure for defining the medial and superior borders of the structure posteriorly. To define the superior border of the amygdala at this level, a straight line was drawn laterally from the superolateral aspect of the optic tract to the fundus of the inferior portion of the circular sulcus of the insula (Figure 2).

This method of defining the superior border of the amygdala is arbitrary and undoubtedly excludes small amounts of the medial and central nuclei. However, it should prevent such structures as the substantia innominata, inferior portion of the putamen and inferior portion of the claustrum from being included in the amygdaloid measurement. At its posterior end, the amygdala occupies the medial half of the roof of the inferior horn of the lateral ventricle, and care must be taken to exclude the tail of the caudate nucleus, the overlying globus pallidus and putamen, and the lateral geniculate body (Figure 3).

In cases in which the border of the putamen cannot be clearly defined, only the medial half of the structures in the roof should be included in the amygdaloid volume at this level.

Hippocampal Volume

It is obviously most difficult to define the boundaries of the hippocampus in its most anterior portion, the hippocampal head. The most reliable structure separating the head of the hippocampus from the amygdala in this region is the inferior horn of the lateral ventricle. This is especially true if the ventricular cavity extends into the deep part of the uncus anterior to the head of the hippocampus, thereby forming the uncal recess of the inferior horn. However,

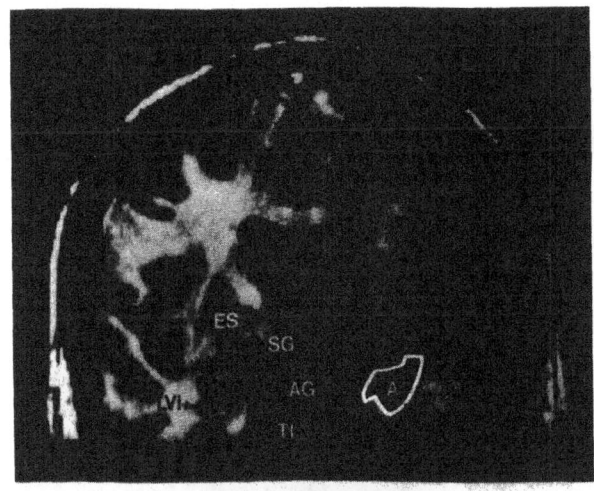

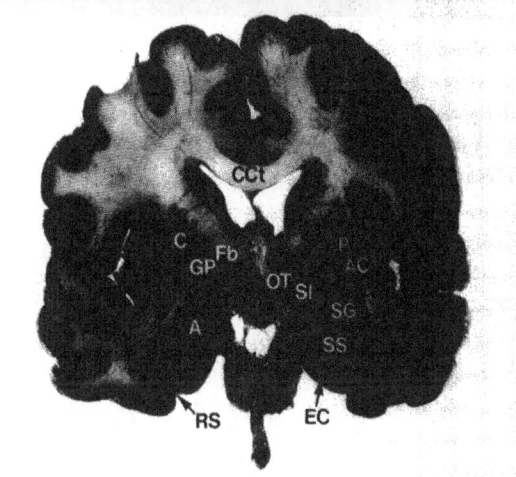

Figure 1. Angled coronal sections of the cerebral hemispheres passing through the anterior segment of the uncus. Upper plate: MRI scan with amygdala outlined on the left (see text for MRI sequence parameters). Lower plate: Brain section stained with the LeMasurier modification of the Mulligan stain.

Abbreviations used in figures:

A	amygdala	Hf	fimbria of hippocampus
AC	anterior commissure	Hh	hippocampus, head (pes)
AG	ambient gyrus	HS	hippocampal sulcus
BG	band (limbus) of Giacomini	Ht	hippocampus, tail
C	claustrum	IF	interventricular foramen
CaS	calcarine sulcus	IG	intralimbic gyrus
CCg	corpus callosum, genu	LGB	lateral geniculate body
CCr	corpus callosum, rostrum	LVct	lateral ventricle, collateral trigone
CCs	corpus callosum, splenium	LVi	lateral ventricle, inferior horn
CCt	corpus callosum, trunk	OT	optic tract
CGi	isthmus of cingulate gyrus	P	putamen
CoS	collateral sulcus	PG	parahippocampal gyrus
CSi	circular sulcus of insula	RS	rhinal sulcus
EC	entorhinal cortex	SC	subicular complex
ES	endorhinal sulcus	SG	semilunar gyrus
Fb	fornix, body	SI	substantia innominata
Fc	fornix, crus	SS	semianular (amygdaloid) sulcus
GP	globus pallidus	TI	tentorial indentation
Hb	hippocampus, body	UC	uncal cleft

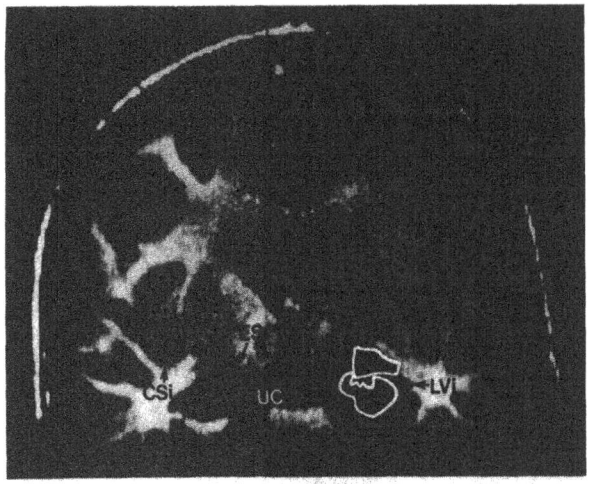

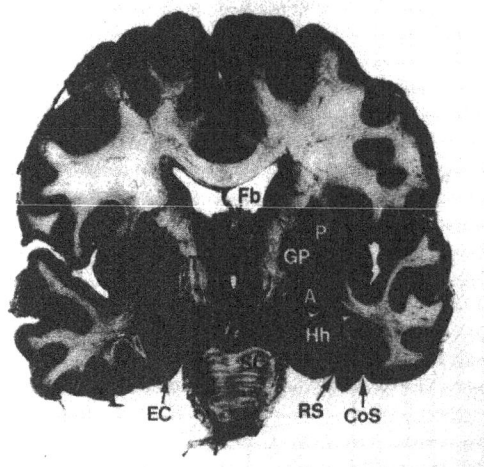

Figure 2. Angled coronal sections of the cerebral hemispheres passing through the posterior segment of the uncus. Upper plate: MRI scan with amygdala and hippocampal head outlined on the left. Lower plate: Brain section.

portions of the uncal recess are often obliterated, especially medially, and the hippocampal digitations are fused to the amygdala across the ventricular cavity. When this was the case, three guidelines were used to outline the hippocampal head and separate it from the adjacent amygdala. If an obvious semilunar gyrus was present on the surface of the uncus, a line was drawn connecting the inferior horn of the lateral ventricle to the sulcus at the inferior margin of the semilunar gyrus (i.e., the semi-annular or amygdaloid sulcus). It was also useful to use the alveus covering the ventricular surface of the hippocampal digitations to distinguish the hippocampus from the amygdala. If neither the semi-anular sulcus nor the alveus was obvious, a straight horizontal line was drawn connecting the plane of the inferior horn of the lateral ventricle with the surface of the uncus. The inferior margin of the hippocampus was outlined to include the subicular complex and the uncal cleft with the border separating the subicular complex from the parahippocampal gyrus being defined as the angle formed by the most medial extent of those two structures. In the normal control population no attempt was made to outline the grey matter on the superior and inferior banks of the uncal cleft as it was usually quite narrow. The grey matter of the entorhinal cortex or parahippocampal gyrus was excluded from this measurement (Figures 2 and 3).

In the hippocampal body, the delineation of the hippocampus included the subicular complex, hippocampus proper, dentate gyrus, alveus and fimbria. The border between the

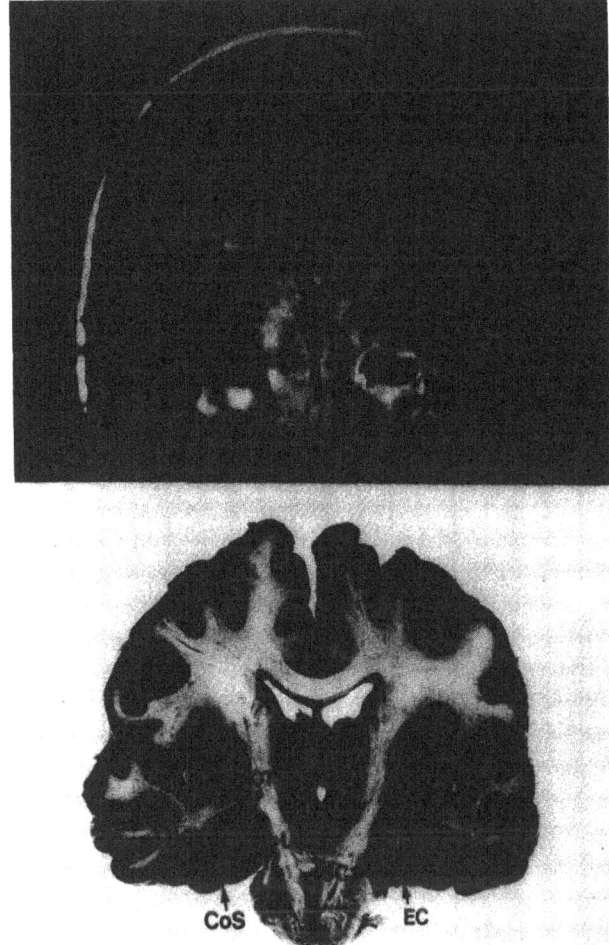

Figure 3. Angled coronal sections of the cerebral hemispheres passing through the posterior segment of the uncus. Upper plate: MRI scan with posterior portion of hippocampal head outlined on the left. Lower plate: Brain section.

subicular complex and the parahippocampal gyrus was defined in the same manner as in the hippocampal head. Therefore, the cortex of the parahippocampal gyrus was once again excluded from the measurement (Figure 4).

In the hippocampal tail, measurement again included the subicular complex, hippocampus proper, dentate gyrus, alveus and fimbria. Excluded at this level were the crus of the fornix, isthmus of the cingulate gyrus (retrosplenial cortex) and parahippocampal gyrus. The most posterior section measured was the section with the crus of the fornix clearly separating from the hippocampus and its fimbria (Figure 5).

This left a small segment of the tail of the hippocampus outside the measured hippocampal volume. As the distance from the anterior end of the hippocampus to the point of separation of the crus of the fornix from the fimbria of the hippocampus was approximately 35–38 mm, we estimate that the entire hippocampus except for its most posterior 2–4 mm was included in the volume measurement. Therefore, assuming a total anterior-posterior length of the hippocampus of approximately 40 mm, these guidelines should result in a volume measurement of 90–95% of the total hippocampal formation.

We used this protocol in 30 patients with intractable temporal lobe epilepsy. Our results corroborate those of others in verifying that volumetric studies of the hippocampus and amygdala are helpful in lateralising the epileptogenic region. We found hippocampal volumes

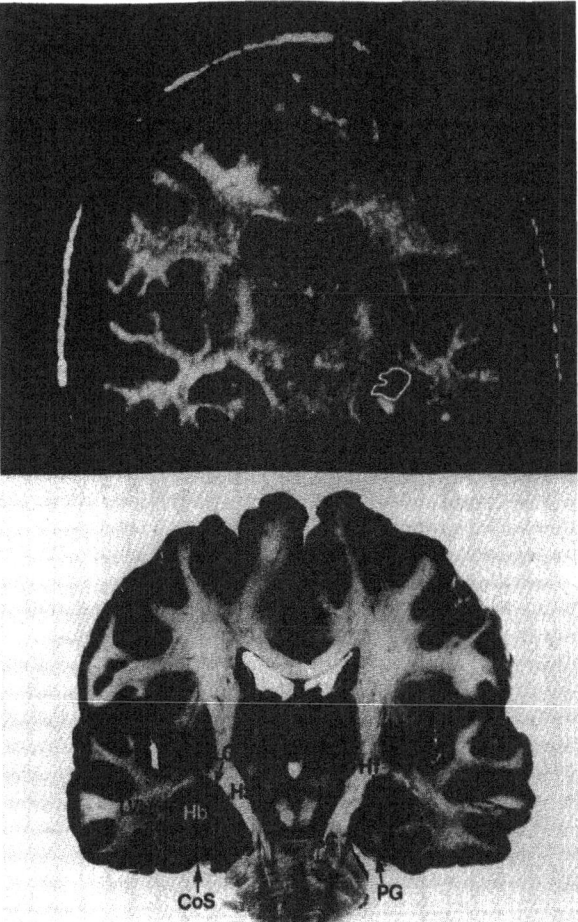

Figure 4. Angled coronal sections of the cerebral hemispheres passing through the lateral geniculate body and the parahippocampal gyrus. Upper plate: MRI scan with hippocampal body outlined on the left. Lower plate: Brain section.

to be more sensitive than amygdaloid volumes (87% vs 67%). However, when both hippocampal and amygdaloid volumes were considered, lateralisation was obtained in 93% of patients (Cendes et al., 1992a; Cendes et al., 1993).

Our preliminary data suggest that amygdaloid and hippocampal volume measurements may be useful in providing supplementary information in patients with bilateral temporal ictal onsets (Figure 6) (Watson et al., 1991; Cendes et al., 1992a; 1993).

We are now in the process of accumulating a large normal control population which will be crucial for the interpretation of patients with bilateral hippocampal and amygdaloid atrophy as well as conducting multicentre inter-rater and intra-rater reliability studies (Cendes et al., 1992b,c).

DISCUSSION

The development of high resolution MRI-based volumetric measurement has proved useful in the pre-operative evaluation of patients with temporal lobe epilepsy caused by unilateral hippocampal sclerosis. Studies have shown significantly reduced hippocampal volumes, which corroborate neurophysiological studies and allow lateralisation of the epileptogenic region, correlation with neuropathological and neuropsychological abnormalities, and

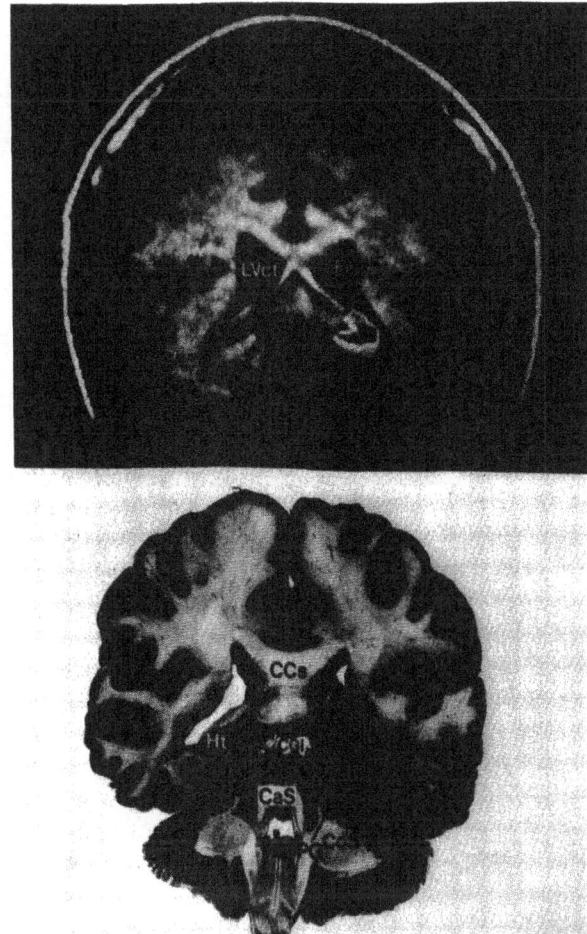

Figure 5. Angled coronal sections of the cerebral hemispheres passing through the splenium of the corpus callosum and isthmus of the cingulate gyrus. Upper plate: MRI scan with hippocampal tail outlined on the left. Lower plate: Brain section showing the transition from fimbria of hippocampus to crus of fornix. (Reproduced with permission of author and publisher.)

correlation with outcome after temporal lobectomy (Jack et al., 1990, 1992; Ashtari et al., 1991; Cascino et al., 1991; Watson et al., 1991; Cendes et al., 1992a; Lencz et al., 1992). We expect that quantitative MRI techniques will reduce the number of patients who require invasive, prolonged and expensive EEG monitoring, thereby allowing more patients to be treated effectively using non-invasive EEG monitoring coupled with non-invasive imaging techniques and neuropsychological studies. The addition of amygdaloid volume measurements to those of the hippocampus may allow assessment of the relative contribution of each of these structures to epileptogenesis. Post-operative quantitation of the amount of amygdaloid and hippocampal resection should yield better understanding of which structures need to be removed and in what volume.

PROBABLE DEVELOPMENT OVER THE NEXT FIVE YEARS

Advances in morphometric and volumetric analysis are likely to be quite useful in the evaluation of patients with bilateral temporal ictal onsets as well as those with unilateral seizure onset (Watson et al., 1991; Cendes et al., 1992a, 1993; Jack et al., 1992). The pattern of hippocampal and amygdaloid involvement (Cook et al., 1992) may become quite useful in

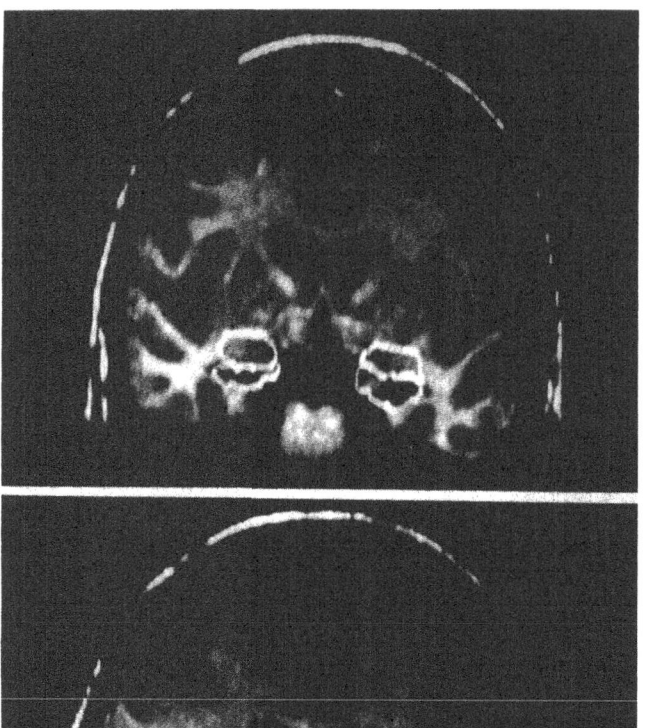

Figure 6. Angled coronal MRI sections from a patient with bilateral, independent temporal ictal onsets that were much more frequent from the right side. MRI-based volumetric studies showed bilateral statistically significant hippocampal atrophy that was much more prominent on the right side. Pathology showed severe hippocampal sclerosis on the right side.

planning surgical approaches which may be more limited than standard operative procedures and allow us to test the outcome of various surgical approaches. With increased spatial resolution we may begin to visualise, in at least an approximate fashion, specific hippocampal sectors and amygdaloid nuclei. This will allow further advances in our understanding of the pathogenesis of hippocampal sclerosis and other basic processes such as memory.

REFERENCES

Ashtari, M., Barr, W.B., Schaul, N., and Bogerts, B., 1991, Three-dimensional fast low-angle shot imaging and computerized volume measurement of the hippocampus in patients with chronic epilepsy of the temporal lobe, AJNR, 12: 941–947.

Cascino, G.D., Jack, C.R., Jr., Parisi, J.E., Sharbrough, F.W., Hirschorn, K.A., Meyer, F.B., Marsh, W.R., and O'Brien, P.C., 1991, Magnetic resonance imaging-based volume studies in temporal lobe epilepsy: pathological correlations, Ann Neurol. 30: 31–36.

Cendes, F., Andermann, F., Watson, C., Evans, A., Gloor, P., Melanson, D., Jones-Gotman, M., Leroux, G., Olivier, A., and Peters, T., 1992a, Volumetric measurements of amygdaloid body (AB) and hippocampal formation (HF) in temporal lobe epilepsy (TLE), Neurology 42 (Suppl 3): 205.

Cendes, F., Andermann, F., Watson, C., Evans, A., Gloor, P., Jones-Gotman, M., Melanson, D., Olivier, A., Leroux, G., and Peters, T., 1992b, MRI volumetric measurements of amygdaloid body and hippocampal formation: inter and intrarater differences, Can J Neurol Sci. 19: 285.

Cendes, F., Cook, M.J., Watson, C., Andermann, F., Peters, T., Free, S.L., Straughan, K., Fish, D.R., Shorvon, S.D., and Stevens, J.M., 1992c, Hippocampal volumes in normal subjects: a multicentre study, Epilepsia 33 (Suppl 3):49.

Cendes, F., Andermann, F., Gloor, P., Evans, A., Jones-Gotman, M., Watson, C., Melanson, D., Olivier, A., Peters, T., Lopes-Cendes, I., and Leroux, G., 1993, MRI volumetric measurement of amygdala and hippocampus in temporal lobe epilepsy, Neurology 43:719–725.

Cook, M.J., Fish, D.R., Shorvon, S.D., Straughan, K., and Stevens, J.M., 1992, Hippocampal volumetric and morphometric studies in frontal and temporal lobe epilepsy, Brain 115: 1001–1015.

Feindel, W., and Rasmussen, T., 1991, Temporal lobectomy with amygdalectomy and minimal hippocampal resection: review of 100 cases, Can J Neurol Sci. 18: 603–605.

Feindel, W., Robitaille, Y., Tampieri, D., Goossens, L., Li, M., and Melanson, D., 1991, Electroencephalography, magnetic resonance imaging, and pathology in patients treated surgically for temporal lobe epilepsy, Can J Neurol Sci. 18: 577–579.

Gloor, P., 1992, Mesial temporal sclerosis: historical background and an overview from a modern perspective, in: "Epilepsy Surgery," H.O. Luders, ed., Raven Press, New York.

Gloor, P., Olivier, A., Quesney, L.F., Andermann, F., and Horowitz, S., 1982, The role of the limbic system in experiential phenomena of temporal lobe epilepsy, Ann Neurol. 12: 129–144.

Jack, C.R., Jr, Sharbrough, F.W., Twomey, C.K., Cascino, G.D., Hirschorn, K.A., Marsh, W.R., Zinsmeister, A.R., and Scheithauer, B., 1990, Temporal lobe seizures: lateralisation with MR volume measurements of the hippocampal formation, Radiology 175: 423–429.

Jack, C.R., Jr, Sharbrough, F.W., Cascino, G.D., Hirschorn, K.A., O'Brien, P.C., and Marsh, W.R., 1992, Magnetic resonance image-based hippocampal volumetry: correlation with outcome after temporal lobectomy, Ann Neurol. 31: 138–146.

Lencz, T., McCarthy, G., Bronen, R.A., Scott, T.M., Inserni, J.A., Sass, K.J., Novelly, R.A., Kim, J.H., and Spencer, D.D., 1992, Quantitative magnetic resonance imaging in temporal lobe epilepsy: relationship to neuropathology and neuropsychological function, Ann Neurol. 31: 629–637.

Watson, C., Andermann, F., Gloor, P., Jones-Gotman, M., Peters, T., Evans, A., Olivier, A., and Leroux, G., 1991, MRI-based volume measurement of the amygdala and hippocampus: description of method and normal control data, Epilepsia 32 (Suppl 3): 76–77.

Watson, C., Andermann, F., Gloor, P., Jones-Gotman, M., Peters, T., Evans, A., Olivier, A., Melanson, D., and Leroux, G., 1992, Anatomical basis of amygdaloid and hippocampal volume measurement by magnetic resonance imaging, Neurology 42: 1743–1750.

THE ROLE OF MRI VOLUMETRIC STUDIES IN THE INVESTIGATION OF PATIENTS WITH INTRACTABLE EPILEPSY

F. Cendes, F. Andermann, P. Gloor, A. Olivier, A. Evans, and T. Peters

Department of Neurology and Neurosurgery
McGill University and the Montreal Neurological Hospital and Institute
3801 University Street
Montreal, Quebec
Canada H3A 2B4

The assessment of intractable epilepsy has traditionally depended on analysis of clinical seizure patterns in association with a searching EEG investigation. EEG recording of seizures is still considered necessary for seizure localisation prior to surgical treatment in patients without an obvious lesion on MRI. Radiological and neuropsychological studies are also essential for pre-surgical investigation. When the findings are not completely congruous, or when there are seeming contradictions in surface and sphenoidal recordings, monitoring with surgically implanted depth electrodes may be required. However, there is a significant risk of morbidity associated with the implantation of depth electrodes. This, together with the limited availability and high costs of the procedure, reduces the number of patients who can benefit from surgical treatment.

Modern neuroimaging techniques, particularly the steady improvement in the quality of MRIs, which may now be acquired faster and with better image quality, have revolutionised this field. The demonstration by MRI of atrophy and signal changes suggesting hippocampal sclerosis has streamlined the pre-surgical evaluation of patients with temporal lobe epilepsy (TLE). Both these findings seem to have a high sensitivity and specificity. As an additional benefit, volumetric studies allow us to quantify and to determine the anatomical extent of the volume loss, important considerations prior to surgery (Sperling et al., 1986; Kuzniecky et al., 1987; Jack et al., 1990; Berkovic et al., 1991; Cascino et al., 1991; Cook et al., 1992; Editorial 1992; Jack et al., 1992; Lencz et al., 1992; Cendes et al., 1993a,b).

Volumetric MRI measurements of temporal lobe structures in patients with TLE accurately detected volume reduction of mesial structures in patients with histologically proven mesial temporal sclerosis (Cascino et al., 1991; Lencz et al., 1992; Cendes et al., 1993a,d). Measuring the amygdala in addition to the hippocampus improves the sensitivity of this non-invasive technique (Cendes et al., 1993a).

Magnetic Resonance Scanning and Epilepsy, Edited by S.D. Shorvon et al.,
Plenum Press, New York, 1994

At our institution, acquisition of MRI data for volumetric study is with coronal views taken perpendicular to the plane of the sylvian fissure obtained with a three-dimensional gradient fast field echo (FFE) sequence, with 3 mm interleaved sections. More recently we have been using MRI acquisition with inversion recovery; this technique allows better assessment of the grey–white matter interface and of cortical gyration. The images are transferred to a Sun SPARC work station (Sun Microsystems, Mountain View, CA, USA). Volumetric measurements are performed with an interactive software program, developed in the Neuroimaging Laboratory of the Montreal Neurological Institute. The regions of interest are outlined using a manual contouring editing function. Once the outline has been defined, the slice volume is calculated automatically by the computer program. Anatomical guidelines for outlining the amygdala and hippocampal formation follow a specific protocol previously described (Watson et al., 1992). Volumes of the amygdala and hippocampus are compared with values from a normal control group. We considered abnormal volumes beyond 2 standard deviations from normal control values.

We studied 100 epileptic patients, using MRI volumetric measurements of amygdala and hippocampus. Seventy-six patients presented with intractable TLE. We found significant atrophy of mesial temporal structures, coinciding with the side of EEG seizure onset, in 92% of those patients having TLE with no foreign tissue lesions. This volume reduction was more pronounced in patients with a history of prolonged febrile convulsion in early childhood (Cendes et al., 1993b). No significant atrophy was demonstrated in the 24 patients who had seizures not originating in the temporal lobe (usually they had frontal or generalised epilepsy) (Cendes et al., 1993a,d).

Mesial temporal sclerosis was the main pathological abnormality in patients who had prolonged febrile convulsions early in life. There was a higher proportion of more severe mesial temporal sclerosis in these patients compared to those with no antecedent of febrile convulsions.

Other pathology, such as gangliogliomas and migration disorders, were found in 10 patients with TLE without antecedent prolonged febrile convulsions. In 80% of these patients with foreign tissue lesions, the amygdala and hippocampus were symmetrical and of normal volume.

Relatively little attention has been paid to the amygdala as an important contributor to epileptogenesis in temporal lobe epilepsy (Gloor, 1992). In our series, volumetric measurements demonstrated more pronounced atrophy of the amygdala in patients who had prolonged febrile convulsions, although the hippocampal volumes were also smaller in this group. All patients who had hippocampal sclerosis had equally severe pathology of the amygdala as shown when tissue from the amygdala was available for analysis. These changes were even more severe than in the hippocampus in three patients with antecedent prolonged febrile convulsions.

When combining the amygdala and the hippocampal volumes, we found lateralisation in 92% of the TLE patients, compared with 87% when using hippocampal volumes alone. This improved discrimination justifies the additional use of amygdala measurements in computerised volumetric studies, and also emphasises the important role played by the amygdala, in addition to the hippocampus, in the genesis of temporal lobe epilepsy (Gloor, 1992; Cendes et al., 1993a,b).

There were six patients in whom no lesion or definite volumetric asymmetry of mesial structures was found, even though the clinical EEG investigation indicated that the origin of seizures was in the temporal lobe. Although in half of these patients there was some asymmetry ipsilateral to the focus, within 1 standard deviation of normal values, we considered these volumetric results as negative. The EEG investigation in these six patients showed maximal abnormalities in the lateral aspects of the temporal lobe, and the amount of slow wave abnormality was much less than in patients with mesial atrophy. Four of these patients were treated surgically, and histopathological investigation showed a mild degree of mesial temporal sclerosis, although there were also pathological changes in the neocortex, mainly gliosis. These patients may represent one extreme of the spectrum of patients with mesial sclerosis, with changes too mild to be detected by MRI volumetric analysis. Another possible explanation for this lack of mesial atrophy is that these patients have developmental lesions, such as subtle neuronal migration disorders, which were not identified.

There were ten patients with TLE who underwent stereotaxically implanted depth EEG (SEEG) because either the extracranial EEG investigation could not define a clear lateralisation or there were discrepancies between inter-ictal and ictal activity, or as a result of other conflicting results. The conclusions of the SEEG investigation were concordant with the lateralisation obtained by volumetric study in all patients. The seizures recorded in the depth studies originated exclusively or predominantly in the smaller amygdala and/or hippocampus. Although these results are encouraging, it is still premature to ignore ambiguities based on scalp EEG recording until greater experience with the clinical significance of volumetrically determined smallness or asymmetry is acquired.

Diminished volumes of amygdala and hippocampus demonstrating mesial temporal atrophy appeared to be specific for patients with seizures that originated in the temporal lobe, because the volumetric studies did not show abnormal size of mesial temporal structures in extra-temporal epilepsy. Furthermore no correlation is found, using regression analysis, between the total duration of the epilepsy and the degree of atrophy of the amygdala and hippocampus as revealed by the MRI volumetric studies (Cendes et al., 1993d). Our data show that patients with early childhood convulsions who had MRI volumetric studies in early adolescence, had greater atrophy than those whose epilepsy was of longer duration but who did not have convulsions in early life. Neither the frequency of partial nor that of generalized attacks considered separately correlated with increased atrophy.

DISCUSSION

According to our observations, and those of others, it was clear that volumetric measurements of mesial temporal structures provide more information than non-quantitative, visually interpreted MRI scans (Jack et al., 1990; Cendes et al., 1993c) (Figures 1 and 2). The difficulty in visually assessing the three-dimensional volume of structures such as amygdala and the hippocampus, presented to the interpreter in serial two-dimensional images, is obvious: the boundaries are irregular, the spatial orientation is complex, the patient's head is not always well positioned and the anatomical variation is considerable. Gross asymmetries may be identified by simple visual impression without difficulty; MRI volumetric measurements, however, help determine the presence of asymmetries which are less obvious. We found that in some patients the visual estimation of volume asymmetry alone was misleading (Cendes et al., 1993c).

Volumetric studies generate numerical values and permit better comparison of the degree of mesial atrophy among various subgroups of patients with epilepsy. The findings can be correlated with different clinical parameters and lead to better discrimination and understanding of the underlying condition.

In conclusion, MRI volumetric studies are useful for the investigation of partial epilepsies, improving the possibility of detecting and lateralising volume loss related to mesial temporal sclerosis. Our findings agree with other reports showing a correlation between the occurrence of prolonged febrile convulsions in infancy and the degree of mesial temporal sclerosis (Meyer et al., 1954; Cavanagh and Meyer 1956; Sperling et al., 1986; Babb and Brown 1987; Kuzniecky et al., 1987; Sagar and Oxbury 1987; Bruton 1988). We have shown that repeated

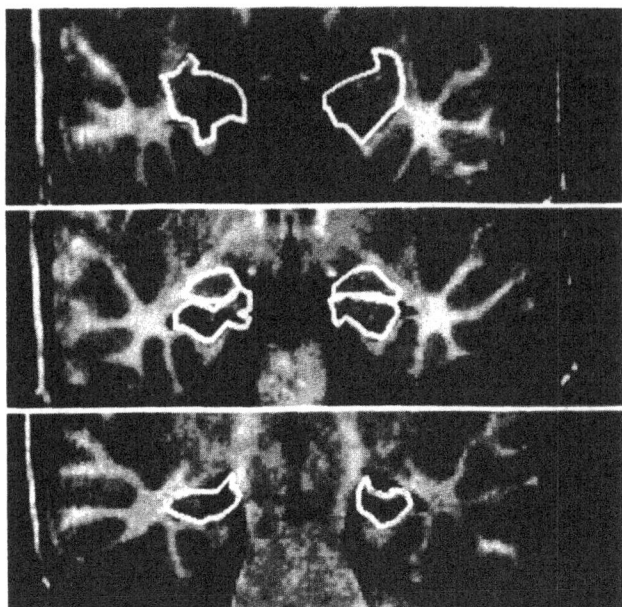

Figure 1. Coronal images with outlines of amygdala (top) and hippocampal formation (HF) (bottom) and of both structures at the level of the head of hippocampus (middle). The visual analysis of the 2 slices showing the hippocampi gives the impression that the left one is smaller. This was due to the position of the patient's head. The volumetric measurements showed symmetrical HFs, but there was an asymmetry of the amygdalae, the right being smaller. The EEG showed a right temporal lobe focus with anterior predominance (equipotentiality at electrode position F8–T4).

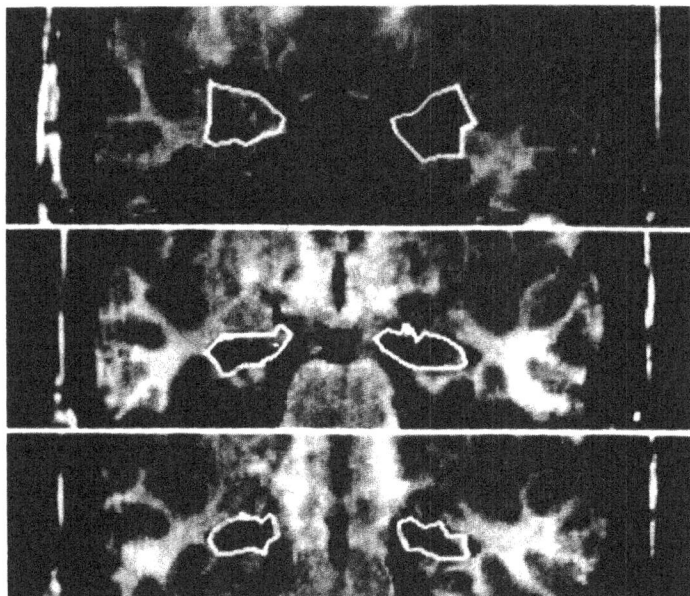

Figure 2. Coronal images with outlines of amygdala (top) and hippocampal formation in a patient with left TLE. On routine MRI no definite asymmetry or smallness could be observed by visual or qualitative interpretation. MRI volumetric measurements showed that both hippocampi and amygdalae were small compared to controls (mean—2 SD). The asymmetry, with left sided smaller mesial structures, correlated with the results of intracranial EEG investigation.

seizures throughout life do not appear to cause an increased measurable atrophy of the amygdala and the hippocampus, and we conclude therefore that the atrophy appears to be the cause rather than the effect of the seizures. However, we recognise that progressive changes of a lesser order of magnitude might also occur which would not be reflected in our studies.

REFERENCES

Babb, T.L., and Brown, W.J., 1987, Pathological findings in epilepsy, in: "Surgical Treatment of the Epilepsies," J. Engel, Jr, ed., Raven Press, New York.

Berkovic, S.F., Andermann, F., Olivier, A., et al., 1991, Hippocampal sclerosis in temporal lobe epilepsy demonstrated by magnetic resonance imaging, Ann Neurol. 29: 175–182.

Bruton, C.J., 1988, "The neuropathology of temporal lobe epilepsy," Oxford University Press, New York.

Cascino, G.D., Jack, C.R., Parisi, J.E., et al., 1991, Magnetic resonance imaging-based volume studies in temporal lobe epilepsy: pathological correlations, Ann Neurol. 30: 31–36

Cavanagh, J.B., and Meyer, A., 1956, Aetiological aspects of Ammon's horn sclerosis associated with temporal lobe epilepsy, BMJ 2: 1403–1407.

Cendes, F., Andermann, F., Gloor, P., et al., 1993a, MRI volumetric measurements of amygdala and hippocampus in temporal lobe epilepsy, Neurology 43: 719–725.

Cendes, F., Andermann, F., Dubeau, F., et al., 1993b, Early childhood prolonged febrile convulsions, atrophy and sclerosis of mesial structures, and temporal lobe epilepsy: an MRI volumetric study, Neurology 43: 1083–1087.

Cendes, F., Leproux, F., Melanson, D., et al., 1993c, MRI of amygdala and hippocampus in temporal lobe epilepsy, J Comp Ass Tomogr. 17(2): 206–210.

Cendes, F., Andermann, F., Gloor, P., et al., 1993d, Atrophy of mesial structures in patients with temporal lobe epilepsy: cause or consequence of repeated seizures?, Ann Neurol. 34: 795–801.

Cook, M.J., Fish, D.R., Shorvon, S.D., Straughan, K., and Stevens, J.M., 1992, Hippocampal volumetric and morphometric studies in frontal and temporal lobe epilepsy, Brain 115: 1001–1015.

Editorial, 1992, Magnetic resonance imaging in epilepsy, Lancet 340: 343–344.

Gloor, P., 1992, Mesial temporal sclerosis: historical background and an overview from a modern perspective, in: "Epilepsy Surgery," H.O. Luders, ed., Raven Press, New York.

Jack, C.R., Sharbrough, F.W., Twomey, C.K., et al., 1990, Temporal lobe seizures: lateralisation with MR volume measurements of the hippocampal formation, Radiology 175: 423–429.

Jack, C.R., Sharbrough, F.W., Cascino, G., et al., 1992, Magnetic resonance image-based hippocampal volumetry: correlation with outcome after temporal lobectomy, Ann Neurol. 31: 138–146.

Kuzniecky, R., de la Sayette, V., Ethier, R., et al., 1987, Magnetic resonance imaging in temporal lobe epilepsy: pathological correlation, Ann Neurol. 22: 341–347.

Lencz, T., McCarthy, G., Bronen, R., et al., 1992, Quantitative magnetic resonance imaging in temporal lobe epilepsy: relationship to neuropathology and neuropsychological function, Ann Neurol. 31: 629–637.

Meyer, A., Falconer, M.A., and Beck, E., 1954, Pathological findings in temporal lobe epilepsy, J Neurol Neurosurg Psychiat. 17: 276–85.

Sagar, H.J., and Oxbury, J.M., 1987, Hippocampal neuron loss in temporal lobe epilepsy: correlation with early childhood convulsions, Ann Neurol. 22: 334–340.

Sperling, M.R., Wilson, C., Engel, J.Jr, et al., 1986, Magnetic resonance imaging in intractable partial epilepsy: correlative studies, Ann Neurol. 21: 57–62.

Watson, C., Andermann, F., Gloor, P., et al., 1992, Anatomical basis of amygdaloid and hippocampal volume measurements by magnetic resonance imaging, Neurology 42: 1743–1750.

THE FUTURE ROLE FOR MR IMAGING IN EPILEPSY

Morphometry and Volume Analysis

P. Schüler and H. Stefan

Department of Neurology
University Erlangen-Nuremberg
Germany

INTRODUCTION

Quantified volume analysis in MRI (qMRI), especially of the hippocampus (Jack et al., 1990), proved to be of great clinical relevance in correct lateralisation of the epileptogenic focus in patients with temporal lobe epilepsy (TLE).

Less is known about the clinical relevance of temporal lobe atrophy frequently found in patients with TLE (Schüler et al., 1991) and of extratemporal atrophies and structural abnormalities.

CURRENT RESEARCH

Volume Analysis

There is no doubt that mesial temporal sclerosis (MTS) is correlated with TLE which is frequently found in patients with prolonged febrile convulsions (Berkovic et al., 1991). It is even correlated with a good post-surgical outcome (Babb et al., 1984; Jack et al., 1992).

Nevertheless, it is not yet clear to what extent MTS is a pre-condition for TLE and whether MTS is always the cause or, perhaps in certain cases, the consequence of TLE.

An additional atrophy of the whole temporal lobe often occurs in patients with TLE (Figure 1): The clinical relevance of this type of temporal lobe atrophy (TLA) is also uncertain. In our study, 17 of 30 patients had unilateral TLE (Figure 2): 11 had a hippocampal atrophy beyond 2 standard deviations (SD), 13 beyond 1 SD; 11 (2 SD) resp. 14 (1 SD) had a temporal lobe atrophy. Both parameters were significantly (2 SD) reduced simultaneously in only 7 cases.

Thus, TLA also seems to be a sensitive parameter to lateralise a temporal epileptogenic focus correctly. TLA is not necessarily concordant with MTS and vice versa.

Magnetic Resonance Scanning and Epilepsy, Edited by S.D. Shorvon et al.,
Plenum Press, New York, 1994

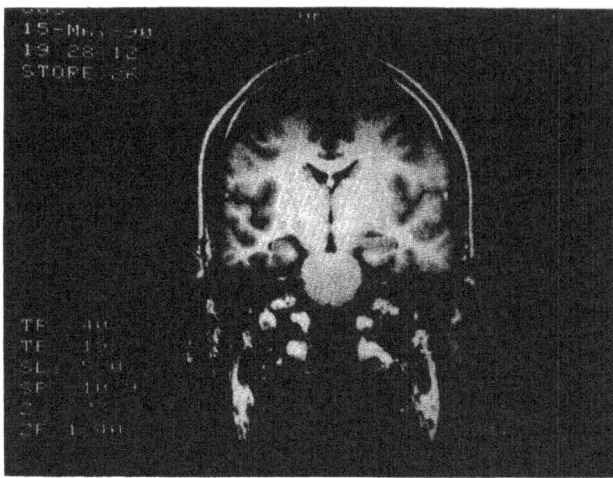

Figure 1. Example of an evident atrophy of the whole right temporal lobe and the right hippocampus: invasive EEG recordings showed ictal onset in mesial structures. The patient became seizure free after a tailored right temporal resection.

Another 13 of these 30 patients had an extra-temporal or a bitemporal epilepsy (bi-TLE): no one in this subgroup showed unilateral abnormalities of both parameters. Thus, TLA can obviously help to differentiate TLE from bi-TLE or non-TLE. In all 30 patients, MTS also affected the opposite side (in the most anterior slice) to a lesser degree (1 SD) in 12 cases, and TLA in 11 cases. Thus atrophy (of hippocampus and/or temporal lobe) is not a problem attributable to only one side of the brain.

TLA was most prominent in the most anterior slice (see Figure 2), a finding also reported after investigations of the hippocampus by Cook et al. (1992). The reason for this finding is still unknown. Whether it has some diagnostic, therapeutic or prognostic relevance will be shown in the future.

In another study of 10 patients with TLE, 40% showed significantly reduced estimated total brain volume, indicating that values in relation to total brain volume are useful. This finding could not be correlated to any anamnestic data except for alcohol abuse (Schüler et al., 1994).

Morphometry

Little work has been done on quantified morphometric analysis. In our group of 10 patients with TLE, the quantification of the number of gyri in four temporal slices was not abnormal on focus side (except the case shown in Figure 3). The same was found in the angle and length of the sylvian fissure. The differentiation of grey and white matter by a signal intensity function (Figure

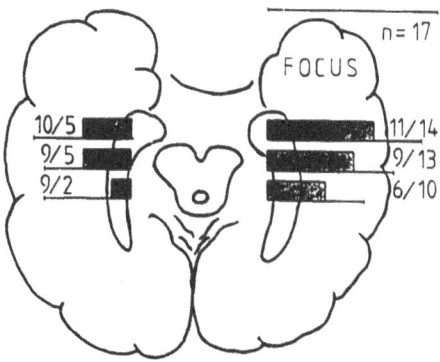

Figure 2. Volumetric analysis of the temporal lobes in patients with unilateral temporal lobe epilepsy: Number of patients with temporal lobe atrophy (in three slices) on temporal focus side (right) and contralateral to focus (left). Total number of patients = 17 (bar on top). Eleven of 17 (65%) have a 2 standard deviation (SD) atrophy, 14 of 17 a 1 SD atrophy in anterior parts on focus side. On the contralateral (non-focus) side, 5 resp. 10 of 17 patients also showed an atrophy. Thick bars = more than 2 standard deviations (SD) from normal; Thin lines = more than 1 SD from normal

3) showed an abnormality in 2 of 10 cases. On the side of epileptic focus, the two peaks for the signals of grey and white matter could not be differentiated, and the single peak indicated a migration abnormality. In one case (Figure 3), this abnormality could be seen by visual inspection of the MRI. In the second case, however, only the signal intensity function was abnormal. Thus this kind of evaluation gives additional information about the structural abnormalities.

DISCUSSION

Without any doubt qMRI has proved to be a helpful and clinically relevant tool that provides additional evidence for the lateralisation of the epileptogenic focus. Nevertheless, the most effective performance of such an analysis in a reasonable time is not yet defined. As it has a high lateralising value, temporal lobe atrophy is of clinical relevance. TLA is not necessarily coexistent with mesial temporal sclerosis. Thus, TLA has its own sensitivity. Likewise, amygdala atrophy also plays a unique role and does not totally coincide with MTS (Watson et al., 1991).

It is currently not known whether the different kinds and patterns of atrophy indicate different types of epilepsies, thus leading to specific therapeutic strategies. For example, it is possible that an atrophy that is more pronounced in neocortical structures of the temporal lobe

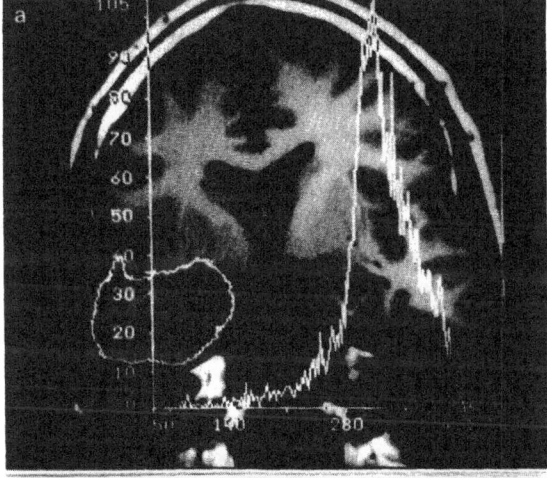

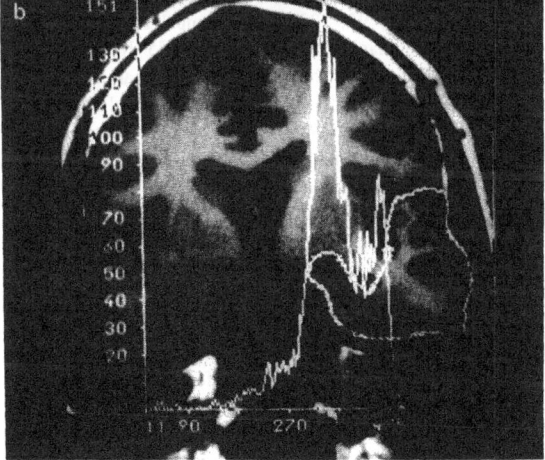

Figure 3. Morphometric analysis of the temporal lobe by signal intensity function (SIF). X-axis: signal intensity; Y-axis: number of pixels. (a) The right temporal lobe shows a migration abnormality, leading to a missing differentiation in the SIF; (b) The two peaks on the normal side which indicate the different signal behaviour of grey and white matter are missing on the focus side

might indicate a focus in the neocortical region. Our results are at too early a stage to support such a hypothesis, and a larger multicentre collection of patients will be necessary to answer this question.

It will also be important to establish the significance of the contralateral atrophy which is frequently found. In order to evaluate both lobes separately, absolute normal values must be available for both sides (and both genders).

Extra-temporal atrophies are more difficult to investigate; however, a reduction in the total brain volume is often seen in epileptic patients. Thus, values of qMRI should be taken in relation to total brain volume to avoid false positive findings.

Abnormalities in morphometry also frequently escape detection. The few abnormalities found are also visible on "bed-side" inspection of the MRI. The only additional abnormality we could detect was a missing second peak in signal intensity function in 1 of 10 patients (in another patient, it was easily visible by eye). This might help to detect migration abnormalities, even in rare cases without an atrophy or MTS.

FUTURE DEVELOPMENTS

Automatic analysis will reduce the time for a quantification procedure. Better and faster three-dimensional sequences will allow a better reformatting of brain substructures. Migration disorders can particularly be detected more easily by such an evaluation method (e.g. by quantifying grey-matter thickness or by signal intensity functions). Because it is not only ipsilateral hippocampi and temporal lobes that are involved in mechanisms leading to an atrophy, "mapping" of volumes of several substructures of the brain will perhaps lead to a better understanding of different epileptic syndromes and to more specific operative strategies. Even if an MRI requires an evaluation time of 2 hours, it should be noted that this is much shorter than the weeks necessary to perform intensive video-EEG monitoring in the course of pre-surgical evaluation. Intensive EEG evaluation has rendered epilepsy surgery possible in some cases and better MRI evaluation will probably allow shorter and less invasive EEG investigations.

REFERENCES

Babb, T.L., Brown, W.J., Pretorius, J., Davenport, C., Lieb, J.P., and Crandall, P.H., 1984, Temporal lobe volumetric cell densities in temporal lobe epilepsy, Epilepsia 25: 729–740.

Berkovic, S.F., Andermann, F., Olivier, A., Ethier, R., Melanson, D., Robitaille, Y., Kuzniecky, R., Peters, T., and Feindel, W., 1991, Hippocampal sclerosis in temporal lobe epilepsy demonstrated by magnetic resonance imaging, Ann Neurol. 29: 175–182.

Cook, M.J., Fish, D.R., Shorvon, S.D., Straughan, K., and Stevens, J.M., 1992, Hippocampal volumetric and morphometric studies in frontal and temporal lobe epilepsy, Brain 11: 1001–1015.

Jack, C.R., Sharbrough, F.W., Twomey, C.K., Cascino, G.D., Hirschhorn, K.A., Marsh, W.R., Zinsmeister, A.R., and Scheithauer, B., 1990, Temporal lobe seizures: lateralisation with MR volume measurements of the hippocampal formation, Radiology 175: 423–429.

Jack, C.R., Sharbrough, F.W., Cascino, G.D., Hirschhorn, K.A., O'Brian, P.C., and Marsh, W.R., 1992, Magnetic resonance image-based hippocampal volumetry: correlation with outcome after temporal lobectomy, Ann Neurol. 31: 138–146.

Schüler, P., Hahn, G., Huk, W., Bauer, J., Neubauer, U., and Stefan, H., 1991, Quantitative and qualitative MRI abnormalities in temporal lobe epilepsy, Nervenarzt 62: 232–236.

Schüler, P., Stefan, H., Kalb, A., and Neubauer, U., 1994, Atrophy of the temporal lobes in patients with temporal and extratemporal epileptogenic foci: a quantified planimetric study in 30 patients, Epilepsia in press.

Watson, C., Anderman, F., Gloor, P., Jones-Gotman, M., Peters, T., Evans, A., Olivier, A., and Leroux, G., 1991, MRI-based volume measurement of the amygdala and hippocampus: description of method and normal control data, Epilepsia 32 (suppl): 76–77.

QUANTITATIVE RELAXOMETRY OF HIPPOCAMPAL SCLEROSIS

J.S. Duncan,[1] G.D. Jackson,[2] A. Connelly,[3] R.A. Grunewald,[1] and D.G. Gadian[2]

[1] Institute of Neurology
Queen Square
London, WC1N 3BG
[2] Institute of Child Health
[3] Hospitals for Sick Children
London
United Kingdom

INTRODUCTION

The non-invasive diagnosis of hippocampal sclerosis (HS) by MRI forms an important part of pre-surgical evaluation and decision making, and is also important in the investigation of the prevalence and evolution of HS. The cardinal qualitative MRI features of HS are atrophy and increased T2-weighted signal intensity (Jackson et al., 1990; Berkovic et al., 1991). Recently, loss of internal structure of the hippocampus and decreased T1-weighted signal intensity have also been described (Jackson et al., 1993a).

A visually evident increase in hippocampal T2-weighted signal intensity has usually been reported in about 30–40% of cases of HS (Jackson et al., 1990; Ashtari et al., 1991; Bronen et al., 1991). In an analogous way to the quantification of atrophy by volumetric analysis (see Chapter 7), T2-weighted signal intensity may be quantified by measurement of the T2 relaxation time, leading to greater sensitivity and precision (Jackson et al., 1993b). T1 and T2 mapping have been shown to be more sensitive than qualitative inspection of T1- and T2-weighted images for the detection of white matter disease (Miller et al., 1989).

CURRENT RESEARCH

T2 maps were constructed in 3 parallel coronal slices from 16 images, with echo times from 22 ms to 262 ms using a Carr–Purcell–Meiboom–Gill sequence. Slices were 8 mm thick and orientated perpendicularly to the hippocampus, minimising partial volume effects. Hippocampal data were derived from the central slice, which was positioned

Magnetic Resonance Scanning and Epilepsy, Edited by S.D. Shorvon et al.,
Plenum Press, New York, 1994

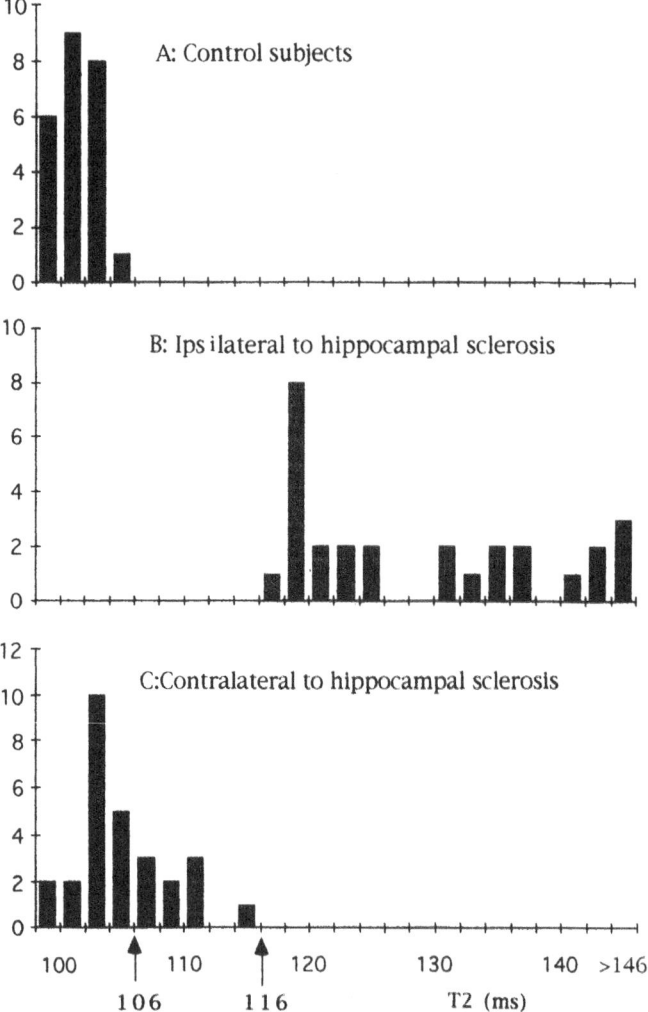

Figure 1. T2 relaxation times (ms) in hippocampi of normal subjects, and in patients with hippocampal sclerosis (from Jackson et al., 1993b).

along the anterior border of the brain stem. Hippocampal T2 times were measured from the calculated T2 map on the largest circular region of interest that could be placed in the hippocampal cross-section.

The range of hippocampal T2 times in control subjects (n = 12) was 99–106 ms, with a maximum side to side difference of 5 ms. There was excellent inter-observer reliability for values obtained from normal subjects and patients. In 41 patients with drug-resistant temporal lobe epilepsy, 28 had unilateral HS on MRI criteria (Jackson et al., 1993a), and resected hippocampal tissue, available in 9, confirmed the diagnosis in these. The range of T2 times in sclerotic hippocampi was 118–154 ms (Figure 1). T2 times in the hippocampus contralateral to HS were outside the normal range in 9 patients (32%) (range: 100–116 ms).

DISCUSSION

T2 relaxation time measurements are a useful identifier of hippocampal pathology, values > 116 ms being associated with HS. In patients with HS there was a visually evident increase in T2-weighted signal intensity in 77% of patients with scans obtained under optimal conditions (Jackson et al., 1993a). Intermediate values of 106–116 ms were seen in (a) patients without MR imaging evidence of HS, (b) contralateral to HS and (c) in some patients with extratemporal seizure onset.

T2 data must be interpreted in the light of high quality anatomical imaging, or misdiagnoses may be made, for example with lesions such as glioma or hamartoma which may also give rise to elevation of T2. It is also important to avoid partial volume effects with CSF, by using oblique coronal scan orientation that is perpendicular to the body of the hippocampus, and by careful region of interest placement.

The data from healthy subjects indicate that there is a narrow range of normal hippocampal T2 relaxation times, resulting in the parameter being a useful absolute measure. This is in contrast to hippocampal volume measurements, for which the wide normal range of absolute values largely limits assessment to identification of asymmetry and may preclude identification of bilateral HS, and lesser degrees of contralateral hippocampal damage.

The pathological correlate of T2 prolongation in HS is probably gliosis and neuronal fall-out. In a rat model, cortical astrocytosis was associated with a 4–9 ms prolongation of T2 time (Jackson et al., 1991). Oedema secondary to seizures and occult partial volume effects are also possible contributory factors.

DEVELOPMENTS OVER THE NEXT FIVE YEARS

Application of hippocampal T2 mapping to longitudinal studies and correlation of T2 times with volumetric data, histological findings and extent of neuronal loss in patients with HS.

- T2 mapping of hippocampus with greater spatial resolution.
- Evaluation of T2 mapping at extratemporal sites.
- Evaluation of T1 mapping of the hippocampus.

ACKNOWLEDGEMENTS

We are grateful to Action Research for project grant support, and to Ms Sandra Powell for the radiography.

REFERENCES

Ashtari, M., Barr, W.B., Schaul, N., and Bogerts, B., 1991, Three dimensional fast low angle shot imaging and computerized volume measurements of the hippocampus in patients with chronic epilepsy of the temporal lobe, AJNR 12: 941–947.

Berkovic, S.F., Andermann, F., Olivier, A., et al., 1991, Hippocampal sclerosis in temporal lobe epilepsy demonstrated by magnetic resonance imaging, Ann Neurol. 29: 175–182.

Bronen, R.A., Cheung, G., Charles, J.T., et al., 1991, Imaging findings in hippocampal sclerosis: correlation with pathology, AJNR 12: 933–940.

Jackson, G.D., Berkovic, S.F., Tress, B.M., Kalnins, R.M., Fabinyi, G., and Bladin, P.F., 1990, Hippocampal sclerosis can be reliably detected by magnetic resonance imaging, Neurology 40: 1869–1875.

Jackson, G.D., Williams, S.F., van Bruggen, N., Williams, S.R., and Duncan, J.S., 1991, Vigabatrin-induced cerebellar and cortical lesions are demonstrated by quantitative magnetic resonance imaging, Epilepsia 32 (suppl 1): 13.

Jackson, G.D., Berkovic, S.F., Duncan, J.S., and Connelly, A., 1993a, Optimizing the diagnosis of hippocampal sclerosis using MRI. AJNR 114: 753–762.

Jackson, G.D., Connelly, A., Duncan, J.S., Grünwald, R.A., and Gadian, D.S. 1993b, Detection of hippocampal pathology in intractable partial epilepsy: Increased sensitivity with quantitative magnetic resonance T_2 relaxometry. Neurology 43: 1793–1799.

Miller, D.H., Johnson, G., Tofts, P.S., Macmanus, D., and McDonald, W.I., 1989, Precise relaxation time measurements of normal-appearing white matter in inflammatory central nervous system disease, Magn Reson Med. 11: 331–336.

THE SIGNIFICANCE OF T2 CHANGES IN THE HIPPOCAMPUS

P. Tofts

Institute of Neurology
Queen Square
London, WC1N 3BG
United Kingdom

MEASUREMENT OF RELAXATION TIMES

Relaxation times T1 and T2 can be measured accurately and reproducibly in the brain (Tofts and Du Boulay, 1990), enabling white matter in different disease groups to be differentiated (Miller et al., 1989). However, scanner performance can degrade both accuracy and reproducibility, and the pathological cause of changes in relaxation times has yet to be established with certainty.

Bilateral changes in relaxation time can be established as genuine, and not artificially caused by poor machine performance, by imaging a uniform phantom under the same conditions. The phantom should be filled with water and doped to produce similar relaxation times to those in the brain at the field strengths being used.

Absolute values of relaxation times can be verified by using a calibrated phantom made from doped water or agarose gel (Tofts et al., 1993). The true relaxation times of the phantom can be established by one of three methods: (1) they can be measured on a spectrometer (which produces accurate values) operating at the same field; (2) commercially produced gels (e.g. Lerski and McRobbie 1992) which are already calibrated can be used; or (3) gels can be made to a published recipe where the relationship between concentration and relaxation time has already been established (e.g. Tofts et al., 1993). Erroneous T1 values may be too long or too short, depending on what aspect of the instrument is at fault. However, T2 values are hardly ever too long, and usually too short, because of poor refocusing by the 180° pulses. Multiple echo sequences often perform poorly in this respect, and a series of single echoes at different echo times, although slow, is likely to be more accurate (Tofts et al., 1993). Poor refocusing causes an artificially fast decay in the transverse magnetisation. A straightforward and cheap test for T2 accuracy is therefore to measure the apparent T2 of distilled water, which has a true T2 of 2.5 seconds. The effect of poor refocusing is to reduce the measured T2, to as low as 200 ms (Tofts et al., 1993). Provided the measured value is above about 1 s, the values for white and grey matter (80–200 ms) will not be significantly in error.

If the scanner is unstable (i.e. drifting or upgraded) during the period that patients and controls are studied (which may be a period of many months), this can produce an apparent difference between the two groups. This can be ruled out in one of two ways:

(1) Phantoms should be measured, possibly as part of a quality assurance scheme (Barker and Tofts, 1992).

(2) The patients and controls should be interleaved and studied over the same time period. If there is a change in the scanner during the duration of the study, the phantom measurements will detect this, but will not necessarily enable the in vivo measurements to be corrected. Interleaving of the patient and controls is the only sure way to avoid a change of scanner performance producing an artefactual difference between patients and controls.

In small structures, partial volume effects can alter the measured change in relaxation time towards that of the surrounding tissue(s), if the voxel size is too large to be entirely contained within the structure of interest. For example, the hippocampus could have an artificially reduced T2 where it is adjacent to white matter (T2 = 103 ms for hippocampus (see Chapter 11), 80 ms for white matter). Adjacent to the CSF it would have an artificially increased T2 (CSF T2 = 2500 ms). CSF contamination can be ruled out in two ways: first, in multi-echo data with good refocusing pulses any CSF in the voxel will appear as a long T2 component. Second, T2 can be correlated against the size of the object. (The partial volume effect means that T2 will increase with reducing size if the object is surrounded by CSF.) The T2 values from the two groups of patients can then be corrected for size, to make a comparison at the same size. The increased T2 values in the hippocampus reported by Duncan et al. (see Chapter 11) could possibly be artefactual, because hippocampal volumes are known to be reduced (see Chapter 7).

PATHOPHYSIOLOGICAL SIGNIFICANCE

Models of relaxation in very simple systems, such as agarose solutions doped with gadolinium-DTPA are good; the correspondence between material structure and relaxation times is well understood. However, models of relaxation in tissue are less developed. It is not currently possible, given a particular tissue structure, to predict quantitatively what its relaxation times will be; nor can we predict what the tissue structure is from the relaxation times. Even alterations in relaxation times are non-specific. For example, increased relaxation times in white matter can be caused by either oedema or gliosis. Simple models of relaxation in tissue do exist (Bottomley et al., 1987; reviewed in Tofts and Du Boulay 1990), and they tell us two ways in which relaxation times can increase. First, an increase in the amount of free water will increase relaxation times. This could arise from an increase in the extracellular space, as in oedema. Second, a decrease in the coupling between bound water and free water will increase relaxation times. Bound water is attached to proteins, macromolecules, myelin, etc., and the coupling (magnetisation transfer) between bound and free water is responsible for relaxation of the free water that is observed by MRI (see Chapter 12). The high magnetisation transfer contrast of white matter suggests that myelin is particularly efficient at relaxing the free water.

The increased rate (i.e. 1/T1) of white matter relative to that of grey matter may be caused by myelin-mediated relaxation.

ANIMAL MODELS AND HUMAN BIOPSY MATERIAL

Because modelling of relaxation in tissue has been relatively unsuccessful so far, the collection of empirical evidence is particularly important. In multiple sclerosis, animal models of the disease have enabled us to correlate pathological changes with MRI changes, and hence we can infer the pathological significance of MRI changes seen in patients. In epilepsy the same approach may be required. In addition, patient tissue, obtained from biopsies or during surgery, may help us verify the pathological significance of NMR changes that we have inferred from animal models.

REFERENCES

Barker, G., and Tofts, P.S., 1992, Semiautomated quality assurance for quantitative magnetic resonance imaging, Magn Reson Imag. 10: 585–595.

Bottomley, P.A., Hardy, C.J., Argersinger, R.E., and Allen-Moore, G., 1987, A review of 1H nuclear magnetic resonance relaxation in pathology: Are T1 and T2 diagnostic?, Med Phys. 14: 1–37.

Lerski, R.A., and McRobbie, D.W., 1992, Instructions for Eurospin II Magnetic Resonance Quality Assessment Test Objects, Diagnostic Sonar Ltd, Livingston.

Miller, D.H., Johnson, G., Tofts, P.S., Macmanus, D., and McDonald, W.I., 1989, Precise relaxation time measurements of normal appearing white matter in inflammatory central nervous system disease, Magn Reson Med. 11: 331–336.

Tofts, P.S., and Du Boulay, E.P.G.H., 1990, Towards quantitative measurements of relaxation times and other parameters in the brain, Neuroradiology 32: 407–415.

Tofts, P.S., Shuter, B., and Pope, J.M., 1993, Ni-DTPA doped agarose gel-a phantom material for Gd-DTPA enhancement measurements, Magn Reson Imag. 11: 125–133.

INVESTIGATION OF EFFECTS OF VIGABATRIN WITH MAGNETIC RESONANCE IMAGING AND SPECTROSCOPY IN VIVO

J.S. Duncan,[1] G.D. Jackson,[2] A. Connelly,[2] R.A. Grünewald,[1] N.E. Preece,[2] N. Van Bruggen,[2] and S.R. Williams[2]

[1]Institute of Neurology
Queen Square
London, WC1N 3BG
[2]Institute of Child Health and Hospitals for Sick Children
London
United Kingdom

INTRODUCTION

MR Imaging

Vigabatrin (gamma vinyl GABA, GVG) is an irreversible inhibitor of gamma-aminobutyric acid (GABA) transaminase, the enzyme that is responsible for degradation of GABA in the CNS. Vigabatrin is effective against partial seizures (Rimmer and Richens, 1984; Mumford and Dam, 1989; Reynolds, 1992). In toxicological studies involving rodents and dogs, high doses of GVG were associated with the development of a site-selective intramyelinic oedema that was accompanied by an astrocytic reaction (Butler et al., 1987; Gibson et al., 1990). A concern has been expressed about whether similar neuropathological changes may develop in human patients receiving long-term GVG therapy. No such changes have been identified in 51 surgical specimens and 13 autopsy cases (Cannon, 1991). Evoked response latencies have been shown to be prolonged in dogs with GVG-associated intramyelinic oedema, and these parameters have not been delayed in GVG-treated patients (Hammond and Wilder, 1985; Tartara et al., 1986). Evoked responses, however, only sample a small part of the neuraxis.

T2-weighted MR images are a sensitive means for the identification of white matter disease, and T2 mapping has been shown to be more sensitive than qualitative inspection of T2-weighted images for the detection of pathological changes (Miller et al., 1989). Visually apparent MRI changes have been noted in dogs given high doses of GVG, with development of intramyelinic oedema (Weiss et al., 1991). Visually apparent MRI changes have not been noted in patients treated with GVG (Chiron et al., 1989). We have used quantitative T2 mapping to demonstrate the neuropathological changes associated with GVG in the rat brain in vivo, and have used the same technique as part of a prospective, double-blind, randomised, parallel group evaluation of human patients dosed with GVG for 20 weeks.

MR Spectroscopy

The elevation of intracerebral GABA concentrations by administration of GVG provides a model in which the ability of proton MR spectroscopy to assess GABA concentrations in vivo may be evaluated (Preece et al., 1994).

CURRENT RESEARCH

MR Imaging

Ten Sprague-Dawley rats received 250 mg/kg per day of GVG orally for 8 weeks. T2-weighted images on these and seven control rats were obtained using a 30 cm bore magnet of 2.35 T. In seven treated and five control rats, T2 relaxation times were obtained on a single parasagittal slice from four images (TE 30, 60, 90, 120 ms, TR 3100 ms, NEX 4, 128 X 256) by exponential regression of image intensities from selected regions of interest. Pathological examination included haematoxylin and eosin staining and immunocytochemical examination with GFAP and ED1 (Prof. Roy Weller; Dr W. Butler). T2-weighted imaging showed an increase in signal intensity in cerebellar white matter. T2 relaxation time was 12 ms longer in cerebellar white matter in treated (78 ± 1.9) than control (66 ± 3.9) rats ($p < 0.002$). In the thalamus, hippocampus and cerebral cortexts there were no visually apparent changes, but T2 relaxation time was prolonged by 4–9 ms in these areas in the GVG-treated as compared with the control rats ($p < 0.02$). The pathological correlate of the visually apparent 12 ms increase in T2 time was intramyelinic oedema, reactive astrocytosis and microglial activation. The pathological correlate of the 4–9 ms increase was reactive astrocytosis and microglial activation, without intramyelinic oedema (Jackson et al., 1991).

The aim of the human study was to assess possible GVG-related changes in the brains of patients with epilepsy, using quantitative MRI with T2 relaxation time mapping. Forty-five patients with refractory partial seizures were studied in a prospective, randomised, placebo-controlled, add-on, parallel group, double-blind trial in which 3 g/day of GVG or matching placebo was added to the patients' usual antiepileptic drug treatment. T1- and T2-weighted scans and T2 maps were obtained using a Siemens 1.5 T Magneton SP63 instrument. T2 relaxometry was carried out at baseline and after 20 weeks' treatment with GVG or placebo. T2 maps were constructed in three parallel coronal 8 mm slices from 16 images, with echo times varying from 22 ms to 262 ms using a Carr-Purcell-Meiboom-Gill sequence. T2 times were measured from the calculated T2 map on circular regions of interest which were placed in the hippocampus, thalamus, frontal, temporal and occipital white matter, cerebellar hemisphere white matter and vermis. No region showed a prolongation of T2 time after GVG treatment. There was a time-dependent fall in T2 relaxation time in cerebellar white matter with no difference between the vigabatrin and placebo groups (Grünwald et al., 1993).

MR Spectroscopy

Five male Sprague-Dawley rats received 250 mg/kg per day of GVG for 3 weeks. These and five control rats were anaesthetised and placed in a 8.5 T magnet interfaced to a Bruker AM-360 spectrometer. A 7 mm surface coil was placed on the scalp for recording ^{1}H spectra.

A 12 mm surface coil was used to record ^{31}P spectra. After the completion of measurements, the brains were removed and, extracted, and single-pulse spectra were obtained at 500 MHz using a JEOL JX-500 spectrometer.

Non-edited ^{1}H spectra were recorded in vivo with a spin-echo sequence. ^{1}H spectra edited for a- and g-GABA resonances were acquired by interleaving two experiments with decoupling irradiation at the b-GABA resonance in one and a control irradiation at 7.5 p.p.m. in the other (Preece et al., 1994). On non-edited spectra the increased intensities attributable to GABA were not adequately resolved from other metabolites. Using edited spectra, GABA could not be adequately detected in vivo in the control group but was clearly seen in GVG treated rats, with a GABA/N-acetyl aspartate signal intensity ratio of 0.1 ± 0.04 and an estimated cerebral GABA concentration of 6.0 ± 2.3 mmol/kg. There were no changes in ^{31}P spectra in rats treated with GVG.

DISCUSSION

MR Imaging

The investigations in the rat confirmed that quantitative T2 mapping was a sensitive method for detecting neuropathological changes associated with GVG. This provided a validation of the technique for the studies of patients in which no prolongation of T2 relaxation time has been found after 4 months of treatment with 3 g/day of GVG.

MR Spectroscopy

In these studies using an 8.5 T instrument, GABA was identified and quantified non-invasively following GVG administration, with a reasonable concordance between GABA concentrations measured in vitro and in vivo. GABA could not be reliably identified on non-edited spectra.

DEVELOPMENTS OVER THE NEXT FIVE YEARS

MR Imaging

Further studies of rats receiving GVG will include examination of the temporal course of the evolution of MRI changes, including quantitative relaxometry and diffusion-weighted imaging, neuropathological abnormalities after commencement of GVG and the resolution of changes after withdrawal.

Further longer-term investigations are necessary in patients to determine whether there is any evidence of abnormalities developing with more prolonged GVG administration. Longitudinal studies of patients with newly diagnosed epilepsy and being treated with GVG or other antiepileptic drugs as monotherapy for 12 months, using quantitative MRI, are in progress.

MR Spectroscopy

The detection of elevated GABA concentrations is now possible in localised regions of the brain at 1.5 T or above using clinical spectroscopy instruments with double irradiation facilities (Rothman et al., 1993). Developments in MR spectroscopy may allow non-invasive investigation in vivo of the relationship between regional cerebral GABA concentrations, epileptic foci and the efficacy of antiepileptic drugs.

ACKNOWLEDGEMENTS

We are grateful to the following for support and encouragement: Marion Merrell Dow and Action Research for project grant support, Professor Roy Weller (Southampton University, UK) and Dr William Butler (BIBRA, UK) for neuropathological examination in the animal studies and Professor David Gadian (Institute of Child Health and Royal College of Surgeons), Rank Foundation, Wellcome Trust, Imperial Cancer Research Fund, Wolfson Foundation, Medical Research Council and Picker International.

REFERENCES

Butler, W.H., Ford, G.P., and Newberne, J.W.A., 1987, Study of the effects of vigabatrin on the central nervous system and retina of Sprague Dawley and Lister-hooded rats, Toxicol Pathol. 15:143–148.

Cannon, D., 1991, No vigabatrin-induced microvacuolation in human brains: Further neuropathologic investigations, Epilepsia 32 (suppl 1): 12.

Chiron, C., Dulac, O., Palacios, L., Mondragon, S., Dinh, T.S., et al., 1989, Magnetic resonance imaging in epileptic children treated with g-vinyl GABA (vigabatrin), Epilepsia 30 (Suppl 1): 736.

Gibson, J.P., Yarrington, J.T., Loudy, D.E., Gerbig, C.G., Hurst, G.H., and Newberne, J.W., 1990, Chronic toxicity studies with vigabatrin, a GABA transaminase inhibitor, Toxicol Pathol. 18: 225–238.

Grünwald, R.A., Jackson, G.D., Connelly, A., Duncan, J.S., 1993, Vigabatrin-related changes in the human brain measured by quantitative MRI, Epilepsia 34(suppl. 6): 97.

Hammond, E.J., and Wilder, B.J., 1985, Effects of g-vinyl GABA on human pattern evoked potentials, Neurology 35: 1801–1803.

Jackson, G.D., Williams, S.F., van Bruggen, N., Williams, S.R., and Duncan, J.S., 1991, Vigabatrin-induced cerebellar and cortical lesions are demonstrated by quantitative magnetic resonance imaging, Epilepsia 32 (suppl 1): 13.

Miller, D.H., Johnson, G., Tofts, P.S., Macmanus, D., and McDonald, W.I., 1989, Precise relaxation time measurements of normal-appearing white matter in inflammatory central nervous system disease, Magn Reson in Med. 11: 331–336.

Mumford, J.P., and Dam, M., 1989, Meta-analysis of European placebo controlled studies of GVG in drug resistant epilepsy, Br J Clin Pharmacol 27 (suppl): 119S-124S.

Preece, N.E., Jackson, G.D., Williams, S.F., Houseman, J.A., Duncan, J.S., and Williams, S.R., 1994, NMR detection of elevated cortical GABA in the Vigabatrin-treated rat in vivo, Epilepsia, in press.

Reynolds, E.H., 1992, Vigabatrin. Rational treatment for chronic epilepsy, BMJ 300: 277–278.

Rimmer, E.M., and Richens, A., 1984, Double-blind study of g-vinyl GABA in patients with refractory epilepsy, Lancet i: 189–190.

Rothman, D.L., Petroff, O.A.C., Behar, K.L., Mattson, R.H., 1993, Localized ^{1}H NMR measurements of γ-amino butyric acid in human brain in vivo. Proc Nat Acad Sci USA 90: 5662–5666.

Tartara, A., Manni, R., Galimberti, C.A., et al., 1986, Vigabatrin in the treatment of epilepsy: a double blind placebo-controlled study, Epilepsia 27: 717–723.

Weiss, K.L., Schroeder, C.E., Kastin, S., Clinton, G., Arezzo, J.C., et al., 1991, Vigabatrin-induced intramyelinic edema II: effects on MRI in dogs, Neurology 41 (suppl 1): 331.

MR OF EPILEPSY

Three Observations

L.C. Meiners,[1] J. Valk,[2] G.H. Jansen,[3] and P.R. Luyten[4]

[1] University Hospital Utrech
Department of Diagnostic Radiology
Utrecht
[2] Free University Hospital Amsterdam
Department of Diagnostic Radiology
Amsterdam
[3] University Hospital Utrecht
Department of Pathology
Utrecht
[4] Philips Medical Systems
Best
The Netherlands

INTRODUCTION

The First Observation

This observation is a reduced grey and white matter distinction in the temporal lobe, described on MRI as a concomitant finding in patients with a high signal intensity in the hippocampus, suggestive of mesial temporal sclerosis (MTS) (Froment et al., 1989; Gates et al., 1990; Jackson et al., 1990).

To study the occurrence and the nature of this abnormality, 23 patients with ictal EEG-confirmed temporal lobe epilepsy were studied using MRI. Only patients with an MRI suggestive of MTS were included.

Fifteen of 23 patients had a reduced grey–white matter distinction in the affected temporal lobe, 13 of whom showed a concomitant increase in signal intensity in the ipsilateral hippocampus (Figure 1). This diminished distinction is best discerned on the first echo of the T2-weighted images using a TR/TE of 2000/50 100. It can not be appreciated on inversion recovery images.

A temporal lobectomy was performed in 13 patients. In 9 cases histology confirmed the presence of MTS.

Magnetic Resonance Scanning and Epilepsy, Edited by S.D. Shorvon et al.,
Plenum Press, New York, 1994

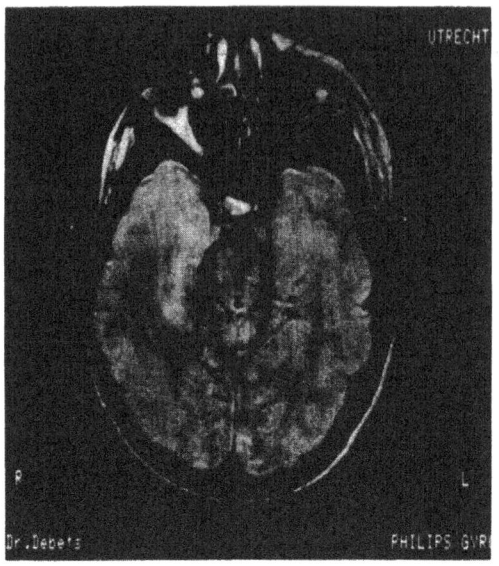

Figure 1. T2-weighted image (TR/TE 2000/50 100) in the transverse plane angulated along the long axis of the hippocampus. A high signal intensity is present in the right hippocampus. In the ipsilateral temporal lobe the grey and white matter demarcation is diminished.

Eight of nine cases showed a high signal intensity in the pathological hippocampus. Six of nine had a decrease of grey and white matter demarcation, and four of six patients a number of oligoglial cell clusters were found in the white matter of the temporal lobe. However, this finding was also present in patients with an abnormal hippocampus without extra-hippocampal changes on MRI. Furthermore one patient with an altered demarcation, a slightly increased signal intensity in the ipsilateral amygdala and an increased number of oligoglial cell clusters was found without hippocampal changes indicating MTS. It is also a frequent finding at post-mortem examination in normal temporal lobe tissue.

Overall the oligoglial cell clusters were seen in the majority of MTS confirmed cases (seven of nine) and this finding may warrant further investigation.

Jackson et al., (1990) have described the presence of corpora amylacea in a case with diminished demarcation. This was seen in only one patient in the presented group. However, the corpora amylacea may also result from the previous presence of depth electrodes.

In view of the fact that the findings are not seen on inversion recovery T2-weighted images, the altered grey–white matter distinction may indicate a chemical alteration in the substance of the white matter, rather than a structural change. Chemical investigation may therefore be of value to explain this observation.

The Second Observation

The second observation concerns acquired dysgyrias. Dysgyrias are the product of interference with the normal development of the cerebral cortex and can be caused by a multitude of factors, such as chromosomal disorders, fetal intoxications, fetal infections, hypoxic-ischaemic insults and inborn errors of metabolism. Dysgyrias may be the result of an encephaloclastic process, occurring either after completion of the formation of the normal structure or during the formative process. In the range of perinatal posthypoxic damage, periventricular leucomalacia (PVL) is the most common expression of posthypoxic-ischaemic encephalopathy (PHIE), usually considered to occur in a periventricular border zone. This may result in parietal dysgyria or sclerotic ulegyria. This type of parietal parasagittal gliosis may also result from border zone infarctions. These forms can be distinguished by their MR

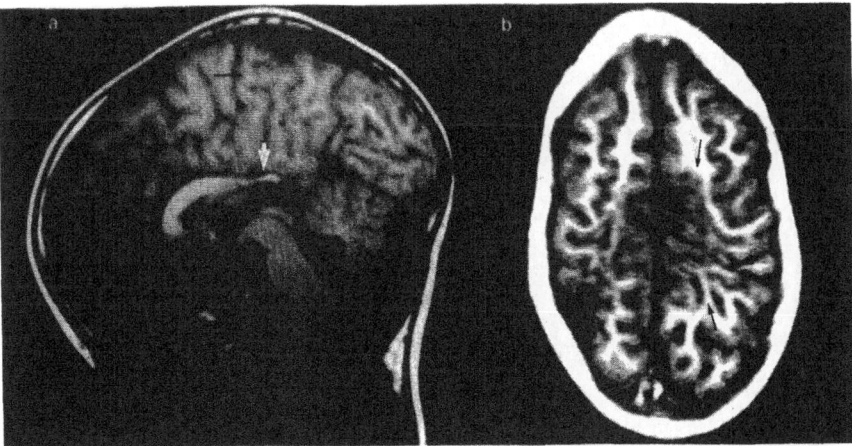

Figure 2. T1 weighted sagittal (a) and transverse (b) image of 5 year old boy with mental retardation, spastic paraparesis and epileptic seizures. Local dysgenesis of the splenium [white arrow in (a)] are corresponding with the parietal ulegyria [black arrows in (a) and (b)]. The distribution of the lesion makes it possible that this is the consequence of a lesion of a primary myelination zone.

appearance (Figures 2 and 3). Cortical changes may also follow cortical laminar necrosis, another expression of PHIE. Infants and children with PVL have spastic para- or tetraparesis and mental handicap. They rarely have epileptic seizures, as opposed to patients with parietal ulegyria and cortical laminar necrosis, who often present with seizures.

The Third Observation

The third observation concerns a ^{1}H spectroscopic image made in a patient with temporal lobe epilepsy (TLE), in whom the EEG registrations and the positron emission tomography (PET) scan indicated the right temporal lobe as being abnormal, whereas the MRI was normal.

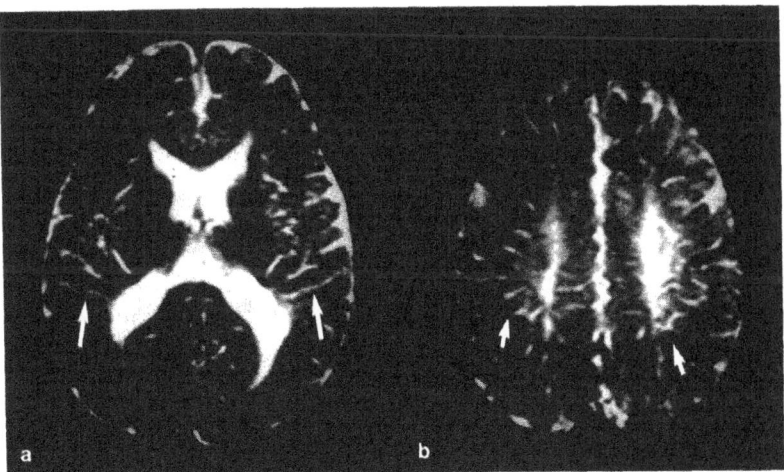

Figure 3. Two T2W transverse images at the ventricular level (a) and the centrum semiovale (b) gliotic retraction of partietal gyri is shown. The parasagittal direction of the higher slice (b) suggests involvement of the border zone between anterior and middle cerebral artery.

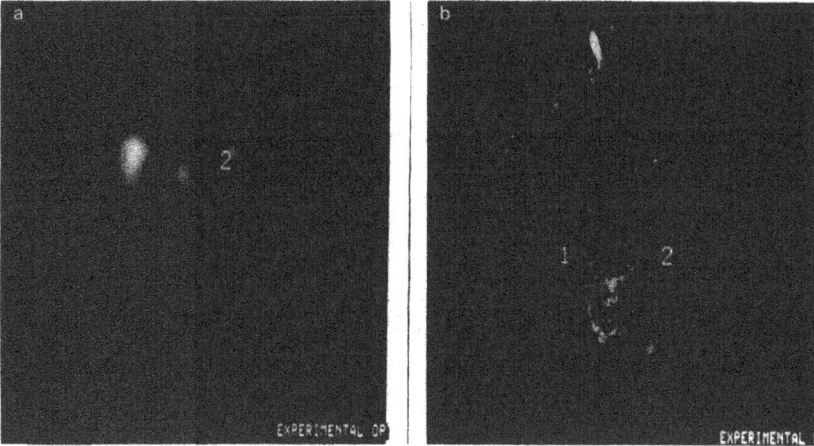

Figure 4. (a) ^{1}H spectroscopic image demonstrating an increase in choline in the mesial area of the right temporal lobe (indicated with the number 1). (b) Transverse T2-weighted image (TR/TE 2000/100) through the plane of the hippocampus showing the volume of the spectroscopic image.

The N-acetyl-aspartate (NAA) image was normal. However, a pathological high signal intensity was observed on the choline (Cho) and creatine (Cr) images in the area of the right uncus (Figure 4a and b). In general the NAA is decreased in pathological processes in the brain. Increased Cho/NAA and Cr/NAA ratios were found in a previous study in a patient with TLE and a histologically proven hamartomatous change in the hippocampus. The increased ratio was, however, partly the result of a local decrease in NAA (Luyten et al., 1990).

REFERENCES

Froment, J.C., Mauguiere, F., Fischer, C., Revol, M., Biemre, T., and Convers, P., 1989, Magnetic Resonance Imaging in refractory focal epilepsy with normal CT scans, J Neuroradiol. 16: 285–291.

Gates, J.R., and Cruz-Rodrigues, R., 1990, Mesial temporal sclerosis: Pathogenesis, diagnosis, and management, Epilepsia 31 (suppl 3): S55-S66.

Jackson, G.D., Berkovic, S.F., Tress, B.M., Klanins, R.M., Fabinyi, G.C.A., and Bladin, P.F., 1990, Hippocampal sclerosis can be reliably detected by Magnetic Resonance Imaging, Neurology 40: 1869–1875.

Luyten, P.R., van Rijen, P.C., Meiners, L.C., Marien, A.J.H., and den Hollander, J.A., 1990, Identifying epileptic foci by 1H NMR Spectroscopic imaging in patients with therapy resistant epilepsy, Society of Magnetic Resonance in Medicine (SMRM), Book of Abstracts, Volume 2.

Section 3

Cortical Dygenesis and Epilepsy

CORTICAL DYSPLASIA AND HETEROTOPIAS

A.J. Barkovich

University of California Medical Center
San Francisco, California

INTRODUCTION

The use of magnetic resonance (MR) imaging has revolutionised our ability to detect small areas of dysplastic grey matter in the cerebral cortex, hemispheric white matter and subependymal regions. Although large areas of dysplastic cortex and grey matter heterotopia were recognised by computed tomography (CT) and, for that matter, pneumoencephalography, the results of subtle derangements of normal neuronal migration have only recently been detected (Barkovich et al., 1987, 1989; Barth, 1987; Smith et al., 1988; Byrd et al., 1989; Kuzniecky et al., 1989; Palmini et al., 1991a,b,c,d; Barkovich and Kjos, 1992a,b,c). In fact, distinctions between the various categories of neuronal migration anomalies are losing their meaning as a result of the knowledge that we have gained through analysis of MR images. For example, band heterotopias (double cortex) seem to be part of a continuum between grey matter heterotopias and type I lissencephaly (Palmini et al., 1991a). Large subcortical heterotopias may, in fact, be deep involuted areas of cortical dysplasia (Barkovich and Kjos, 1992a).

CURRENT RESEARCH

The development of gradient echo techniques using gradient spoilers to give T1-weighted images has allowed the acquisition of extremely thin-section, contiguous MR images in a timely fashion (Brant-Zawadzki et al., 1992). As a result of their extremely thin (less than 1 mm) slice thickness and the contiguity of the slices, these images can be reconstructed with extremely high resolution in any plane. As a result, extremely high-resolution analysis of cortical thickness and regularity of the cortical white matter junction (Figures 1–3) can be performed, without having to worry about the obliquity of the imaging slice with respect to the cortex. Thus, artefactual cortical thickening as a result of obliquity of the plane of section with respect to the orientation of the gyri ceases to be a problem. This technique is now being used to analyse some rather complex anomalies of neuronal migration in an attempt to understand the anatomy of these distorted brains better. In addition, these three-dimensional Fourier transformer (3DFT) techniques can be used in areas where the brain may be subtly or

Magnetic Resonance Scanning and Epilepsy, Edited by S.D. Shorvon et al.,
Plenum Press, New York, 1994

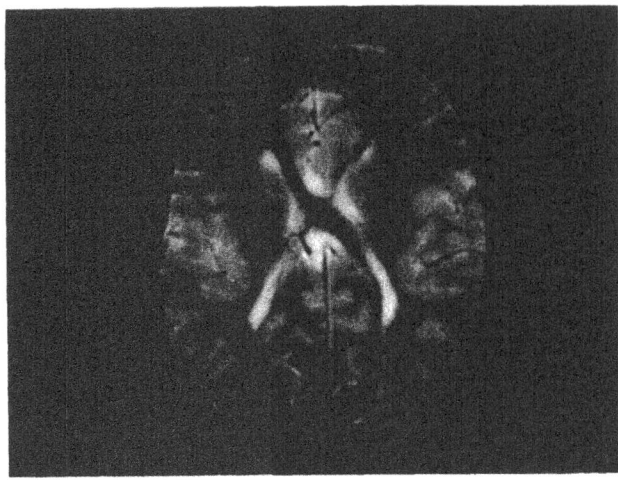

Figure 1. Axial 5 mm T2-weighted MR shows abnormal ventricular configuration resulting from callosal hypogenesis. The posterior sylvian cortex is questionably thickened.

questionably abnormal in an attempt to differentiate artefactual cortical dysplasia from true cortical dysplasia.

DISCUSSION

It has become very obvious over the past decade that a wide spectrum of neuronal migration anomalies can cause epilepsy. The Montreal group has shown that patients with focal anomalies of neuronal migration can be treated surgically with excellent results (Palmini et al., 1991b,c). We have had similar excellent results at the University of California, San Francisco. Moreover, it has become dear that clinical outcome correlates best with resection of the area of anatomical distortion, as opposed to the area with electrical anomalies (Palmini et al., 1991b,c). Therefore, it has become imperative to identify the extent of the anatomical distortion. 3DFT GRE techniques provide the highest anatomical resolution and the ability to analyse the data in any plane and, therefore, should be the optimal way to image these patients. In addition, the high-resolution images allow more accurate analysis of the anatomy of the

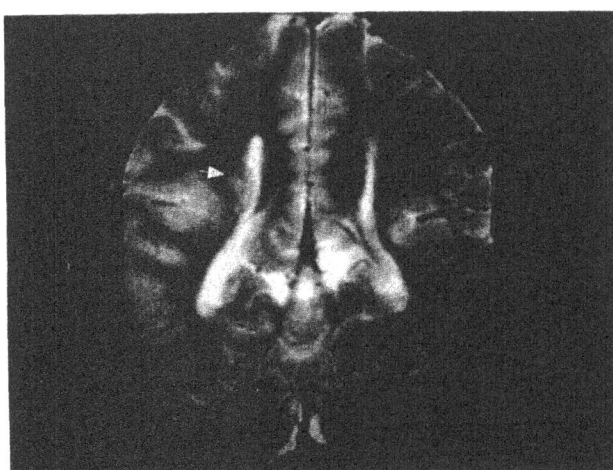

Figure 2. Coronal 5 mm T2-weighted MR image shows heterotopic grey matter (white arrow) along the lateral margin of the right ventricular atrium. No definite cortical dysplasia is identified. The left sylvian cortex, in particular, looks normal.

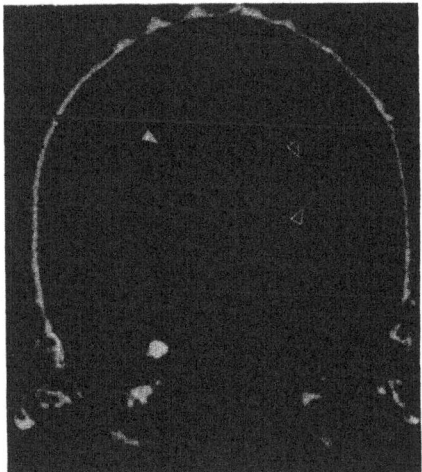

Figure 3. Coronal 0.9 mm SPGR image shows thickened, irregular cortex (open arrow) in the left posterior sylvian region. The right atrial heterotopia (closed arrow) is also identified.

distorted brain, which should help in the classification of these disorders, and, ultimately, in a better understanding of the aberrations of the underlying developmental processes.

PROBABLE DEVELOPMENT OVER THE NEXT FIVE YEARS

With the high resolution available using 3DFT gradient echo techniques and the ability to create cortical maps using these techniques, the techniques should aid in the localisation and surgical treatment of focal anomalies of neuronal migration. Fetal MR in utero (Girard and Raybaud, 1992) may enable us to detect these anomalies, allowing earlier surgical intervention and maybe better outcome due to the plasticity of the infant brain.

REFERENCES

Barkovich, A.J., and B.O. Kjos, 1992a, Gray matter heterotopias: MR characteristics and correlation with developmental and neurological manifestations, Radiology 182: 493–499.

Barkovich, A.J., and Kjos, B.O., 1992b, Non-lissencephalic cortical dysplasia: correlation of imaging findings with clinical deficits, AJNR 13: 95–103.

Barkovich, A.J., and Kjos, B.O., 1992c, Schizencephaly: correlation of clinical findings with MR characteristics, AJNR 13: 85–94.

Barkovich, A.J., Chuang, S.H., et al., 1987, MR of neuronal migration anomalies, AJNR 8: 1009–1017.

Barkovich, A.J., Jackson, D.E. Jr, et al., 1989, Band heterotopias: a newly recognized neuronal migration anomaly, Radiology 171: 455–458.

Barth, P.G., 1987, Disorders of neuronal migration, Can J Neurol Sci. 14: 1–16.

Brant-Zawadzki, M., Gillan, G., et al., 1992, MP RAGE: a three-dimensional, T1-weighted, gradient-echo sequence-initial experience in the brain, Radiology 182: 769–775.

Byrd, S., Osborn, R., et al., 1989, The CT and MR evaluation of migration disorders of the brain. Part II. Schizencephaly, heterotopia, and polymicrogyria, Pediatr Radiol. 19: 219–222.

Girard, N., and Raybaud, C., 1992, In vivo MRI of fetal brain cellular migration, J Comput Assist Tomogr 16: 265–267.

Kuzniecky, R., Andermann, F., et al., 1989, Bilateral central macrogyria: epilepsy, pseudobulbar palsy, and mental retardation—a recognizable neuronal migration disorder, Ann Neurol 25: 547–554

Palmini, A., Andermann, F., et al., 1991a, Diffuse cortical dysplasia, or the "double cortex" syndrome: the clinical and epileptic spectrum in 10 patients, Neurology 41: 1656–1662.

Palmini, A., Andermann, F. et al., 1991b, Focal neuronal migration disorders and intractable partial epilepsy: results of surgical treatment, Ann Neurol 30: 750–757.

Palmini, A., Andermann, F., et al., 1991c, Focal neuronal migration disorders and intractable partial epilepsy: a study of 30 patients, Ann Neurol 30: 741–749.

Palmini, A., Andermann, F., et al., 1991d, Neuronal migration disorders: a contribution of modern neuroimaging to the etiologic diagnosis of epilepsy, Can J Neurol Sci 18: 580–587

Smith, A.S., Weinstein, M.A., et al., 1988, Association of heterotopic gray matter with seizures: MR imaging, Radiology 168: 195–198.

16

CORTICAL DYSGENESIS IN ADULTS WITH EPILEPSY

A.A. Raymond, M.J. Cook, D.R. Fish, and S.D. Shorvon

National Hospital for Neurology and Neurosurgery
Queen Square
London, WC1N 3BG
United Kingdom

INTRODUCTION

Gross cortical dysgenesis (CD) is a well-recognised cause of epilepsy. Affected patients present with epilepsy in infancy or early childhood, are often severely mentally handicapped, and more often than not exhibit bilateral motor deficits. Recently, subtle forms of CD have been identified in adults with previously designated cryptogenic epilepsy (Raymond et al., 1992, 1993). Unlike children with CD, affected adults may have normal intelligence and rarely exhibit fixed neurological signs.

High-resolution MRI of 100 adults with chronic epilepsy at the National Hospital revealed that CD was the second most common cause of epilepsy after hippocampal sclerosis, accounting for 24% of the cases.

Cortical dysgenesis is abnormal development and maturation of the cerebral cortex. Normal corticogenesis begins with the generation of neuroblasts and glioblasts in the germinal matrix which line the lateral ventricles around the sixth gestational week, proceeds through a series of precisely timed steps and ends with axonal myelination which continues well into postnatal life (Sarnat, 1991). The most common forms of CD result from insults to the brain between the 7th and 16th gestational weeks, which is the period of maximal neuronal migration, although migration is known to continue until the fifth postnatal month (Angevine and Sidman, 1961). Neuroblasts migrate mainly radially from the ventricular germinal matrix to the cortical plate along radially oriented glial fibres. They migrate in an orderly but inside-out fashion so that earlier generated neurons come to lie deeper to those that are generated later in the cortical plate (Angevine and Sidman, 1961; Rakic, 1978). Recent evidence, however, suggests that there may also be lateral migration and/or dispersion of neuroblasts during corticogenesis (Walsh and Cepko, 1992). Insults to the brain during this stage of corticogenesis (e.g. ischaemia, exposure to drugs or irradiation, infections) or genetic factors may result in neuroblasts being arrested somewhere along their migratory pathways, giving rise to a disorganised and thickened cortex. Indeed a thickened cortical ribbon and loss of the normal six-layered organisation of the cortex are characteristic of most forms of CD.

Magnetic Resonance Scanning and Epilepsy, Edited by S.D. Shorvon et al.,
Plenum Press, New York, 1994

As gyration of the cerebral cortex is to a large extent dependent upon normal neuroblast migration (Richman et al., 1975), it is often also abnormal in CD. In fact, the various forms of CD derive their names not from the structure of the abnormal cortex but from the associated gyral pattern abnormalities or the morphology or histological appearance of the arrested nests of neurons. Thus, agyria or lissencephaly is the name given when there is complete absence of gyri, pachygyria or macrogyria, when there are few broad and shallow gyri and polymicrogyria, in which there are many small, incompletely separated gyri. Agyria is a diffuse form of CD. Macrogyria differs from agyria only in degree and is thus usually more localised. Hemimegalencephaly is used to describe a brain with an enlarged hemisphere associated with diffuse macrogyria on the affected side. Polymicrogyria may be either diffuse or localised. An abnormal pial-ependymal cleft, often lined with polymicrogyria and which may be bilateral is known as schizencephaly. When gyration is not affected, CD is usually more subtle, more focal or more localised, and is often only diagnosed post mortem or at surgery. This may take the form of heterotopic grey matter, focal cortical dysplasia or microdysgenesis. Heterotopias vary in location and morphology. They may occur in the subcortical white matter where they either form bands of grey matter (band or laminar heterotopia) or, nodules (nodular heterotopia). Nodular heterotopia may also be found subependymally or rarely, occur as meningeal glioneuronal heterotopias. When laminar heterotopia is bilateral, they should be considered as diffuse CD. Different forms of CD may coexist, a common occurrence being the coexistence of agyria or macrogyria with heterotopias.

The subependymal and cortical lesions of tuberous sclerosis are also forms of CD (Barkovich et al., 1992). The basic defect appears to be an inability of neurons and glial cells to integrate themselves into the brain (Stefansson et al., 1988). Those cells that remain in the germinal matrix and proliferate form subependymal hamartomas and giant-cell tumours whereas those that migrate to the cortex but fail to differentiate form cortical tubers. Forme fruste of tuberous sclerosis is the term applied when similar lesions are found in the brain but extracranial stigmata of tuberous sclerosis are lacking (Andermann et al., l989).

Dysembryoplastic neuroepithelial tumour (DNT) is a newly described lesion, pathologically and prognostically distinct from other benign brain tumours (Raymond et al., 1994; Daumas-Duport et al., 1988). First described by Daumas-Duport et al., (1988), these lesions have a heterogeneous cellular composition (consisting of both neuronal and glial elements); they are frequently associated with foci of cortical dysplasia, they are often intracortical and they invariably present in early childhood with intractable epilepsy. Although there is still debate as to whether or not these lesions are hamartomas or true tumours, these features would suggest that DNT might fit into the general scheme of CD. However, unlike some other forms of CD, DNT carries a good prognosis when surgically removed (Raymond et al., 1994; Daumas-Duport et al., 1988).

Although CD can often be detected on MRI, the diagnosis of microdysgenesis and very small focal cortical dysplasias requires histological examination.

Current classification of CD is unsatisfactory and has traditionally been based on morphology and pathology. A classification scheme used at our centre is shown in Table 1.

As current generations of MRI have resolutions high enough to demonstrate gross pathology, there is obviously a need to revise the current classification of CD to incorporate radiological criteria. This is also important from the point of view of treatment planning.

CURRENT RESEARCH

The purpose of the current study is to determine the clinical, neuropsychological, neurophysiological, neuroradiological and pathological characteristics of CD in adults with epilepsy in order to offer information regarding early diagnosis, treatment and prognosis.

Table 1. One Hundred Adults with Cortical Dysgenesis and Epilepsy

	No. of patients
Focal localised cortical dysgenesis	
Focal macrogyria/polymicrogyria	18
Other gyral abnormalities	8
Dysembryoplastic neuroepthelial tumour	20
Focal cortical dysplasia	5
Microdysgenesis	3
Tuberous sclerosis/forme fruste of tuberous sclerosis	7
Subependymal/subcortical nodular heterotopia	20
Bilateral peri-sylvian syndrome	2
Schizencephaly	5
Hemimegalencephaly	0
Diffuse cortical dysgenesis	
Agyria/lissencephaly	4
Bilateral band heterotopia	8
Diffuse polymicrogyria	0

To date we have identified 100 adult patients with CD and epilepsy. Diagnosis of CD was established at neuroimaging in just over 75% of the patients, and by histological examination of surgical or postmortem material in the remaining patients. MRI was performed on a 1.5 T General Electric (GE) signa unit which included 1.5 mm section volume acquisitions and multiplanar reformatting in the majority of the patients. Age at seizure onset ranged from 3 weeks to 41 years (n = 98). Forty patients were male and sixty female. Various forms of CD were seen but there were no patients with diffuse polymicrogyria or hemimegalencephaly (Table 1). CD was focal in 88 cases and diffuse in only 12. The lesions were scattered throughout the brain but were extra-temporal in most cases (70%) with the exception of DNT where 19 of the 20 cases were temporal. DNT was the single most common lesion in our series, accounting for one-fifth of the cases.

Routine neuropsychological assessment showed a wide variation in IQ scores but only seven patients were mentally handicapped and 40% of the patients had an IQ of 90 or greater. The mean IQ was 88. All except two patients presented with medically refractory epilepsy and were previously designated as cryptogenic cases. There was no correlation between seizure type, seizure frequency, secondary generalisation or occurrence of status epilepticus and type of CD. Risk factors for both epilepsy and cortical dysgenesis were looked at. Although postnatal risk factors were unlikely to cause CD, they may in some way contribute to the genesis of epilepsy. Risk factors were identified retrospectively in 41 patients of whom 12 had more than one risk factor: family history of epilepsy (19 cases), family history of other neurological diseases (mental handicap, hyperekplexia, neurofibromatosis, psychiatric disease (six cases), intrauterine exposure to drugs/infections (two cases), pre-eclampsia (five cases), polyhydramnios (one case), other congenital defects (dysmorphic features, cardiac and skeletal abnormalities) (seven cases), major birth injury (24 cases), febrile seizures (8 cases), encephalitis/meningitis (four cases) and severe head injury (three cases).

EEGs were available for review in 94 patients and were abnormal in all except 4 patients. All patients with diffuse CD except one had background abnormalities, being diffuse in 88% and localised in 12% of patients. In contrast, only 60% of patients with focal CD had background abnormalities and these were focal in the majority of cases.

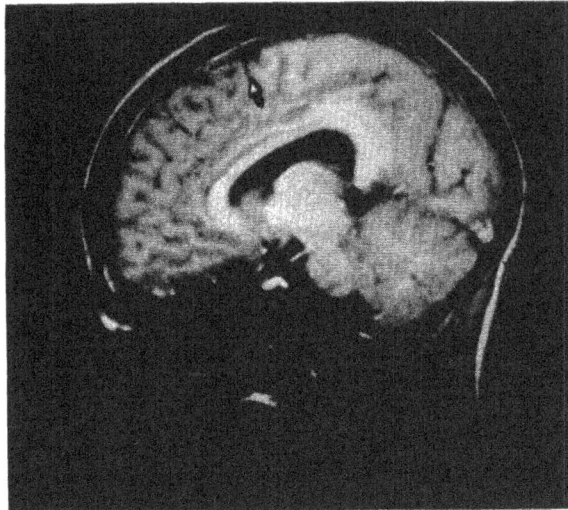

Figure 1. Parasagittal T1-weighted MR image of the brain showing focal macrogyria posterior to the central sulcus (arrow). Previous routine MRI was normal.

Inter-ictal spiking was seen in 78 patients (83%), being less extensive than or concordant with the lesion in 55%, more extensive than and overlapping the lesion in 24%, and distant to the lesion in 21% of cases.

The majority of cases had previously had one or more routine MR scans which were either normal or reported as normal. Examples of such cases are shown (Figures 1 and 2). Some of the features of DNT often observed on MRI are illustrated in Figure 3.

DISCUSSION

Cortical dysgenesis is an important cause of epilepsy in adults and must be considered in all patients with medically refractory epilepsy, particularly in those in whom there are prenatal risk factors and epilepsy is extra-temporal. More importantly, the presence of additional postnatal risk factors for the development of epilepsy does not preclude the diagnosis of CD.

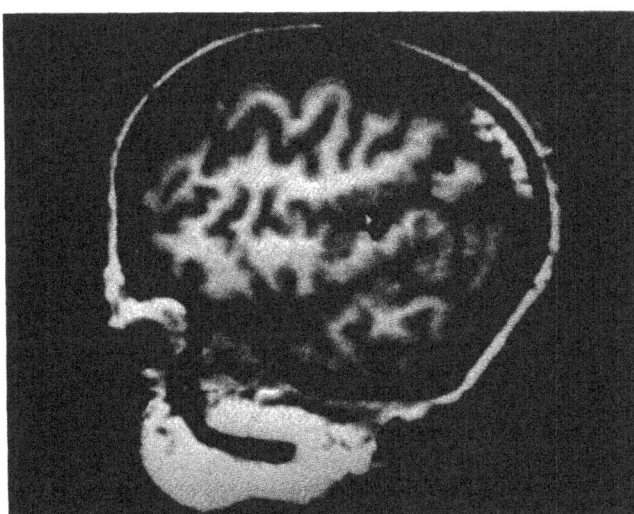

Figure 2. Reformatted oblique T1-weighted MR image through the superolateral surface of the right hemisphere showing extensive perirolandic polymicrogyria (arrow). This was not previously detected on routine MR imaging.

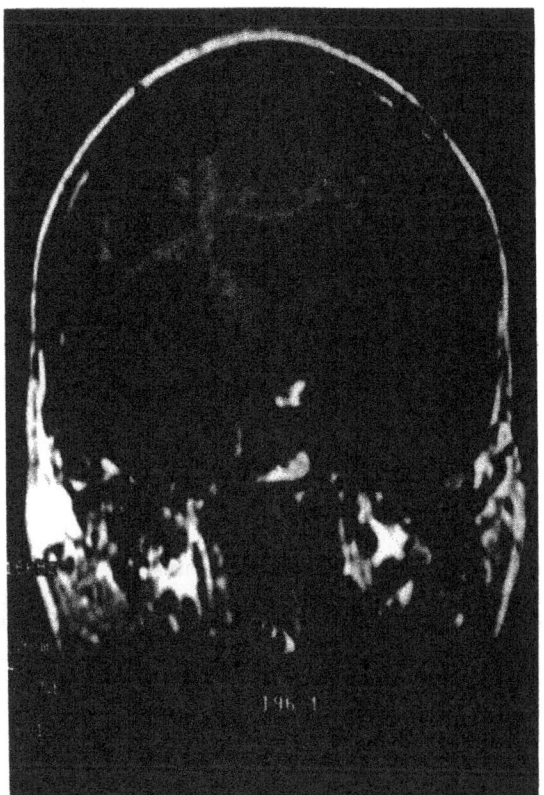

Figure 3. T1-weighted coronal MR image showing a large hypointense, intracortical and well-circumscribed mass lesion in the right temporal lobe, anterior to the hippocampus, affecting the mid-temporal gyrus and superior temporal sulcus and expanding the overlying calvarium. A diagnosis of DNT was made on histological examination. This scan also illustrates another uncommon feature of DNT, namely, bilaterality—there is a clear but smaller hypointense lesion in the left temporal lobe affecting the uncus, anterior and inferior to the amygdala.

It may be that in some patients with CD, the presence of such factors may contribute to the genesis of subsequent epilepsy.

The mechanism by which CD causes epilepsy is unknown. The two prevailing hypotheses are that (1) there is associated synaptic dysgenesis (Becker, 1991) and (2) there is abnormal distribution and morphology of local circuit inhibitory neurons (Ferrer et al., 1992). Whether abnormalities of neurotransmitter balance or abnormalities of circuitry beyond the anatomical lesion exist remains to be investigated. Similarly, little is known about the neurophysiological properties of dysgenetic lesions.

The pre-surgical detection of CD has been greatly improved by the availability of high-resolution MRI, particularly using thin-section volume acquisition techniques and multiplanar reformatting. Routine 5 mm slices, owing to overlapping effects, are likely to miss subtle dysgenetic lesions which may not exceed the thickness of the cortical ribbon. This is particularly true of adults who are more likely to have subtle rather than gross CD. A slice thickness of 1.5 mm or less is more appropriate for the detection and description of CD.

In this preliminary report, it has been shown that CD is pathologically heterogeneous and exhibits a great variation in expression—not only is there a wide variation in size and site but also in surgical outcome.

LIKELY DEVELOPMENT IN THE NEXT FIVE YEARS

There are three main areas of interest in the future.

(1) There is a need to further improve detection of CD. Possible methods include performing even thinner MRI slices, using different MR sequences, for example suppressing the CSF signal, devising post-processing techniques to look closer at gyral patterns, using three-dimensional reformatting, novel analytical methods such as fractal analysis, and possibly using functional MR imaging.

(2) There is a need to address the question of aetiology of CD. Obviously, there is a need to look more closely at antenatal records to identify possible prenatal risk factors. Family and genetic studies are also required; MRI of family members, even when asymptomatic, must be considered.

(3) With the throughput of surgical cases, there will be opportunities to perform neurophysiological studies and immunocytochemistry on sliced dysgenetic tissue, and to use immunocytochemical techniques so that we may learn why these lesions are epileptogenic and perhaps why surgical outcome is poor for most forms of CD.

REFERENCES

Andermann, F., Olivier, A, Melanson,D., and Robitaille, Y., 1989, Epilepsy due to focal cortical dysplasia with macrogyria and the forme fruste of tuberous sclerosis: a study of 15 patients, in: "Advances in Epileptology" Vol. 16, P. Wolf, M. Dam, D. Janz, F.E. Dreifuss, FE, eds, Raven Press, New York.

Angevine, J.B., Jr, and Sidman, R.L., 1961, Autoradiographic study of cell migration during histogenesis of cerebral cortex in the mouse, Nature 192: 766–768.

Barkovich, A., Gressens, P., and Evrard, P., 1992, Formation, maturation, and disorders of brain neocortex, AJNR 13: 423–446.

Becker, L.E., 1991, Synaptic dysgenesis, Can J Neurol Sci. 18: 170–180.

Daumas-Duport, C., Scheithauer, B.W., Chodkiewicz, J.P., Laws, E.R., and Vedrenne, C., 1988, Dysembryoplastic neuroepithelial tumor: a surgically curable tumor of young patients with intractable partial seizures: report of thirty-nine cases, Neurosurgery 23: 545–546.

Ferrer, I., Pineda, M., Tallada, M. et al., 1992, Abnormal local-circuit neurons in epilepsia partialis continua associated with focal cortical dysplasia, Acta Neuropathol. 83: 647–652.

Rakic, P., 1978, Neuronal migration and contact guidance in the primate telencephalon, Postgrad Med J 54 (suppl): 25–40.

Raymond, A.A., Fish, D.R., Cook, M.J., Sander, J.W.A.S., and Shorvon, S.D., 1992, Adult patients with cortical dysgenesis and epilepsy, Epilepsia (suppl 3); 33: 74–75 (abstr).

Rayrnond, A.A., Fish, D.R., Cook, M.J., and Shorvon, S.D., 1993, The EEG features in adults with cortical dysgenesis and epilepsy, Electroencephalogr Clin Neurophysiol; 86: 34P (abstr).

Raymond, A.A., Halpin, S.F.S., Alsanjari, N. et al., 1994, Dysembryoplastic neuroepithelial tumour: features in 16 patients, Brain; in press.

Richman, D.P., Stewart, R.M., Hutchinson, J.W., and Caviness, V.S., 1975, Mechanical model of brain convolutional development: pathologic and experimental data suggest a model based on differential growth within the cerebral cortex, Science 189: 18–21.

Sarnat, H.B., 1991, Cerebral dysplasias as expressions of altered maturational processes, Can J Neurol Sci 18: 196–204.

Stefansson, K., Wollmann, R., and Huttenlocher, P., 1988, Lineages of cells in the central nervous system, in: "Tuberous Sclerosis," M. Gomez, ed., 2nd ed, Raven Press, New York.

Walsh, C., and Cepko, C.L., 1992, Widespread dispersion of neuronal clones across functional regions of the cerebral cortex, Science 255: 434–440.

HEMIMEGALENCEPHALY

C. Diebler[1] and O. Dulac[2]

[1]Centre Medico-Chirurgical Foch
92151 Suresnes
[2]Hôpital Saint-Vincent-de-Paul
75674 Paris
France

Hemimegalencephaly is a variant of cortical dysplasia involving the whole hemisphere (Robain et al., 1988). There is no clear border between the two types of malformation because from one to several lobes can be involved whereas the rest of the hemisphere is spared. The histological findings are similar in both types of malformation and consist of disappearance of cortical lamination and presence of giant neurons, giant glial cells with Rosenthal's fibres and occasionally calcifications. The white matter underlying the abnormal cortex is also involved.

Aetiology remains unknown. To our knowledge, no familial case has been reported. Rare cases are combined with neurocutaneous syndromes including sebaceous naevus linearis (Vigevano et al., 1984), Sturge-Weber disease (Oi et al., 1987) and neurofibromatosis (Cusmai et al., 1990). A genetic disorder with somatic mutation may therefore be involved.

Epilepsy, mental handicap and focal neurological signs are the main symptoms. Seizures are usually the first clinical manifestation, appearing in the first weeks of life; they take a focal form or manifest in clusters of spasms, soon becoming intractable (Vigevano and Di Rocco, 1990). In rare cases, they occur later in the first year of life. In cases with early onset of partial seizures the EEG shows triphasic spikes on the malformed side; in cases with clusters of spasms, it shows an asymmetrical suppression burst pattern; in cases with later onset, or later in the course of the disease in patients with early onset, EEG shows a fast pseudo-alpha rhythmic activity over the malformed hemisphere (Palladin et al., 1989). Functional imaging shows ictal hyperperfusion or hypermetabolism in the malformed hemisphere during the first months of the epilepsy (Chiron et al., 1991a). Later, the whole malformed hemisphere shows inter-ictal hypoactivity. Removal (Vigevano and Di Rocco, 1990) or disconnection (Delalande et al., 1992) of the malformed areas is increasingly indicated as the surgical procedures improve. For this reason, the major problem is to demonstrate, based on EEG recordings and functional imaging, that the contralateral hemisphere is not involved.

Magnetic Resonance Scanning and Epilepsy, Edited by S.D. Shorvon et al.,
Plenum Press, New York, 1994

RADIOLOGICAL FINDINGS

In its classic form (Araki et al., 1987) radiological features of hemimegalencephaly are: enlargement of one cerebral hemisphere, with a thick, dense, pachygyric cortex and a disorganisation of the white matter with areas of heterotopias alternating with areas disorganisation of an increased signal in T2-weighted views suggesting glial lesions. The homolateral ventricle is generally enlarged and there may be calcifications and vascular abnormalities (Kalifa et al., 1987).

Clinical and pathological findings, however, suggest that the spectrum of hemimegalencephaly is larger than previously believed. Variants exist with:

- Smaller areas of cortical dysplasia, showing the same histological lesions and resulting in the same clinical presentation.
- Dysplastic areas which may be multiple, bilateral.
- Focal hypoplasia instead of hypertrophy.

Precise location and delineation of the dysplastic areas is of major importance, because there is increasing evidence that the extent of surgical removal should be guided by anatomical lesions, not EEG abnormalities (Palmini et al., 1991).

OTHER ASPECTS

Molecular biological studies on cell culture of cells obtained from the abnormal hemisphere may help elucidate the pathogenesis of this condition (Ronnet et al., 1990). As there are giant glial cells and the white matter is often involved, it is likely that the malformation is not merely the consequence of a neuroblastic disease. In mild cases, the epilepsy may be controlled by anti-epileptic drug treatment, particularly vigabatrin, even when occurring very early with clusters of spasms and suppression bursts (Chiron et al., 1991b). However, at that stage, radiological diagnosis of such cases is difficult, and EEG features may be more contributory.

In intractable cases, pre-surgical evaluation needs to determine both the extent of the malformed area and whether the contralateral hemisphere is spared. It is critical to determine involvement of the rolandic area but this is particularly difficult to establish based on clinical examination before the age of 6 months. As the surgical procedure may be indicated very early in life resulting from the severity of the epilepsy, there is a need to refine the radiological criteria which help identify the extent of cortical involvement. This is a major challenge.

The timing and extent of surgical removal or disconnection have to take into account two opposing requirements. On the one hand, seizures should be controlled as early as possible to protect the rest of the brain, and permit plasticity to assure partial recovery of the functions previously held by the dysplastic hemisphere. On the other hand, it is currently necessary to wait until the child is sufficiently mature in order to assess cortical functions, to avoid removing areas that are still effective, and unlikely to benefit from brain plasticity, such as the motor strip.

REFERENCES

Araki Y., Mori, S., Kanoh, M., et al., 1987, Congenital hemicerebral arterial ectasy complicating unilateral megalencephaly, Br J Radiol. 60:3 95–400.
Chiron, C., Raynaud, C., Jambaque, I., Dulac O., Zilbovicius, M., and Syrota, A., 1991a, A serial study or regional cerebral blood flow before and after hemispherectomy in a child, Epilepsy Res 8: 232–240.

Chiron, C., Dulac, O., Beaumont, D., Palacios, L., Pajot, N., and Mumford, J., 1991b, Therapeutic trial of vigabatrin in refractory infantile spasms, J Child Neurol 6 (suppl): 2S52–2S59.

Cusmai, R., Curatolo, P., Mangano, S., Cheminal, R., and Echenne, B., 1990, Hemimegalencephaly and neurofibromatosis, Neuropediatrics 21: 179–182.

Delalande, O., Pinard, J.M., Basdevant, C., Gauthe, M., Plouin, P., and Dulac, O., 1992, Hemispherectomy: a new procedure for central disconnection (abstract), Epilepsia 33: 99.

Kalifa, G.L., Chiron, C., Sellier, N., et al., 1987, Hemimegalencephaly: MR imaging in five children, Radiology 165: 29–33.

Oi, S., Urvi, S., and Matsumoto, S., 1987, Hemiventriculomegaly and hemicranial expansion in Klippel-Trenaunay-Weber syndrome, J Pediatr Neurosci 3: 21–27.

Palladin, F., Chiron, C., Dulac, O., et al., 1989, Electroencephalographic aspect of hemimegalencephaly, Develop Med Child Neurol.31: 377–383.

Palmini, A., Andermann, F., Olivier, A., Tampieri, D., and Robitaille, Y., 1991, Focal neuronal migration disorders and intractable partial epilepsy: results of surgical treatment, Ann Neurol.30: 750–757.

Robain, O., Floquet, J., Heldt, N., and Rozenberg, F., 1988, Hemimegalencephaly. a clinicopathological study of four cases, Neuropathol Appl Neurobiol 14: 125136.

Ronnet, G.V., Hestler, L.D., Nye, J.S., Connors, K., and Snyder, S.H., 1990, Human cortical neuronal cell line: establishment from a patient with unilateral megalencephaly, Science 248: 603–605.

Vigevano, F., and Di Rocco, C., 1990, Effectiveness of hemispherectomy in hernimegalencephaly, Neuropediatrics 21: 222–223.

Vigevano, F., Aicardi, J., Lini, M., et al., 1984, La sindrome del nevo sebaceo lineare: presentazione di una casistica multicentrica, Boll Lega It Epil 45/46: 59–63.

AGENESIS OF THE CORPUS CALLOSUM

O. Dulac[1] and C. Diebler[2]

[1] Hôpital Saint-Vincent-de-Paul
75674 Paris
[2] Centre Medico-Chirurgical Foch
92151 Suresnes
France

Seizures, mental handicap and axial hypotonia are often the first symptoms of agenesis of the corpus callosum (CA). The clinical pattern varies according to the anatomical findings and aetiology. Indeed, there is a wide spectrum of brain malformations which involve CA. CA is by no means a clinical diagnosis on its own but its recognition is the first step towards a more precise aetiological diagnosis and prognosis. The clinical relevance of this concept grows as prenatal diagnosis of CA becomes more and more accurate. Prenatal diagnosis is presently often made by means of ultrasonography and it is a real challenge in these cases to determine the prognosis.

A few case reports have mentioned CA as a consequence of exogeneous factors: maternal diabetes (Probst, 1979), maternal hypertension (Probst, 1979), suspected rubella (Friedma and Cohen, 1947), fetal alcohol syndrome (Jones and Smith, 1973), arterial thrombosis (De Morsier and Mozer, 1935). However, the most commonly identified causes of CA are related to genetic factors including various chromosomal aberrations: trisomies 18, 11q2, 13, 8, F, translocations 2–13, 4–15, deletions 1, 18, monosomy 1—for review, see Diebler and Dulac (1987); over 22 families with recurrence of CA and with various modes of inheritance have been reported (Kaplan, 1983). CA may be an unusual finding in genetically determined diseases such as the orodigitofacial syndrome (Townes et al., 1976). Aicardi's syndrome which comprises cortical dysplasia mainly in the rolandic area, retinal lacunae and extracerebral malformations (Aicardi et al., 1969) is likely to be genetically determined. However, in most cases of CA no aetiology can be disclosed.

Mental handicap is observed in 9 of 10 of the cases, axial hypotonia can be misleading in early life and focal neurological signs are rare. Peripheral neuropathy is part of the Andermann syndrome, an autosomal recessive disease which does not involve epilepsy (Andermann et al., 1975).

In a series of 110 patients with CA, 51% had seizures (Kaplan, 1983). They appeared early in life: before 6 months in 26%, before 2 years in 45%, and before 5 years in 47%. Ten per cent had a single seizure; in all the other cases, the second seizure appeared in the first year

Magnetic Resonance Scanning and Epilepsy, Edited by S.D. Shorvon et al.,
Plenum Press, New York, 1994

following the first fit. Seizures were generalised tonic-clonic in half the cases. They consisted of clusters of spasms in 30% of patients. Twenty-seven (48.9%) had partial motor seizures, five of whom had hemiconvulsion-hemiplegia syndrome. Epilepsy was present and usually severe in all cases with the combination of diffuse cortical atrophy, agyria (clusters of spasms), hamartoma of the tuber cinereum (gelastic seizures), lipoma of the corpus callosum (partial seizures), or as part of the Aicardi malformation (clusters of spasms combined with partial seizures). In isolated CA, epilepsy was unusual and relatively benign, focal and eventually associated with rolandic spikes. The combination of CA and partial benign epilepsy including ages of onset and cessation of seizures, and rapid response to antiepilepsy medication has been reported (Santanelli et al., 1989).

The clinical and EEG characteristics of Aicardi's syndrome are the best studied in the spectrum of CA. Focal seizures occur before 3 months of age, and usually precede the occurrence of spasms which are asymmetrical. The ictal event at that stage is very characteristic of the kind of clusters of spasms observed in any type of brain malformations: the focal discharge initiates and drives the cluster of asymmetrical spasms, thus demonstrating that the whole cluster consists of a single seizure and involves a cortical discharge combined with periodic subcortical events (Bour et al., 1986). The inter-ictal EEG initially consists of a unilateral suppression-burst pattern and later multifocal spikes or highly modified hypsarrhythmia.

RADIOLOGICAL FINDINGS

Diagnosis of CA generally shows no difficulty, but confirmation or elimination of other cerebral malformations is not easy because of the changing configuration of the brain with normal maturation and the architectural modifications due to CA itself.

Associated cranial and cerebral malformations are very varied and frequent. In a series of 110 cases essentially disclosed on CT, only 20% of them were considered to have isolated CA (Diebler and Dulac, 1987), and it is most likely that cases of apparently isolated CA will become still more rare with MRI investigation.

Associated malformations of CA, as heterotopias and rolandic cortical dysplasia, may suggest a precise aetiology, but do not allow definite confirmation of any given aetiology. Some are easily detected including hydrocephalus, lipoma of the corpus callosum (Kazner et al., 1980), hamartoma (Diebler and Ponsot, 1983), or posterior fossa malformations, such as cerebellar hypoplasia (Van Epps, 1953), cystic dilatation of the cisterna magna or Dandy-Walker malformation. Large hemispheric malformations as hemiatrophy or intracerebral cysts and calcifications, or extensive areas of pachygyria (Josephy, 1944) are relatively rare in CA, but small malformations as subcortical or periventricular heterotopias, or limited areas of polymicrogyria, are more frequent. These small hemispheric malformations are particularly difficult to detect, even on MRI.

OTHER ASPECTS

The following improvements are envisaged:

(1) Progression in technology with faster sequences, better adapted sequences for the neonatal period and high definition will certainly allow a rapid improvement in the detection of small malformations combined with CA.

(2) A better understanding of aetiology is necessary for any prevention to become possible. Better comprehension will not only be obtained from advancing technology but also from more precise clinico-radiological correlation on a large scale. Determi-

nation of the correlations between identifiable aetiology, various types of malformation complexes and clinical characteristics will also contribute to understanding of
outcome and prognosis.

(3) Now the prenatal diagnosis of CA is possible, at about 20 weeks of gestation, by
systematic sonography and confirmed on prenatal MRI. However, at present, it is
generally impossible to give precise prognosis concerning mental handicap and
seizures. The latter may become increasingly reliable based on the prenatal use of
MRI.

REFERENCES

Aicardi, J., Chevrie, J.J., and Rousselie, F., 1969, Le syndrome spasmes en flexion, agénésie calleuse, anomalies
    choriorétiniennes, Arch Fr Pediatr 26: 1103–1120.
Andermann, E., Andermann, F., Joubert, M., et al., 1975, Three familial midline malformation syndromes of the
    central nervous system: agenesis of the corpus callosum and anterior horn-cell disease; agenesis of the
    cerebellar vermis; and atrophy of the cerebellar vermis, Birth Defects 11: 269–293.
Bour, F., Chiron, C., Dulac, O., et al., 1986, Caractères électro-cliniques des crises dans le syndrome d'Aicardi.
    Rev, EEG Neurophysiol Clin 16: 341–353.
De Morsier, G., and Mozer, J.J., 1935, Agenesie complete de la commissure calleuse et troubles du developpement
    de l'hémisphere gauche avec hémiparésie droite et intégrité mentale, Schweiz Arch Neurol Neurochirur
    Psychiatr 35: 64–80.
Diebler, C., and Dulac, O., 1987, "Pediatric Neurology and Neuroradiology: Cerebral and Cranial Diseases",
    Springer-Verlag, Berlin, New York.
Diebler, C., and Ponsot, G., 1983, Hamartomas of the tuber cinereum, Neuroradiology 25: 93–102.
Friedma, M., and Cohen P., 1947, Agenesis of the corpus callosum as a possible sequel to maternal rubella during
    pregnancy, Am J Dis Child 73: 178- 185.
Jones, K.L., and Smith, D.W., 1973, Recognition of the fetal alcohol syndrome in early infancy, Lancet ii:
    999–1001.
Josephy, M., 1944, Congenital agyria and defect of corpus callosum, J Neuropathol Exp Neurol 3: 63–68.
Kaplan, P., 1983, X-linked recessive inheritance of agenesis of the corpus callosum, J Med Genet 20: 122–124.
Kazner, E., Stochdorph, O., Wende, S., et al., 1980, Intracranial lipoma, J Neurosurg 52: 234–245.
Probst, F.P., 1979, "The Prosencephalies", Springer, Berlin, Heidelberg, New York.
Santanelli, P., Bureau, M., Magaudda, A., Gobbi, G., and Roger, J., 1989, Benign partial epilepsy with
    centrotemporal (or Rolandic) spikes and brain lesion, Epilepsia 30: 182–188.
Townes, P.L., Wood, B.P., and McDonald, J.V., 1976, Further heterogeneity of the oral-facial digital syndromes,
    Am J Dis Child 130: 548–554.
Van Epps, E.F., 1953, Agenesis of the corpus callosum with concomitant malformations, including atresia of the
    foramen of Luschka and Magendi, Am J Roentgenol 70: 47–60.

THE CONGENITAL BILATERAL PERI-SYLVIAN SYNDROME

Imaging Findings

R. Kuzniecky, F. Andermann, R. Guerrini, and the CBPS Multicenter
Collaborative Study[1]

UAB Epilepsy Center
Department of Neurology
University of Alabama at Birmingham
UAB Station
Birmingham, Alabama 35294

INTRODUCTION

Advances in diagnostic imaging techniques, particularly magnetic resonance (MR) imaging, have permitted the recognition of developmental malformations of the central nervous system with a high degree of accuracy (Barth, 1987; Friede, 1989; Byrd et al., 1989; Barkovich and Kjos, 1992). Recent clinico-radiological correlative studies have demonstrated the broad spectrum of these malformations and have contributed to the recognition that some of these disorders have common pathogenic mechanisms (Graff-Radford et al., 1986; Kuzniecky et al., 1988; Palmini et al., 1991; Barkovich and Kjos, 1992a,b).

Kuzniecky et al., (1989) described four patients with congenital facio-pharyngo-masticatory diplegia, epilepsy and cognitive deficits. On imaging studies, all had bilateral peri-sylvian structural abnormalities best characterised as dysplastic in nature. It has emerged, that similar patients had been seen in several countries but had not been recognized as a distinct entity. In this report, we present the clinical and imaging findings in 31 patients with this condition that we have termed the "congenital bilateral peri-sylvian syndrome".

PATIENTS AND METHODS

Thirty-one patients were entered in this study. Ten international centres participated in this study. Recruitment from the participating investigator was carried out through a stand-

---

[1] The investigators and institutions that participated in this study are listed in the acknowledgments section.

Magnetic Resonance Scanning and Epilepsy, Edited by S.D. Shorvon et al.,
Plenum Press, New York, 1994

ardised protocol. All patients underwent physical and neurological examinations. A standardised detailed questionnaire emphasising pregnancy, development, associated malformations and family history was used to acquire information. Particular attention was also paid to
the seizure history, seizure type, frequency, response to treatment and course.

Investigations included routine electroencephalographic (EEG) studies, chromosomal
high-resolution banding, metabolic screening (six patients) and neuropsychological testing
when possible (Benton and Van Allen, 1968; Leiter, 1980; Wechsler, 1981).

All patients had imaging studies including computed tomography (CT) scan and 28 of
the 31 had MR examinations. Because of the international collaborative nature of the study,
patients were imaged with different MR units. Imaging studies included a variety of T1- and
T2-weighted pulse sequences. Coronal, axial and sagittal images, with slice thickness varying
from 3 to 8 mm, were obtained in the majority of patients. More recently some patients
underwent studies using inversion recovery (IR) sequences in the coronal and axial planes (TI
= 300, TE = 20, TR = 1200, field strength 1.5 T). The configuration of the sylvian and opercular
regions was studied particularly. In addition, the anteroposterior extension of the dysplastic
malformations was evaluated using axial images. Cortical thickness was measured using a
previously reported technique (Barkovich and Kjos, 1992a). Neuropathological material was
available in two patients. Macroscopic examination and histological sections were obtained
using routine techniques.

RESULTS

Clinical Features

Twenty of the 31 patients were female. Their ages at the time of study ranged from 1
month to 41 years (mean: 18 years). No particular prevalence of ethnic or racial origin was
observed, but the study group included only European and North American centres.

Family histories revealed no instance of known consanguinity. A positive family history
of epilepsy was present in one sibling and, in another family, an older brother who died at birth
was reported to have had multiple congenital malformations. The occurrence of the syndrome
was documented in two families; in one family, identical monozygotic male twins affected by
the syndrome were studied. In the other family, an affected sister and brother with a deceased
maternal uncle possibly affected were documented. Chromosomal and metabolic studies were
normal in all those tested (17 of 31).

Pregnancies were normal in all but 6 patients. Deliveries were normal in 20 patients, but
11 patients were born by breech presentation. Associated malformations were present in 30%
of patients. Language milestones were delayed in all. Deglutition problems were evident in all
patients when solid food was introduced into the diet.

Neurological manifestations common to all patients consisted of severe dysarthria and
nasal speech. Two patients were mute with normal comprehension. The degree of dysarthria
varied between moderate to severe. Tongue movements were consistently restricted with very
limited protrusion and lateral movements. Intellectual assessment showed that 75% of patients
had mild to moderate cognitive deficits, with an average full scale intelligence quotient (FSIQ)
in those tested of 70, with a range of 52–77. Five patients exhibited low average intelligence
(FSIQ = 82–91). Language testing revealed normal comprehension in those tested.

Seizures were documented in 28 of the 31 patients (90%). The seizures in the majority of
cases consisted of atypical absence and rare generalised tonic-clonic (GTC) attacks. In addition,
atonic and tonic drop attacks were also documented. Five patients (19%) had partial seizures
with or without secondary generalisation, and three patients had bilateral clonic contractions

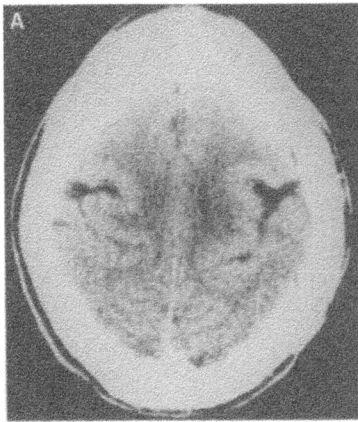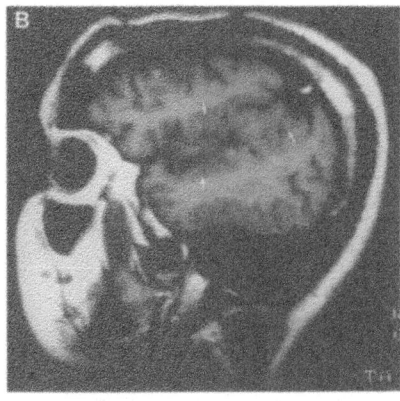

Figure 1. Patient B-6. (A) CT scan section demonstrating bilateral centroparietal cortical malformations. Note slight asymmetric distribution posteriorly. (B) Sagittal image (500/15/2) shows abnormal cortex involving the insula and sylvian fissure and extending posteriorly into the parietal lobe. The malformation involves the superior temporal gyrus (arrow), subcentral gyrus (arrowhead) and supramarginal gyrus (small arrows).

of the lips or perioral seizures with secondary generalisation. The frequency of seizures varied between individuals, but 55% of patients had almost daily seizures.

Imaging Studies

CT scan revealed symmetrical, bilateral, peri-sylvian, cortical thickening. The abnormal cortex appeared thick and smooth, and the sylvian fissures were slightly enlarged in all patients. On CT, the malformations extended into the centroparietal regions with minor asymmetries (Figure 1A). MR confirmed the bilateral peri-sylvian involvement but, with higher resolution, demonstrated some variability in the extent of the abnormalities among patients. In the sagittal plane, the malformations were centred in the insular region with variable extension into the pars opercularis. The subcentral gyrus was invariably involved with limited extension into the transverse temporal gyrus (Figure 1B). The insula appeared exposed and the long insular gyrus was invariably thick. Posterior extension with involvement of the supramarginal gyrus and associated atrophy of the angular gyrus was prevalent. In some cases, the malformations involved the opercular and peri-sylvian regions alone, whereas in others the malformations extended into the parietal and superior temporal regions. Cortical thickness in the abnormal regions ranged from 8 to 10 mm (Figure 2). At the most posterior aspect of the malformations, increased subarachnoid space was common. Using IR sequences, the abnormal cortex showed increased interdigitations between white and grey matter overlaid by small fused gyri, suggesting polymicrogyria (Figure 3). Nodular heterotopias or other abnormalities were not present on MRI. An absent septum pellucidum was observed in one patient.

Of the 28 patients with MR examinations, 20 had primary involvement of the insulo-opercular region. In three others, the abnormal thick cortex was restricted to the insular region. In the remaining five, extension into the superior temporal and parietal regions was observed. Detailed evaluation of the MRIs using axial images revealed that the extent of the malformations was symmetrical in 80% of patients. In 20%, the MRIs demonstrated minor asymmetry in the anteroposterior extension of the malformations.

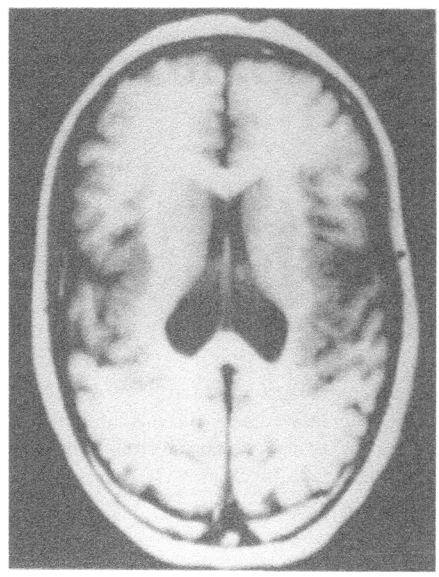

Figure 2. Patient F-14. Axial image (400/20/2) shows symmetrical bilateral malformations involving the insular region. Note small gyri and shallow sulci (arrows).

Neuropathological Findings

Two brains were available for examination. Macroscopic examination of the brain revealed asymmetrical opercularisation in one and symmetrical bilateral opercular hypoplasia resulting in exposure of the insula in the other. No periventricular heterotopias were found, and the rest of the brain was normal in both. Histological sections revealed four-layered polymicrogyria in the insular and opercular region extending into the inferior frontal and parietal regions (Figure 4).

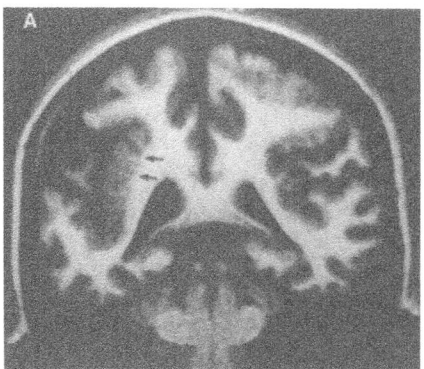 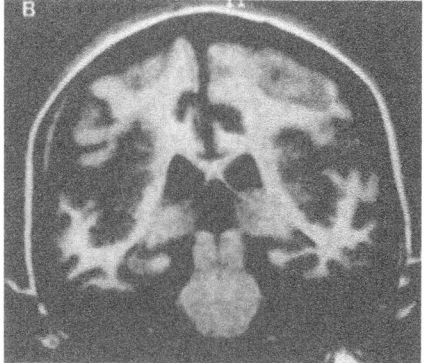

Figure 3. Patient I-4. Coronal IR sequences. Contiguous slices demonstrating asymmetrical malformations. Densely packed small gyri with thin grey–white matter digitations are observed within the malformations (arrows).

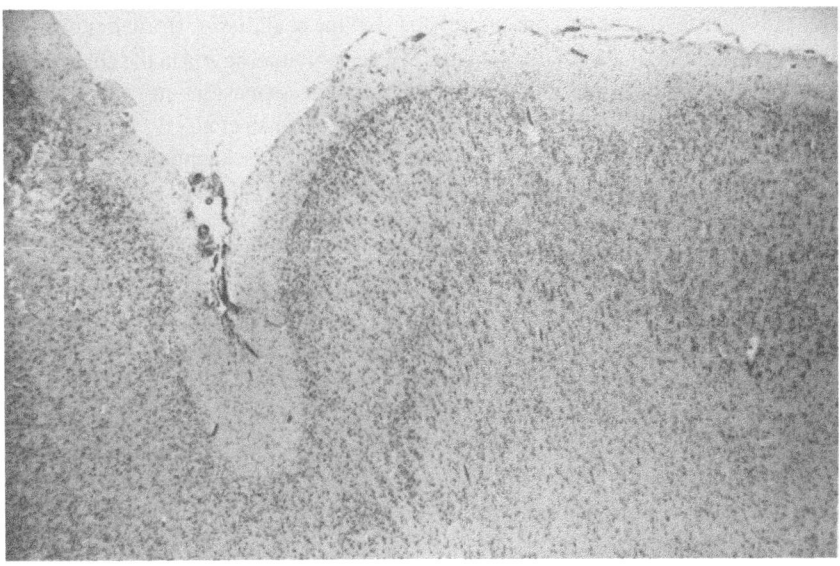

Figure 4. Patient M-31. Histological section through the right operculum showing polymicrogyric cortex. Magnification x 2.

DISCUSSION

The 31 patients described in this study share a congenital syndrome with remarkable similarities. The syndrome includes developmental delay, variable cognitive deficits, prominent cortical pseudobulbar symptoms, and variable pyramidal signs. Seizures were common, and all patients shared the presence of bilateral peri-sylvian cortical malformations on imaging studies. These clinical and imaging features are sufficiently consistent to suggest a rather homogeneous entity.

These patients have prominent cortical pseudobulbar symptoms, especially variable dysarthria, orofacial paresis and, most strikingly, the inability to protrude or move the tongue from side to side. Similar acquired symptoms have been described in adults as the Foix-Chavany-Marie syndrome due to bilateral anterior opercular infarctions (Foix et al., 1926; Mariani et al., 1980). It is clear that the prominent pseudobulbar symptoms are the direct result of involvement of the insular and opercular regions. The degree of oromotor dysfunction, however, did not correlate with the extension of the malformations on MR imaging, but depended on their symmetrical distribution; those with asymmetrical opercular and insular abnormalities tended to have milder forms of dysarthria. Conversely, those with pyramidal limb motor dysfunction had evidence on MR of extended malformations into the prefrontal and central regions when compared to those patients with no or mild pyramidal signs.

Imaging studies revealed the presence of bilateral peri-sylvian and peri-rolandic abnormalities in all patients. CT scans demonstrated thick smooth cortex in the opercular region, but MR imaging revealed that some cortical areas had multiple small gyri. Furthermore, using IR sequences, we were able to demonstrate multiple small gyri and absence of normal white matter digitations within the lesions in some patients. Therefore, contrary to the early suggestion that the lesions represent pachygyria or macrogyria, we believe that the imaging features are representative of polymicrogyria in the opercular and peri-sylvian regions (Barkovich and Kjos, 1992a). The insular distribution and the well-known predilection of the parasylvian region for polymicrogyria support our impression (Levine et al., 1974; Bordarier et al., 1991).

Histological studies in two of our patients revealed polymicrogyria in the abnormal cortex involving the opercular regions bilaterally, with variable extension into the frontal lobes (Figure 4). The aetiology of polymicrogyria is variable (Norman et al., 1958; Hamilton et al., 1962; Levine et al., 1974; Barth, 1987; Bordarier et al., 1991). Ischaemia has been postulated as a possible mechanism. Histopathological studies have suggested that polymicrogyria may be the result of a post-migration insult (20–24 weeks' gestation) (Norman et al., 1958; Hamilton et al., 1962; Levine et al., 1974; Williams and Caviness, 1976; Bordarier et al., 1991). Conversely, experimental work in rodents (Dvorák and Juránková, 1978; Humphreys et al., 1991) and case studies on fetal pathology (Barth and van der Harten, 1985) have suggested that early migration accidents (12–16 weeks' gestation) may be responsible for the microgyric cortex, and therefore polymicrogyria represents a disorder of neuronal migration. Irrespective of the exact timing of the injury, and considering that both early and late ischaemic injuries may induce similar macroscopic peri-sylvian malformations (open operculum), it is likely that, in our patients, the lesions are the result of a restricted ischaemic injury during development.

Many of these patients are presently unrecognised. Appropriate evaluation of the speech abnormality and identification of the prominent pseudobulbar signs should be sufficient to make a tentative diagnosis. This can be confirmed with CT scan or MR imaging.

ACKNOWLEDGEMENTS

The following investigators and institutions participated in this study. Investigators: Ruben Kuzniecky, MD, Study Chairman (UAB Epilepsy Center, University of Alabama at Birmingham); Frederick Andermann, MD, Study Co-Chairman (Montreal Neurological Institute, McGill University, Montreal); Renzo Guerrini, MD (INPE-IRCCS, Stella Maris, Pisa); Donnatela Tampieri, MD, Eva Andermann, MD, PhD, Andre Palmini, MD, Andre Olivier, MD, Denis Melanson, MD, Bernard Rosenblatt, MD, Michael Shevell, MD (Montreal Neurological Institute and Montreal Children's Hospital, McGill University, Montreal); Lucia Fusco, MD, Federico Vigevano, MD (Hospedale Bambino Gesu, Rome); Neill Graff-Radford, MD (University of Iowa); Suzanne Christie, MD, Peter Humphreys, MD, Sharon Whiting, MD (University of Ottawa); Jean Aicardi, MD (Hopital des Enfants Malades, Paris); G. Ambrosetto, MD, Carlo A. Tassinari (Università di Bologna); Bernardo Dalla Bernardina, MD, Vito Colamaria, MD (Università di Verona); Edward Faught, MD, Richard Morawetz, MD (University of Alabama at Birmingham); Charlotte Dravet (Centre St. Paul, Marseille).

REFERENCES

Barkovich, A., and Kjos, B., 1992a, Nonlissencephalic cortical dysplasias: Correlation of imaging findings with clinical deficits, AJNR 13: 85–103.

Barkovich, A., and Kjos, B., 1992b, Schizencephaly: Correlation of clinical findings with MR characteristics, AJNR 13: 85–94.

Barth, P., 1987, Disorders of neuronal migration, Can J Neurol Sci. 14: 1–16.

Barth, P., and van der Harten, J., 1985, Parabiotic twin syndrome with topical isocortical disruption and gastroschisis, Acta Neuropathol. 67: 345–349.

Benton, A., and Van Allen, M., 1968, Impairment in facial recognition in patients with cerebral disease, Cortex 4: 344–358.

Bordarier, C., Robain, O., and Ponsot, G., 1991, Bilateral poroencephalic defect in the newborn after injection of Benzol during pregnancy, Brain Dev. 13: 126–129.

Byrd, S., Osborn, R., Bohan, T. and Naidich, T., 1989, The CT and MR evaluation of migrational disorders of the brain. Part II. Schizencephaly, heterotopia and polymicrogyria, Pediatr Radiol. 19: 219–222.

Dvorák, K., Feit, J., and Juránková, Z., 1978, Experimentally induced focal microgyria and status verrucosis deformis in rats: Pathogenesis and interrelation, histological study, Acta Neuropathol. 44: 121–129.

Foix, C., Chavany, J., and Marie, J., 1926, Diplegie facio-linguo-masticatrice d'origine cortico-sous-cortical sans paralysie des membres, Rev Neurol. 33: 214–219.

Friede, R., 1989, Dysplasias of the cerebral cortex, in: "Developmental Pathology," R. Friede, ed., Springer-Verlag, Vienna.

Graff-Radford, N., Bosh, E., Stears, J. and Tranel, D., 1986, Developmental Foix-Chavany-Marie syndrome in identical twins, Ann Neurol. 20: 632–635.

Hamilton, W., Boyd, J., and Mossman, H., 1962, Human embryology, Williams and Wilkins, Baltimore, 350.

Humphreys, P., Rosen, G., Press, D., Sherman, G., and Galaburda, M., 1991, Freezing lesions of the developing rat brain: A model for cerebrocortical microgyria. J Neuropathol Exp Neurol. 50: 145–160.

Kuzniecky, R., Berkovic, S., Andermann, F., Melanson, D., Olivier, A., and Robitaille, Y., 1988, Focal cortical myoclonus and rolandic cortical dysplasia: Clarification by MRI, Ann Neurol. 23: 317–325.

Kuzniecky, R., Andermann, F., Tampieri, D., Melanson, D., Olivier, A., and Leppik, T., 1989, Bilateral central macrogyria: Epilepsy, pseudobulbar palsy and mental retardation—A recognizable neuronal migration disorder, Ann Neurol. 25: 547–554.

Leiter, G., 1980, Leiter International Performance Scale (Revised), Stoeling, Chicago.

Levine, D., Fisher, M., and Caviness, V., 1974, Porencephaly with microgyria: a pathologic study, Acta Neuropathol (Berl)., 99–113.

Mariani, C., Spinnler, H., Sterzi, R., and Vallar, G., 1980, Bilateral peri-sylvian softenings: Bilateral anterior opercular syndrome (Foix-Chavany-Marie syndrome), J Neurol. 223: 269–284.

Norman, R., Urich, H. and Woods, G., 1958, The relationship between prenatal porencephaly and the encephalomacias of early life, J Ment Sci. 104: 758–771.

Palmini, A., Andermann, F., Olivier, A., Tampieri, D., and Melanson, D., 1991, Focal neuronal migration disorders and intractable epilepsy: A study of 30 patients, Ann Neurol. 30: 741–749.

Wechsler, D., 1981, "Wechsler Adult Intelligence Scale (Revised)," Psychological Corporation, New York.

Williams, R., and Caviness, V., 1976, The cellular pathology of microgyria. A Golgi analysis, Acta Neuropathol. 36: 269–283.

FOCAL CORTICAL DYSPLASIA IN TEMPORAL LOBE EPILEPSY

The Role of Magnetic Resonance Imaging

R. Kuzniecky

UAB Epilepsy Center
Department of Neurology
University of Alabama at Birmingham
UAB Station
Birmingham, Alabama 35294

INTRODUCTION

Magnetic resonance imaging (MRI) has proved to be extremely useful in the detection of central nervous system pathology (Brant-Zawadzki et al., 1983). Its value in the investigation of patients with epilepsy has been confirmed by our studies (Kuzniecky et al., 1988; Berkovic et al., 1991) and by those of others (Jack et al., 1990; Bronen et al., 1991; Theodore, 1986; Duncan, 1990). In the majority of patients with intractable temporal lobe epilepsy the underlying pathological substrate is mesial temporal sclerosis (MTS). This abnormality can be detected by MRI in almost all cases, if the appropriate techniques are used (Kuzniecky et al., 1987). The typical imaging findings consist of hippocampal and amygdaloid atrophy, increased T2-weighted signal from the abnormal hippocampi and loss of internal structure of the hippocampal formation. Other pathological abnormalities include glial and non-glial neoplasms, vascular malformations, post-traumatic changes and other conditions (Avrahami et al., 1987; Altman, 1988; Bracchi, 1988). A less common pathological entity encountered in patients with intractable partial seizures is focal cortical dysplasia (Kuzniecky et al., 1991). It is characterised by a lack of cortical organisation associated with abnormal giant neurons and increased astrocytosis (Taylor et al., 1971; Kuzniecky et al., 1991). Although this anomaly was originally reported in 1971 by Taylor et al., it was not until recently that other investigators reported similar findings in surgical specimens from other brain regions. As high-resolution MRI is sensitive in the detection of subtle lesions, it has been possible to detect pre-operatively these developmental lesions in some patients selected for resective surgery. Recognition of these peculiar and often subtle abnormalities in patients with intractable temporal lobe epilepsy has increased the value of MRI in the pre-surgical investigation of these patients.

Magnetic Resonance Scanning and Epilepsy, Edited by S.D. Shorvon et al.,
Plenum Press, New York, 1994

METHODS

All patients with refractory partial seizures of temporal lobe origin admitted to the UAB Epilepsy Center for surgical intervention were examined using a standardised MRI protocol. Of the patients investigated and operated on, 12 were selected on the basis of histological confirmation of cortical dysplasia. All patients were evaluated with prolonged EEG-video monitoring, neuropsychological studies and more recently with inter-ictal SPECT. MRI examinations were performed using different 1.5 T units. Spin echo studies (TR: 2000–2500 ms; TE: 25–100 s) were performed in the axial and coronal planes. T1-weighted images (TR: 500; TE:15) were also obtained in all planes. More recently, inversion recovery sequences (TR:1200 TE:20 TI:300) were used. Three patients received gadolinium-DTPA (diethylenetriamine pentaacetic acid) intravenous contrast. Temporal lobe resections were carried in all patients. The resections were guided by the imaging and findings on electro-corticography, but in general they included the mesial structures and the inferior and middle temporal gyrus, sparing the superior temporal convolution unless this was involved on MRI. Histological studies were carried out after staining with haematoxylin and eosin, cresyl violet, glial fibrillary acid protein (GFAP) antisera and silver impregnation. Tissue sections were examined and classified into two groups. Group 1 consisted of mild dysplasia and group 2 included those specimens with severe dysplastic changes. The histopathological classification has been described in detail previously (Kuzniecky et al., 1991). Qualitative visual analysis of the MRIs was performed by one observer. Localisation by visual analysis was compared to the EEG data and the surgical procedure.

RESULTS

The mean age of the 12 patients entered in this study was 22 years (range 7–36). The mean age of onset for the epilepsy was 4.1 years (0.7–13). The mean seizure frequency was 8.8 seizures per month (range 6–22). All patients had complex partial seizures and in 9 secondary generalisation occurred. The inter-ictal and ictal EEG studies indicated a left temporal focus in 9 of the 12 patients, and MRI studies revealed abnormalities in 9 of the 12 patients. The pattern observed was variable but was unilateral. In five patients, MRI revealed non-homogeneous abnormal signal from the temporal lobe on T2-weighted scans (Figure 1). The abnormal signal involved the anterior, inferior and middle temporal regions. In three of these patients, the abnormality extended into the mesial structures (Figure 2 A,B). In one patient, the dysplastic cortex involved all of the temporal convolutions and extended into the parietal lobe (Figure 3). Contrast studies with gadolinium-DTPA did not reveal any changes in these patients. Four patients had subtle abnormalities of cortical organisation. The changes consisted of an abnormal grey–white matter pattern. The cortex appeared thick and the underlying white matter digitations were short and indistinct (Figure 4). In one patient, the temporal horn was unilaterally large. Pathological analysis subclassified six patients in group 1. In this group, MRI was abnormal in three patients. The abnormalities were always subtle without T2 changes. Of the six patients in group 2, all had changes of varying severity ranging from T1 and T2 abnormalities to subtle cortico-white matter changes (Figure 5). In some, the entire temporal lobe was abnormal whereas, in others, the changes were restricted to one temporal gyrus or the white matter. In all, however, the MRIs were abnormal. EEG correlation revealed focal abnormalities corresponding to the MRI abnormality in all patients.

DISCUSSION

Excellent anatomical definition of the temporal lobes is essential for recognising subtle abnormalities in patients with temporal lobe epilepsy. This can be achieved by using imaging

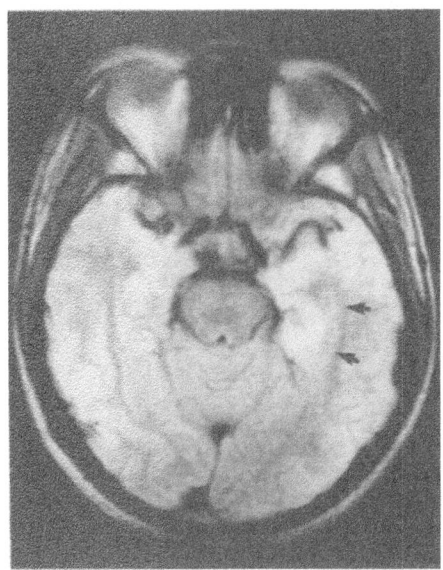

Figure 1. Axial MRI (TR 2500 mg; TE 30 mg) demonstrate abnormal signal and configuration of left temporal lobe. Note involvement of left mesial structures and abnormal white matter (arrow).

sequences that provide high resolution between grey and white matter such as T1-weighted or inversion recovery (IR) sequences and by using multiplanar imaging, in particular angulated coronal slices. In our experience, IR studies have occasionally revealed subtle but definite changes when T1-weighted images were of questionable significance. The excellent contrast offered by IR sequences allowed recognition of cortico-white matter abnormalities. Although IR studies may increase scanning time, we believe that the information obtained warrants its use in selected patients. Additionally, T2-weighted images may confirm the presence of pathology by demonstrating tissue signal changes. The T2-weighted abnormalities observed in cortical dysplasia are often less circumscribed when compared to small tumours or hamartomas. The use of contrast agents, such as gadolinium-DTPA, does not appear warranted unless one is attempting to rule out the possibility of a malignancy. Recent studies have confirmed the sensitivity and specificity of MRI in the recognition of different forms of cortical developmental malformations (Kuzniecky et al., 1992). Cortical dysplastic lesions appear to

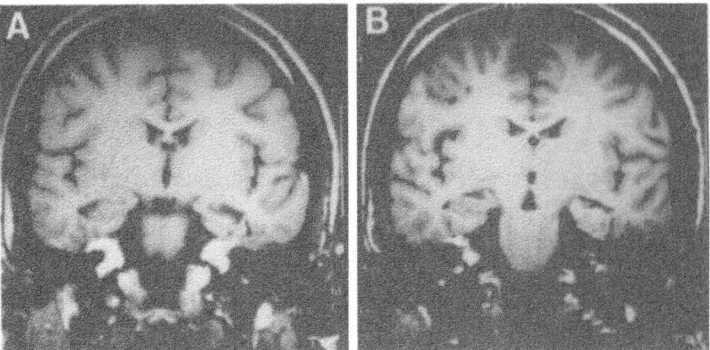

Figure 2. A–B. Coronal MRI (TR 70 mg; TE 20 mg). Two consecutive images showing involvment of the left parahippocampal gyrus and temporal lobe. See text. Refer to Figure 5 for corresponding pathology.

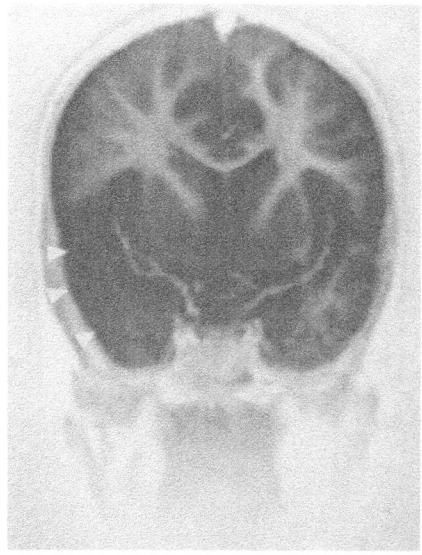

Figure 3. Coronal MRI (IR). Note extensive involvment of left temporal lobe including all temporal convolutions. Note abnormal cortico-white matter organization (arrowheads).

be more frequent in the frontal and parietal lobes, and the pre- and post-central regions have a particularly high incidence of these malformations. The imaging features consist of cortical gyral abnormalities with variable signal changes. Similar imaging features were observed in our cases of temporal lobe dysplasia with variable cortical and white matter changes. An interesting observation is the paucity of involvement of the mesial structures by these lesions; in only 3 out of the 12 patients, was there some evidence of mesial involvement by MRI. In one patient, the MRI showed an abnormally thin parahippocampal gyrus but the hippocampus and dentate gyrus, although slightly smaller, had normal configuration (Figure 2A,B). It is well established that the organisation and formation of the hippocampus is a slow process which possibly extends into the first postnatal year. However, the process of hippocampal inversion

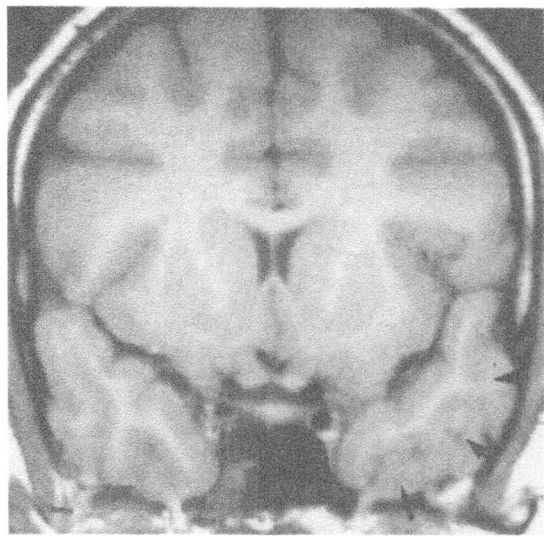

Figure 4. Coronal MRI (TR 50 mg; TE: 15). The left temporal lobe is abnormal. Note thick temporal gyri with thin white matter (arrows).

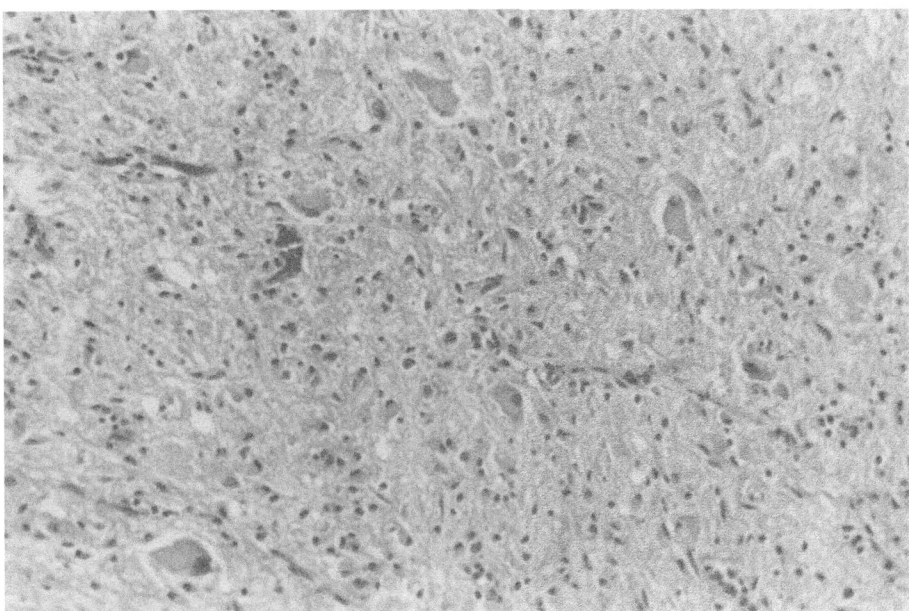

Figure 5. Example of one of the several histological abnormalities; cortical dyslamination, abnormally large neurons and astrocytocis (H-E × 400).

occurs early in the prenatal period. The appearance of a small and vertical (non-inverted) hippocampus in patients with lissencephaly, holoprosencephaly and agenesis of the corpus callosum point out to early arrest of migration (Baker and Barkovich, 1992). In cortical dysplasia, normal horizontal morphological orientation is present. Our findings, although in a few patients, would support the concept of a limited and late insult causing abnormal neuronal migration in the mesial temporal structures (Baker and Barkovich, 1992). Classical focal cortical dysplasia and the subtle forms described in this chapter and by other investigators (Hardiman et al., 1988) should be differentiated from mesial temporal sclerosis and other pathologies by using MRI. The typical features of MTS have been well described (Kuzniecky et al., 1987; Jack et al., 1990; Berkovic et al., 1991; Bronen et al., 1991). Atrophy and increased signal from the hippocampus should not be mistaken for other lesions. Small tumours and hamartomas usually present with well-defined borders or mass effect and, therefore, should be differentiated from cortical dysplasia. We believe that the presence of a thick, poorly defined, cortical ribbon and underlying white matter within a temporal convolution should raise the diagnosis of focal cortical dysplasia. The pre-operative identification of dysplastic lesions by MRI is important for several reasons. First, these lesions are common in patients with medically resistant seizures. Second, these lesions often become symptomatic early in life, remain intractable and have a profound impact on the quality of life of young children. Third, visualisation by MRI should allow early diagnosis and surgical intervention, thus preventing the potentially devastating effect of medically intractable seizures. MRI studies in a larger number of cases will be necessary to establish the imaging spectrum of these malformations in temporal lobe epilepsy.

REFERENCES

Altman, N.R., 1988, MR and CT characteristics and gangliocytoma: a rare cause of epilepsy in children, AJNR 9: 917–921.

Avrahami, E., Cohn, D., Neufeld, M., et al., 1987, Magnetic resonance imaging (MRI) in patients with complex partial seizures and normal computerised tomography (CT) scan, Clin Neurol Neurosurg. 89: 89–94.

Baker, L., and Barkovich, A., 1992, The large temporal horn: MR analysis in developmental brain anomalies versus hydrocephalus, AJNR 13: 115–122.

Berkovic, S.F., Andermann, F., Ethier, R., et al., 1991, Hippocampal sclerosis in temporal lobe epilepsy demonstrated by magnetic resonance imaging, Ann Neurol. 29: 175–182.

Bracchi, M., 1988, MR in epilepsies: methodological aspects, Boll Lega Ital Epilessia 63: 47–50.

Brant-Zawadzki, M., Davis, P., Crooks, L., et al., 1983, NMR demonstration of cerebral abnormalities: Comparison with CT, AJNR 4: 117–124.

Bronen, R., Chevny, G., Charles, J., et al., 1991, Imaging findings in hippocampal sclerosis: correlation with pathology, AJNR 12: 933–940.

Duncan, R., et al., 1990, CT, MR and SPECT imaging in temporal lobe epilepsy, J Neurol Neurosurg Psychiat. 53: 11–15.

Hardiman, O., Burke, T., Phillips, J., et al., 1988, Microdysgenesis in resected temporal neocortex: incidence and clinical significance in focal epilepsy, Neurology 38: 1041–1047.

Jack, C., Sharbrough, F., Twomey, C., et al., 1990, Temporal lobe seizures: lateralisation with MR volume measurements of the hippocampal formation, Radiology 175: 423–429.

Kuzniecky, R., de La Sayetle, Ethier R., et al., 1987, Magnetic resonance imaging in temporal lobe epilepsy: pathological correlations, Ann Neurol. 22: 341–347.

Kuzniecky, R., Berkovic, S., Andermann, F., et al., 1988, Focal cortical myoclonus and rolandic cortical dysplasia: clarification by magnetic resonance imaging, Ann Neurol. 23: 317–325.

Kuzniecky, R., Faught, E., and Garcia, J., 1991, Cortical dysplasia in temporal lobe epilepsy: magnetic resonance correlations, Ann Neurol. 29: 293–298.

Kuzniecky, R., Murro, A., King, D., et al., 1992, MRI in intractable epilepsy of childhood: pathological correlations, Epilepsia 33: 102.

Taylor, D., Falconer, M., Bruton, C., 1971, Focal dysplasia of the cerebral cortex in epilepsy, J Neurol Neurosurg Psychiat. 34: 369–387.

Theodore, W.H., 1986, Neuroimaging, Neurol Clin. 4: 645–668.

MR IN CONGENITAL AND HEREDITARY METABOLIC DISORDERS ASSOCIATED WITH EPILEPSY

F. Vigevano, G. Fariello, A. Bartuli, E. Bertini, C. Dionisi-Vici, and L. Fusco

Section of Neurophysiology
Children's Hospital and Scientific Research Institute "Bambino Gesu'"
Rome
Italy

INTRODUCTION

Metabolic disorders result in various types of brain lesion. The commonest neurological symptoms are developmental delay, movement disorders and epileptic seizures. In some metabolic disorders, epilepsy is the most prominent symptom; in others it is one of several associated symptoms, and in other forms seizures are rare. This depends on the degree of disruption of normal brain structure. In general, the severity of epilepsy reflects the degree of cortical grey matter involvement and the level of maturity of the brain. The latter is relevant because metabolic disorders often become manifest during the early phases of development. MR imaging is invaluable for defining the underlying neuropathology. In this chapter we examine correlations between the brain lesion, type of epilepsy and MR appearances.

CURRENT RESEARCH

Metabolic disorders cause epilepsy through one of three pathogenetic mechanisms:

The Metabolic Disorder Interferes with the Nervous System during the Prenatal and Neonatal Stages of its Development

The characteristic pathological patterns include delayed and defective myelination, white matter spongiosis and gliosis, cerebral atrophy, thinning of the corpus callosum, and neuronal migration disorders. Even though the cortical grey matter is often spared, epilepsy is one of the predominant symptoms, probably a consequence of a deficiency of inhibitory systems.

This group includes amino acidopathies (non-ketotic hyperglycinaemia, methylmalonic and propionic acidaemia, maple syrup urine disease, tyrosinaemia, phenylketonuria, hyper-beta-alaninaemia) and some peroxisomal disorders.

Magnetic Resonance Scanning and Epilepsy, Edited by S.D. Shorvon et al.,
Plenum Press, New York, 1994

The disease becomes clinically evident in the neonatal period, the predominant abnormalities being lethargy, severe developmental delay and convulsions. Within days of birth the infant presents partial seizures and myoclonic jerks. The EEG contains the pattern known as "suppression-burst". MR imaging may show progressive atrophy, thinning of the corpus callosum and delayed myelination. T2-weighted images are particularly useful for demonstrating the state of myelination (Press et al., 1989).

Metabolic Defects Provoking Progressive Degeneration of an Apparently Well-formed Nervous System

In this heterogeneous group of diseases, enzymatic deficiency and metabolic product accumulation lead to the destruction of cerebral neurons. Epilepsy is particularly frequent and severe in disorders which predominantly affect the grey matter, including the lipidoses and the ceroid lipofuscinoses, or conditions affecting grey and white matter, for example the peroxisomal and mitochondrial disorders. Epilepsy is less common in the leucodystrophies, with the exception of Krabbe's disease.

In these metabolic disorders epileptic seizures start at any age, and may be partial or generalised. Because neuronal damage is generally diffuse, the seizures are polymorphic. In ceroid lipofuscinosis, myoclonic epilepsy and ragged red fibers disease (MERFF) and the other conditions with a slowly progressive course, epilepsy may be the only symptom for years, with unusual clinical and EEG appearances (Dalla Bernardina et al., 1982). MR imaging provides useful diagnostic information. The various neuroradiological appearances have been described in detail and correlate closely to the neuropatholoy (Becker, 1992; Kendall, 1992). In patients with disorders that are exceptionally difficult to identify, for example some cases of Alper's disease, MR imaging will often provide key diagnostic information.

Metabolic Diseases Related to an Acute, Diffuse or Focal Brain Lesion

In some organic acidaemias (glutaric aciduria type II, pyruvate dehydrogenase deficiency), an energy deficit may lead to severe, acute cerebral oedema, followed by diffuse cerebral atrophy with consequent grey and white matter damage.

In the acute phase of the disease severe convulsions occur, with a subsequent lesional epilepsy. In other cases, the lesions involve particularly the basal ganglia (methylmalonic and propionic acidaemia). Mitochondrial encephalopathy, lactic acidosis and stroke-like episodes (MELAS) and ornithine carbamyl transferase deficiency provoke stroke-like lesions that are isolated or multiple. These changes may cause epilepsy with partial seizures sometimes taking the form of epilepsia partialis continua (Chevrie et al., 1987).

DISCUSSION

The field of metabolic disorders is one of constant discovery, in which new biochemical defects continue to be identified. Many of these advances have been made possible by MR imaging, which has proved far superior to other neuroradiological imaging techniques. Its superiority is particularly marked in abnormalities affecting the white matter, in neuronal migration disorders, and in acute lesions of the basal ganglia. Our schematic distinction is certainly not complete and many metabolic disorders still defy classification. Despite such drawbacks, attempting a correlation between the type of epilepsy and the MR imaging appearances is worthwhile. Not only does it help us to understand the neuroimaging data, it also provides a clearer description of the underlying neuropathology.

PROBABLE DEVELOPMENT OVER THE NEXT FIVE YEARS

In many cases today, a metabolic disorder is suspected, but the biochemical defect remains unknown. In the future, larger case studies are required to make a better definition of the neuroimaging appearances of the range of metabolic disorders. MR imaging is likely then to become a fundamental tool in the diagnosis of metabolic diseases affecting the nervous system.

REFERENCES

Becker, L.E., 1992, Lysosomes, peroxisomes and mitochondria: function and disorder, AJNR 13: 609–620.

Chevrie, J.J., Aicardi, J., and Goutires, F., 1987, Epilepsy in childhood mitochondrial encephalomyopathies, in: "Advances in Epileptology," P. Wolf, M. Dam, D. Janz, F.E. Dreifuss, eds, Raven Press, New York.

Dalla Bernardina, B., Lombardi, A., and Tassinari, C.A., 1982, Aspetti EEG e neurofisio-logici delle malattie dismetaboliche con epilessia dell'et a pediatrica, Bol Lega It Epil. 39: 143–148.

Kendall, B.E., 1992, Disorders of lysosomes, peroxisomes, and mitochondria, AJNR 363: 621–653.

Press, G.A., Barshop, B.A., Haas, R.H., Nyhan, W.L., Glass, R.F., and Hesselink J.R., 1989, Abnormalities of the brain in nonketotic hyperglycinemia: MR manifestations, AJNR 10: 315–321.

MRI IN THE DELINEATION OF GENETIC METABOLIC DISORDERS

P.G. Barth[1] and J. Valk[2]

[1] Division of Paediatric Neurology
University Hospital Amsterdam

[2] Department of Neuroradiology
Free University Hospital Amsterdam
Amsterdam
The Netherlands

INTRODUCTION

Genetic metabolic disorders may interfere with early morphogenesis of the brain. Generalised peroxisomal disorders (GPD) called Zellweger's syndrome (ZS), infantile Refsum's disease (IRD) and neonatal adrenoleucodystrophy (NALD), although biochemically very similar, differ in clinical expression (De Leon et al., 1977; Evrard et al., 1978; Torvik et al., 1988; Wanders et al., 1990). ZS has the poorest prognosis, and IRD the best. ZS has the highest degree of external dysmorphia, underlining its early prenatal onset. Abnormal gyration has been consistently described in ZS, but not in IRD or NALD. We tried to correlate external features of the brain as found either post mortem or on MRI with clinical diagnosis.

Pontocerebellar hypoplasias represent another group of prenatal-onset neurodegenerations (Barth et al., 1992). At least two autosomal recessive disorders, one combined with anterior horn cell depletion, similar to spinal muscular atrophy type I, and the other with microcephaly, mental handicap, epilepsy and dyskinesia, are known. A first publication on this disorder was followed by further cases from non-related families. MRI has an important part in this ongoing research.

L-2-Hydroxyglutaric acidaemia represents a recently described inherited neurometabolic disease with characteristic findings on MRI, knowledge of which even should allow a specific diagnosis in any patient prior to confirmation of by gas chromatography of organic acids.

Magnetic Resonance Scanning and Epilepsy, Edited by S.D. Shorvon et al.,
Plenum Press, New York, 1994

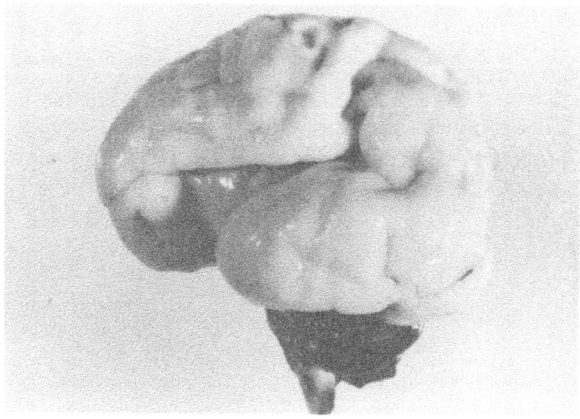

Figure 1. Lateral view of brain of premature (29 weeks) newborn with Zellweger's syndrome showing abnormal vertical sulcus joining the sylvian fissure with the vertex.

CURRENT RESEARCH

Generalised Peroxisomal Disorders

Patients previously diagnosed as ZS who died before 12 months of age were catalogued as severe GPD (sGPD); the others who survived beyond this age and were previously diagnosed as mild ZS or infantile Refsum's disease were catalogued as moderate GPD (mGPD). No cases of NALD were available for study. Five patients with sGPD were studied post mortem and all had prominent neocortical dysplasia, especially a prominent vertical-oriented sulcus extending or branching from the Sylvian fissure (Figure 1).

Five patients with mGPD were studied, one post mortem and the others by MRI. Prominent neocortical dysplasia was present in two. Neocortical anatomy therefore does not rigorously differentiate sGPD and mGPD.

Genetic complementation studies have led to eight complementation groups within the total group of GPD. Therefore (until now), eight genes are involved in peroxisomal assembly. A deficiency of any of these genes will result in GPD (Yayima et al., 1992). Complementation did not solve phenotypic variability of GPD. On the contrary, three complementation groups each include more than one phenotypic variant, e.g. ZS and also NALD or IRD or both. The need for family counselling as well as the emergence of new therapies prompts clear definition of clinical subtypes related to prognosis. A relationship between brain structure at an early age and prognosis in GPD is likely. Therefore further, more detailed, larger studies which make use of MRI could be helpful. The study of neocortical dysplasia is one approach. Other features, especially myelination which is often delayed and degree of ventricular dilatation, may provide additional criteria for phenotyping. Myelination in GPD is delayed, but comparison between sGPD and mGPD in this regard could not be made by us because only a limited number of MRIs of both groups at the same early age were available. MRI could be of benefit in the diagnosis of NALD where demyelination is prominent. For the study of neocortical dysplasia lateral sagittal sections which expose the whole sylvian fissure are likely to give the best approach in GPD.

Pontocerebellar Hypoplasias

On the basis of pathology and clinical features two main types are well delineated, both of which are inherited as autosomal recessives. These include (1) pontocerebellar hypoplasia, congenital contractures and anterior horn degeneration, with early death (Barth et al., 1992) and (2) pontocerebellar hypoplasia with microcephaly, severe mental handicap, extrapyrami-

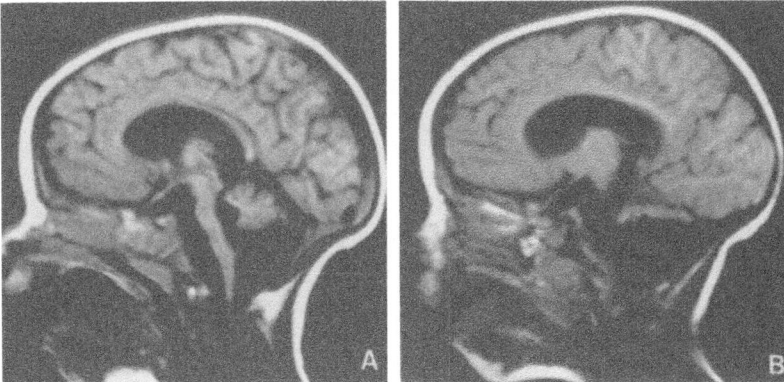

Figure 2. Pontocerebellar hypoplasia in a 6-month-old female patient. T1-weighted images. (A) Vermal and pontine hypoplasia. (B) Severe hypoplasia of cerebellar hemisphere.

dal dyskinesia and epilepsy (Barth et al., 1990). Six families have been detected so far, two outside the Netherlands. Present investigations aim at defining the second disorder on the basis of clinical and MRI findings. Distinguishing MRI features include: severe cerebellar hypoplasia with relative sparing of the vermis; hypomyelination of the cerebellar hemispheres in some, attenuation of the pons; and various degrees of (sub)cortical atrophy (Figure 2a,b). MRI has been found to be superior for diagnosis of this genetic disorder. Other types of pontocerebellar hypoplasia probably exist. A relatively large number of children are born with vermal malformations, such as Dandy–Walker syndrome, Chiari type 2 and isolated vermis hypoplasia. They may occur as part of genetic or chromosomal disorders, but they often occur in isolated cases with no clue to their origin. By contrast pontocerebellar hypoplasias predominantly affect the cerebellar hemispheres, and the finding of pontocerebellar hypoplasia should be strongly suspected as part of a genetic syndrome. This point of view is underlined by the fact that neocerebellar hypoplasia and hypoplasia of the pons, in these disorders, appear to be caused by regressive changes.

L-2-Hydroxyglutaric Acidaemia

L-2-Hydroxyglutaric acidaemia is a recently defined autosomal recessive metabolic disorder. L-2-Hydroxyglutaric acid accumulates in urine, blood and CSF of affected patients who display progressive ataxia and (progressive) mental deficiency, as well as generalised epileptic seizures or febrile seizures. MRI findings are very characteristic; they include subcortical demyelination, and cerebellar atrophy and signal changes on T2-weighted images in the caudate and dentate nuclei.

All cases identified until now have the described pattern on MRI (Barth et al., 1992) (Figure 3).

PROBABLE DEVELOPMENT OVER THE NEXT FIVE YEARS

Generalised Peroxisomal Disorders

Imaging studies of these disorders may further help in defining the phenotypes which belong to each of the genetic deficiencies that cause GPD. It is advocated that a view of the

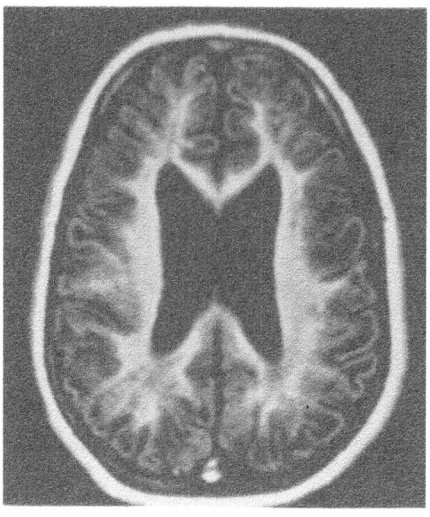

Figure 3. L-2-Hydroxyglutaric acidaemia in a 16-year-old male patient. Tl-weighted image showing severe subcortical myelin loss.

sylvian area on a sagittal scan is included because it provides the best view of neocortical dysplasia in GPD.

Pontocerebellar Hypoplasia

MRI should be helpful in identifying patients to aid in gene-mapping studies for identifying the lesion in this serious disease. Other types of pontocerebellar hypoplasia may be identified by routine MRI studies on mentally handicapped patients.

L-2-Hydroxyglutaric Acidaemia

MRI will aid in detecting those patients, on whom further metabolic studies (gas chromatography, mass spectrometry) should be done. Further refinement in MRS might be helpful in detecting the compound, and probably other organic acids in the brain of affected patients.

REFERENCES

Barth, P.G., 1992, Inherited progressive disorders of the fetal brain: A field in need of recognition, in: "Fetal and perinatal neurology", Y. Fukuyama, Y. Suzuki, S. Kamoshita, P. Casaer, eds, Karger, Basel, pp. 299–313.

Barth, P.G., Vrensen, G.F.J.M., Uylings, H.B.M., Oorthuys, J.W.E., and Stam, F.C., 1990, Inherited syndrome of microcephaly, dyskinesia and pontocerebellar hypoplasia: a systemic atrophy with early onset, J Neurol Sci. 97: 25–42.

Barth, P.G., Hoffmann, G.F., Jaeken, J., Lehnert, W., Hanefeld, F., van Gennip, A.E.H., Duran, M., Valk, J., Schutgens, R.B.H., Trefz, F.K., Reimann, G., and Hartung, H-P., 1992, L-2-Hydroxyglutaric acidemia: a novel inherited neuro-metabolic disease, Ann Neurol. 32: 66–71.

De Leon, G.A., Grover, W.D., Huff, D.S., Morinigo-Mestre, G., Punnett, H., and Kistenmacher, M.L., 1977, Globoid cells, glial nodules, and peculiar fibrillary changes in the cerebro-hepato-renal syndrome of Zellweger. Ann Neurol. 2: 473–484.

Evrard, P., Caviness, V.S. Jr, Pratts-Vinas, J., and Lyon, G., 1978, The mechanism of arrest of neuronal migration in the Zellweger malformation: An hypothesis based upon cytoarchitectonic analysis, Acta Neuropathol (Berl). 41: 109–117.

Torvik, A., Torp, S., Kase, B.F., Ek, J., Skjeldahl, O., and Stokke, O., 1988, Infantile Refsum's disease - A generalised peroxisomal disorder. Report of a case with postmortem examination, J Neurol Sci. 85: 39–53.

Wanders, R.J.A., van Roermund, C.W.T., Schutgens, R.B.H., Barth, P.G., Heymans H.S.A., van den Bosch, H., and Tager, J.M., 1990, The inborn errors of peroxisomal oxidation, J Inher Metab Dis. 113: 4–36.

Yayima, S., Suzuki, Y Shimozawa, N., Yamaguchi, S., Orii, T., Fujiki, Y., Osumi, T., Hashimoto, T., and Moser, H.W., 1992, Complementation study of peroxisome- deficient disorders by immunofluorescence staining and characterization of fused cells, Hum Genet. 88: 491–499.

MINIMAL DEVELOPMENTAL DISTURBANCES IN EPILEPSY AND MRI

H.J. Meencke

Neurologische Abteilung
Klinikum Rudolf Virchow
Free University Berlin
Augustenburger Platz 1
1000 Berlin 65
Germany

INTRODUCTION

Developmental disturbances in epilepsy can be discussed on a macroscopic, microscopic and even a morphometric level. This chapter about minimal developmental disturbances in epilepsy deals with changes predominantly visible only at the microscopic or morphometric level.

We predominantly focus on migrational disturbances, as these are the most frequent findings of developmental disturbances in epilepsy. In our study of 591 brains of epilepsy patients (Meencke and Veith, 1992) we found 46.5% of migration disturbances in epilepsy, compared to 1.7% in normal controls. Migration disturbances are also the most important change on the microscopic or morphometric level.

Very often the term "cortical dysplasia" is synonymously used when minimal migrational disturbances of the brain are mentioned in epilepsies. We have to be aware of the fact, that the term "dysplasia" is a summarising term which includes a large variety of migration disturbances with macroscopic and microscopic changes (Table 1).

CURRENT RESEARCH

Macroscopy

A schematic drawing demonstrates the systematic interrelationship between the different migrational disturbances (Figure 1). The upper half of the scheme shows the predominantly macroscopically identifiable changes. They include microgyria, pachygyria and the different types of heterotopias. The proportional rates of migration disturbances (Table 2)

Magnetic Resonance Scanning and Epilepsy, Edited by S.D. Shorvon et al.,
Plenum Press, New York, 1994

Table 1. Dysplasias of the Cerebral Cortex

• Agyria (lissencephaly)	• Leptomeningeal glioneuronal heterotopias
• Pachygyria	
• Heterotopia	• Persistence of Cajal cells
Nodular	• Columnar arrangement
Laminar	• Abnormal laminar architecture
• Polymicrogyria	• Focal dysplasia of the cerebral cortex
• Nodular cortical dysplasia	

Table 2. Prortional Rates of Migrational Disturbances (%)

	Controls (n = 7374)	Epilepsies (n = 591)
Microdysgenesis	6*	37.7
Microgyria	1	4.7
Heterotopia	0.6	9.3
Pachygyria	0.25	1.9

*n = 150

indicate that heterotopias are the second most frequent finding after microdysgenesis in epileptic brains.

It is now possible to demonstrate macroscopically visible heterotopias with MRI. We can separate laminar heterotopias from nodular heterotopias. In Figures 2 and 3 laminar heterotopias are demonstrated in the frontal lobe. There is a clearly distinguishable subcortical grey substance in the MRI. Figure 3 shows a pathological specimen which also indicates some pathological changes of the overlying cortex; it is important to note that almost all cases have some cortical pathological changes. Laminar heterotopias are correlated most frequently with pachygyria.

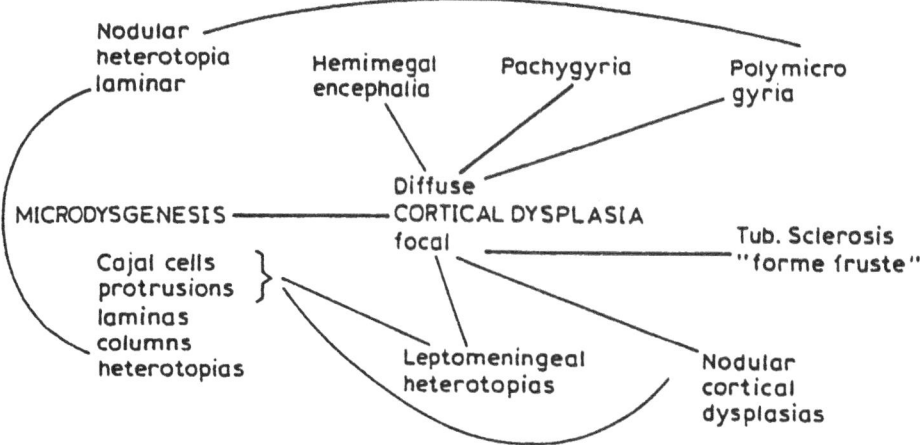

Figure 1. Phenomenological transitions between different migrational disturbances.

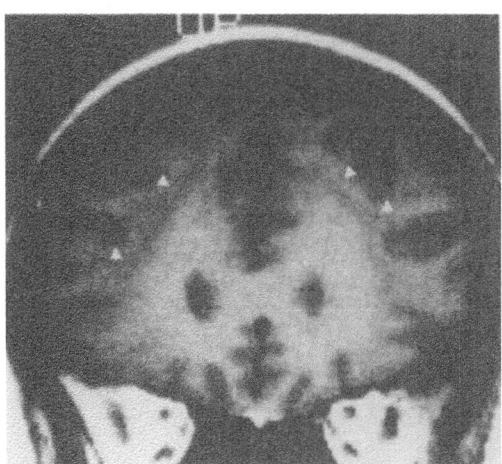

Figure 2. Laminar heterotopia in the frontal lobes. MRI, spin echo, T1-weighted.

In Figures 4 and 5 a nodular type of heterotopia is shown. The subcortical grey masses are especially well shown in the inversion recovery mode of Figure 4. The pathological specimen of Figure 5 demonstrates the additional microgyral changes of the overlying cortex. In our study of 43 cases with heterotopias, only 8 cases had no cortical changes. Six had deep periventricular nodular heterotopias which are, in most of the cases, pathologically irrelevant normal variants. This finding supports the view that the cortical changes in laminar and nodular heterotopias are different.

Agyria and pachgyria, as the partial type of agyria, as well as microgyria, each have a four-layered cortex with different internal organisation (Table 3).

Some cases of microgyria are not migrational disturbances in the narrow sense, but result from early ischaemic lesions which affect the primarily normal developed cortex. This type of microgyria is often associated with false porencephaly which allows us to separate it from that due to migrational disturbances.

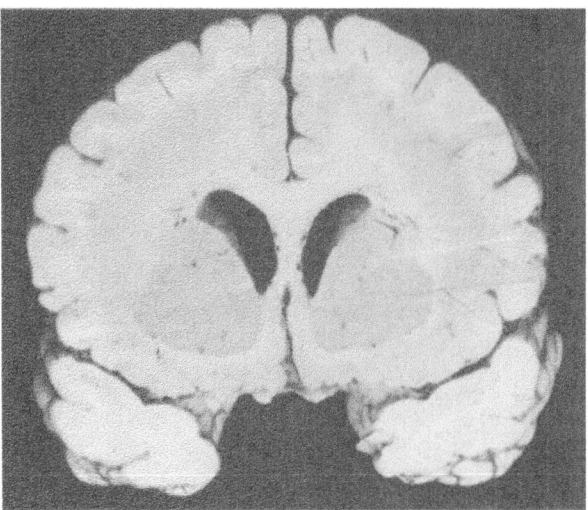

Figure 3. Bifrontal laminar heterotopia. Formalin-fixed brain.

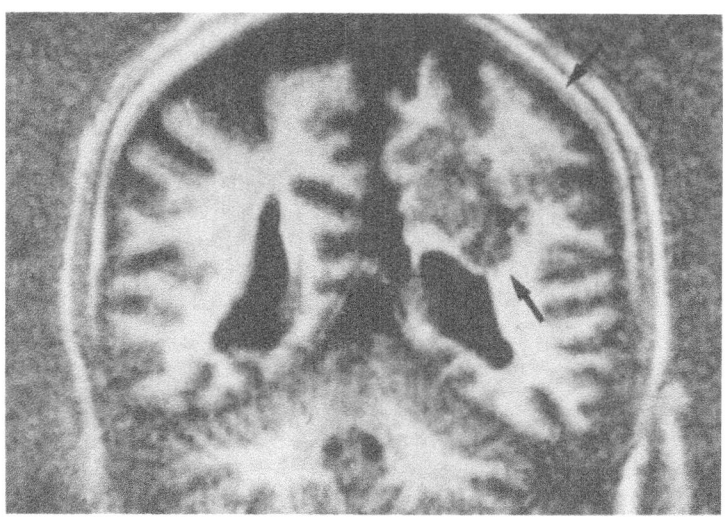

Figure 4. Nodular heterotopia. MRI, inversion recovery.

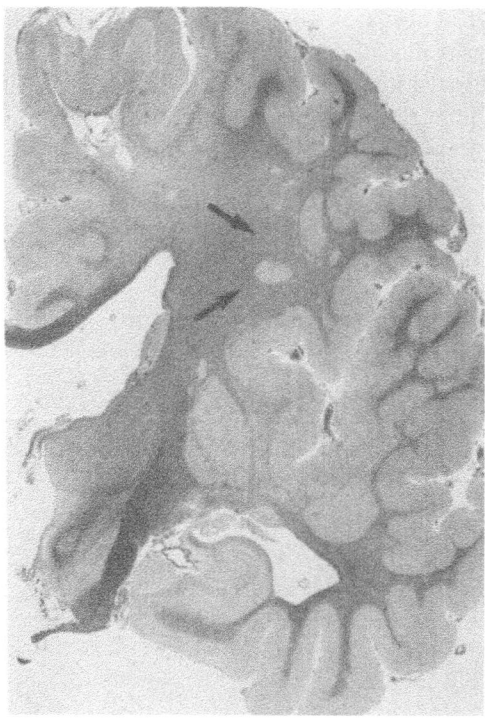

Figure 5. Nodular heterotopia and microgyria. Formalin fixed, paraffin.

Table 3. Internal Organisation of Pathological Cortex

Pachygyria (Four layers)	Microgyria (Four layers)
Molecular layer	Molecular layer
Granular layer	Dense cell layer
Tangential myelinated fibers	Low dense cell layer
Internal thick cell layer	Deep cell layer

Microscopy

The lower part of Figure 1 shows the minimal developmental disturbances in the more narrow sense. It includes different types of cortical dysplasias and microdysgenesis with single neuron heterotopias or changes of the internal architectural organisation of the cortex.

The term "cortical dysplasia" is very often misused in this context. The original paper from Taylor et al. (1971) used the term "focal dysplasia of cerebral cortex". The authors demonstrated histological changes with slight localised architectural disturbances within a macroscopically normal cortex. Ranke (1910) and also Morel and Wilde (1952) used the term "nodular cortical dysplasia" to describe macroscopically abnormal cortical areas.

Figure 6 shows occipital cortical changes which are often described as focal dysplasias but better characterised by the term "pachygyria". Figure 7 shows a macroscopically normal histological specimen of real focal dysplasia with ballooned neurons which are clustered and show no laminar organisation.

Figure 8 shows the variance of microdysgenesis in minimal disturbances of cortical architecture. These slight developmental disturbances are the current challenge for MRI technology, which are to date invisible to in vivo imaging methods.

Microdysgenesis includes localised protrusion of neurons (Figure 9) with the architectural disturbances of the deeper cortical region, disruption of lamination and also very slight single

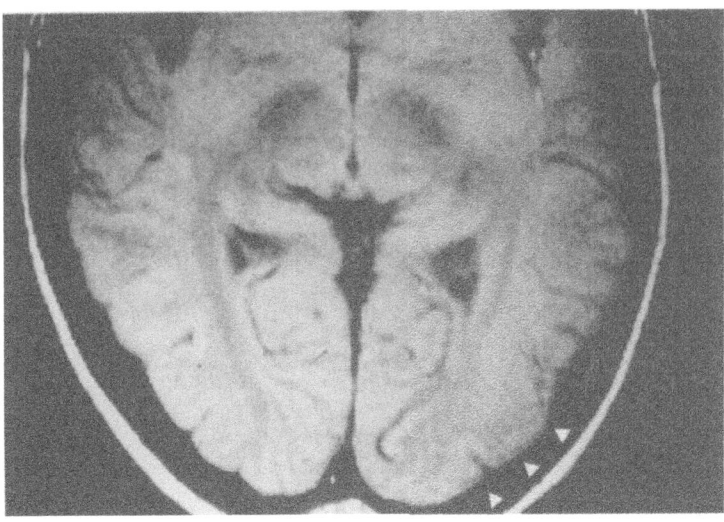

Figure 6. Localised pachygyria. MRI, spin echo, Tl-weighted.

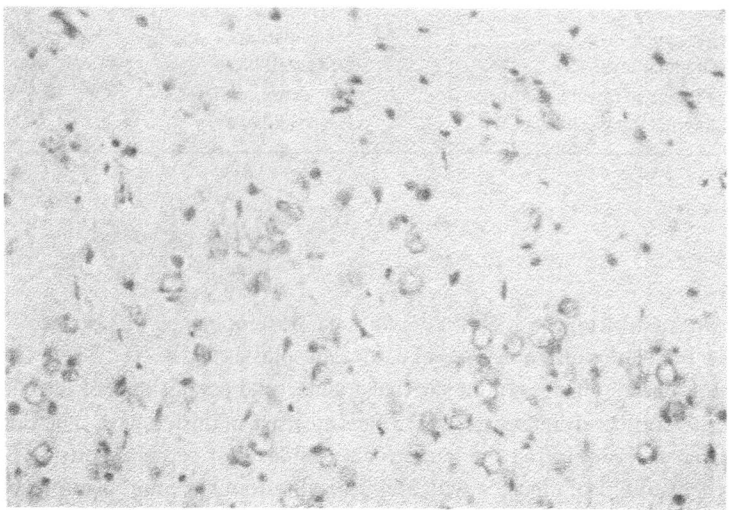

Figure 7. Focal dysplasia of the cerebral cortex. Formalin fixed, paraffin.

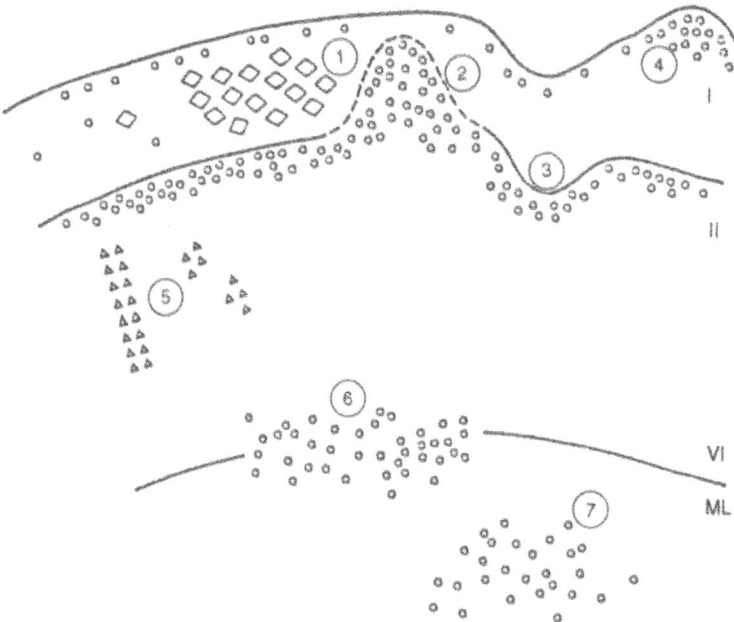

Figure 8. Variation of microdysgenesis. (1) Diffuse or focal increase of dystopic neurons; (2) protrusions of nerve cells; (3) pits and hollows; (4) subpial groups of nerve cells; (5) architechtural disturbances of deeper cortical layers; (6) diffuse border zones; and (7) dystopic nerve cells in the white matter.

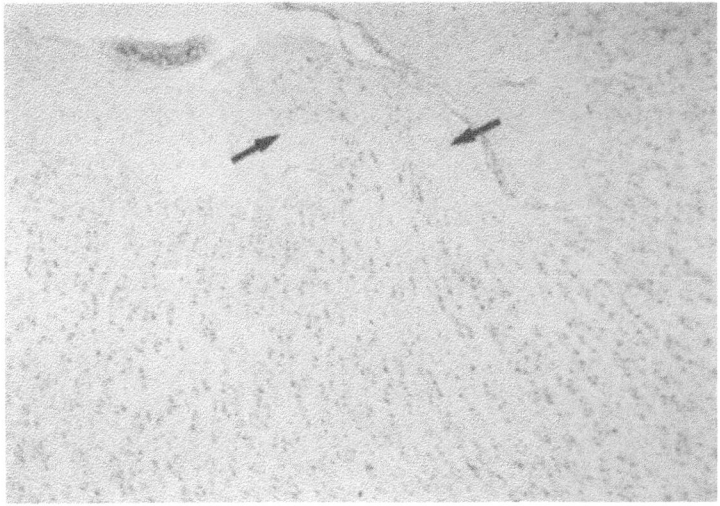

Figure 9. Large localised protrusion of neurons. Paraffin, Nissl.

neuron heterotopias (Figure 10). Other cases showed clustering of neurons found, for example, in secondary generalised epilepsies such as West syndrome (Meencke and Gerhard, 1985) as well as in temporal lobe epilepsies (Figure 11).

In primary generalised epilepsies we have diffuse dystopic neurons in the stratum moleculare (Figure 12) and also in the subcortical white matter (Figure 13).

These findings of minimal migration disturbances with no macroscopic correlation are a challenge to MRI technology.

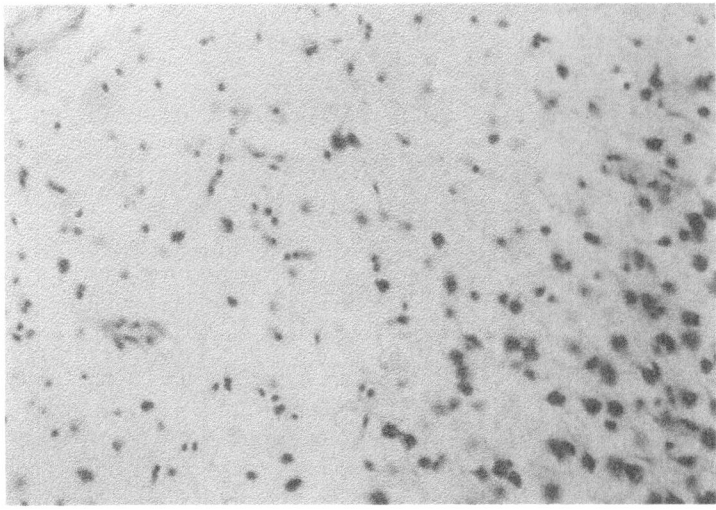

Figure 10. Slight single neuron heterotopias. Paraffin, Nissl.

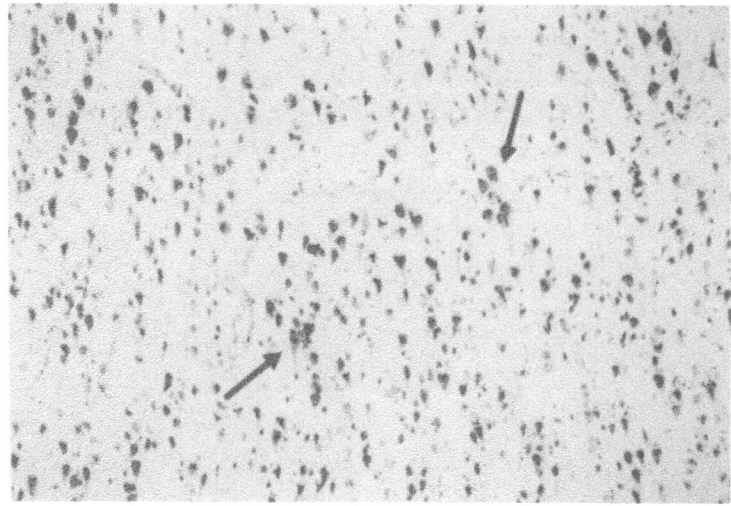

Figure 11. Clustering of intracortical neurons. Paraffin, Nissl.

DISCUSSION

It seems unlikely, in the near future, that these slight developmental disturbances can be visualised, with current restrictions on image resolution. The question arises of whether other indirect parameters, that are related to these minimal developmental disturbances, could be demonstrated more easily.

Four aspects seem to be important: (1) thickness of the cortex; (2) density of the cortex; (3) pattern of gyration; (4) larger dystopic masses: (a) within the cortex; and (b) outside the cortex.

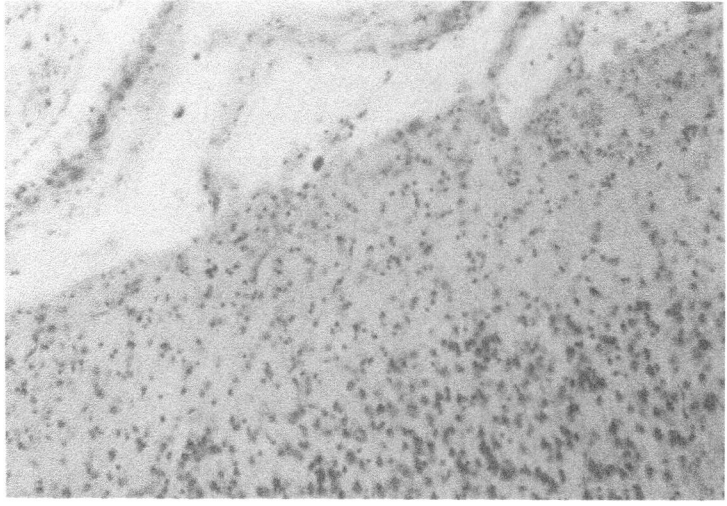

Figure 12. Diffuse dystopic neurons in the stratum moleculare. Celloidin, Nissl.

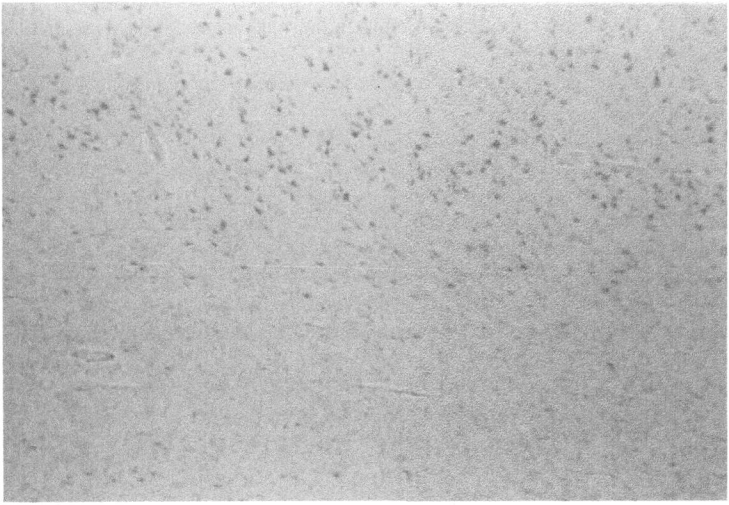

Figure 13. Dystopic neurons in the subcortical white matter. Paraffin, Nissl.

Even for these aspects, the image resolution is critical. Extremely thin (less than 1 mm) slices are required to allow high-resolution analysis of cortical areas, and of the cortex and white matter junction.

Pathological specimens demonstrated that the thickness of the cortex can be changed in cases with more prominent microdysgenesis with secondary generalised or focal epilepsies (Meencke and Janz, 1984; Meencke, 1985a).

In contrast, pathological examinations of patients with primary generalised epilepsies show no alteration of cortical thickness, compared with non-epileptic controls (Meencke, 1983). The high-resolution scanning will also allow better delineation of grey and white matter and the grey–white matter transition, changes that have been demonstrated in pathological specimens (Meencke, 1983).

Slight changes in neuron density could result in changes of the density in cortex imaging, which could possibly be identified by high-resolution scanning. Difficulties in the aetiological differentiation may arise, because ischaemic changes also result in similar pathological relaxation times.

Changes in gyration pattern are easily visible in patients with the more severe changes of pachygyria and microgyria. Even extremely localised changes could be demonstrated if imaging is made done using sections. Slight changes in the gyration pattern might be identified by fractal analysis.

Larger dystopic neuronal masses outside the cortex are easily visible with MRI imaging. Dystopic masses within the cortex, like the focal protrusions of whole cortical laminae (see Figure 9), are likely to be demonstrated using thin sections. So far the demonstration of single dystopic neurons or swarms of single dystopic neurons (see Figure 10), cortical and subcortical, are limited.

In general, MRI is an adequate technique to demonstrate the large variety of migration disturbances. Nevertheless, the minimal developmental disturbances are still a real challenge for this method.

REFERENCES

Meencke, H.J., 1983, The density of dystopic neurons in the white matter of the gyrus frontalis inferior in epilepsies, J Neurol. 230: 171–181.

Meencke, H.J., 1985a, Neuron density in the molecular layer of the frontal cortex in primary generalised epilepsy, Epilepsia, 26: 450–454.

Meencke, H.J., 1985b, Pathology of childhood epilepsies, Clev J Med. 56: 111–120.

Meencke, H.J., and Janz, D., 1984, Neuropathological findings in primary generalised epilepsies: a study of eight cases, Epilepsia 25: 8–21.

Meencke, H.J., and Gerhard, C., 1985, Morphological aspects of aetiology and the course of infantile spasms (West Syndrome), Neuropediatrics 16: 59–66.

Meencke, H.J., and Veith, G., 1992, Migration disturbances in epilepsy, Epilepsy Res. (suppl 9): 31–40.

Morel, F., and Wilde, E., 1952, Dysgenesie nodulaire dissemine de l'encorce frontale, Rev Neurol. 87: 251–270.

Ranke, O., 1910, Beitrege zur Kenntnis der normalen und pathologischen Hirnrindenbildung, Beitr Pathol Anat., 471: 51–125.

Taylor. D.C., Falconer, M.A., Bruton, C.J., and Corsellis, J.A.N., 1971, Focal dysplasia of the cerebral cortex in epilepsy, J Neurol Neurosurg Psychiat. 34: 369–387.

Section 4

Correlation of Imaging with Other Investigative Modalities

CORRELATION OF MRI AND EEG

S.S. Spencer and D.D. Spencer

Yale University School of Medicine
New Haven, Connecticut 06510

INTRODUCTION

Space-occupying lesions have a high correlation with localization of seizure onset in patients with intractable epilepsy, as judged by cessation of seizures after their removal (Rich et al., 1985; Spencer et al., 1984). Atrophy on MRI may also be considered a criterion of the site of seizure onset (Spencer et al., 1991; Spencer, 1993). Some recent studies have used MRI quantitative methods to assess atrophy in temporal lobe (Jack et al., 1990; Lencz et al., 1992). These show nearly 100% specificity and sensitivity of quantitative MRI demonstration of hippocampal atrophy in the prediction of mesial temporal sclerosis, a pathological finding associated with excellent seizure control after temporal lobectomy (Berkovic et al., 1991; Cascino et al., 1991, 1992) and therefore implying medial temporal lobe seizure onset. Despite these observations, however, most investigations have failed to prove a high correlation between MRI and EEG localisation of epileptiform abnormalities (Boon et al., 1991; Dowd et al., 1991), at least in other cerebral regions.

The highly predictive value of MRI in the above studies was derived from retrospective analysis of rigorously selected patients who already carried a diagnosis of temporal lobe epilepsy and subsequently underwent surgery (Berkovic et al., 1991; Cascino et al., 1991, 1992). A recent study suggests that hippocampal atrophy is not a specific sign of temporal lobe epilepsy. In a review of 31 MRI scans with qualitative evidence of hippocampal atrophy, 3 of the patients never had seizures, 4 had complex partial seizures, 2 focal motor seizures and 12 had various types of generalised seizures only (Diaz-Arrastia et al., 1992). Not all studies have quantified MRI, and most EEG data were obtained from surface recording. These methodological irregularities prevent adequate conclusions about the correlation of MRI and EEG.

We sought to clarify the relationship between MRI and EEG, at least in the temporal lobe, by defining the sensitivity and specificity of quantitative hippocampal measurements done by MRI in predicting electrophysiological evidence for medial temporal lobe seizure localisation, in a group of refractory epileptic patients without space-occupying lesions who were studied with intracranial EEG. This approach allows use of more sensitive MRI and EEG techniques than used in the previous studies which found poor correlation between MRI and EEG, while

Magnetic Resonance Scanning and Epilepsy, Edited by S.D. Shorvon et al.,
Plenum Press, New York, 1994

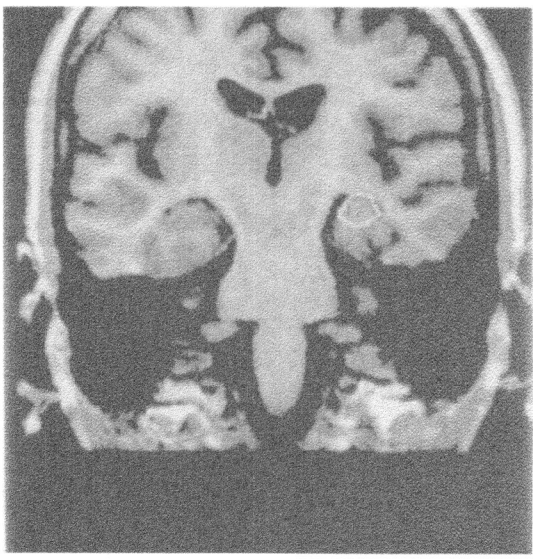

Figure 1. MRI with a qualitative and quantitative evidence of marked left hippocampal atrophy.

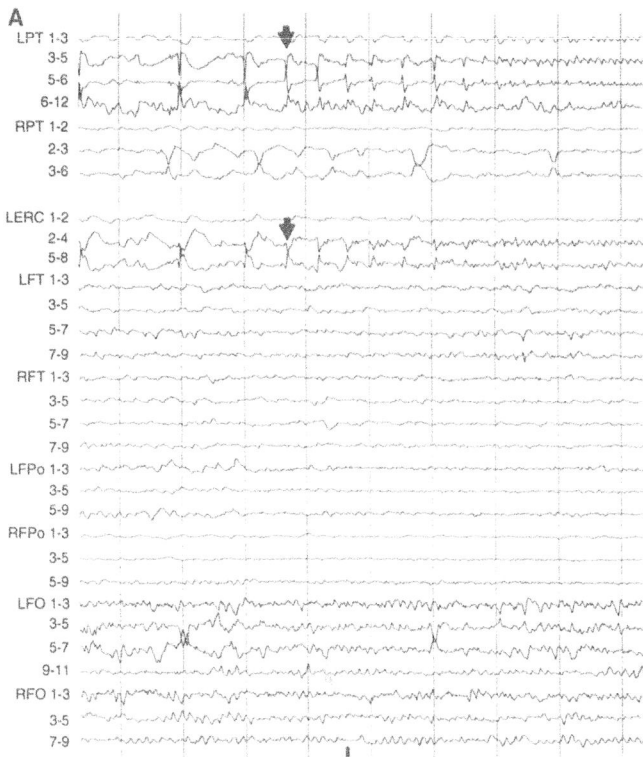

Figure 2. Spontaneous seizure recorded shows left medial temporal onset in hippocampal depth electrode (LPT) contacts 3–5 and 5–6 (arrows), and entorhinal depth electrode (LERC) contacts 2–4 and 5–8 (arrows), corresponding to marked left medial temporal atrophy by quantitative MRI in same patient. EEGs pictured in A, B, and C are continuous 10 second epochs, full scale = 750 μV.

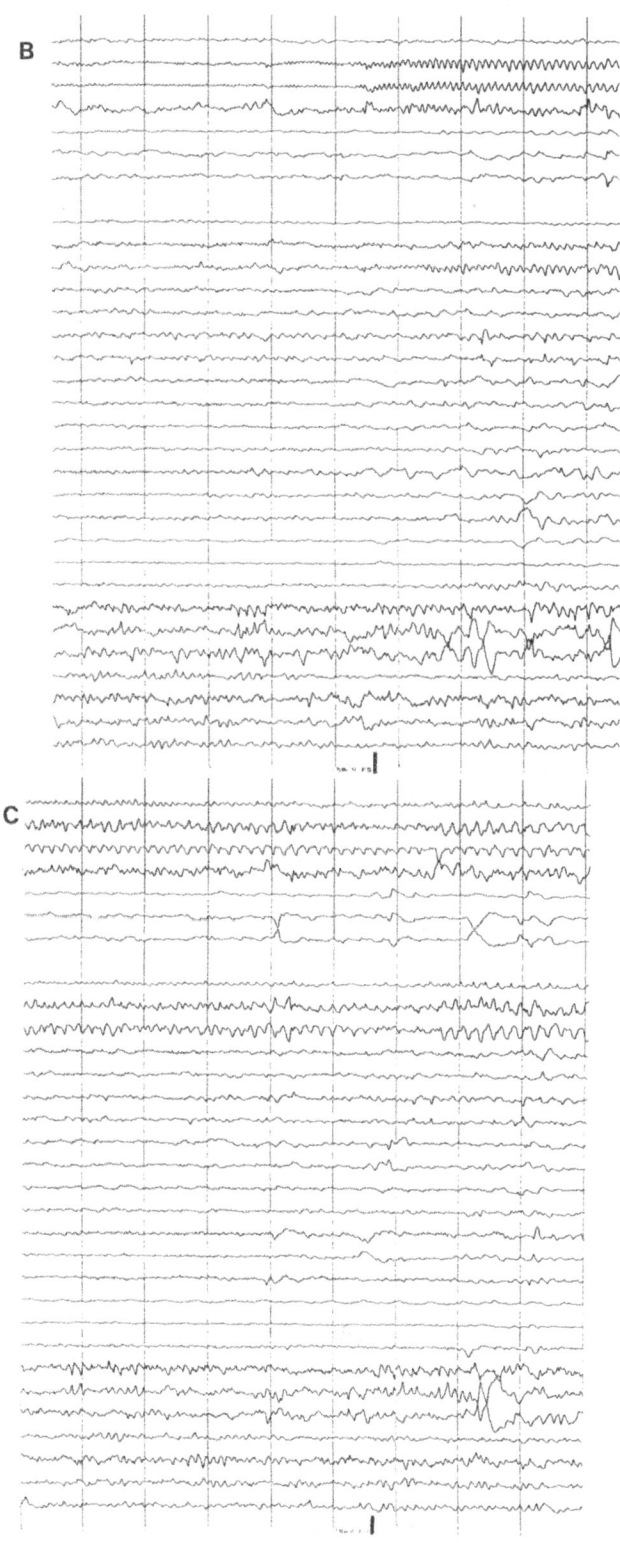

including a more heterogeneous population than the studies that found MRI to be consistently predictive of mesial temporal sclerosis.

CURRENT RESEARCH

All patients who underwent intracranial EEG study at our institution between late 1987 and 1991, and who had pre-operative MRI with quantitative measurement of hippocampal volumes, were included. Hippocampal symmetry was expressed as a dimensionless ratio of left and right measures $(L - R)/(L + R)$. Localising and demographic information were collected and analysed with respect to one another and to hippocampal measurements.

Of 56 patients who fulfilled the criteria for inclusion, 32 had hippocampal volumetric ratios felt to indicate significant unilateral hippocampal atrophy (> 2 standard deviations from normal controls) (Figure 1). Of these 32 patients, 21 had unilateral hippocampal seizure onset concordant with the side of the atrophy (Figure 2), 2 had hippocampal seizure onset contralateral to the side of atrophy and 2 had bilateral independent hippocampal seizure onset. The remaining 7 patients had extrahippocampal seizure onset (as did 14 others without hippocampal atrophy). Of 29 patients who had pure unilateral hippocampal seizure onset recorded by depth electrodes, 21 had concordant unilateral hippocampal atrophy whereas 2 had contralateral atrophy and 6 had none. Those patients with hippocampal seizure onset and hippocampal atrophy had significantly longer duration of epilepsy than those who had hippocampal seizure onset but no atrophy ($t = 3.02$, $p < 0.01$). Our method of expressing hippocampal atrophy was predictably insensitive to bilateral atrophy: in six patients with bilateral independent hippocampal seizure onset, four had hippocampal measurements not distinguishable from control values.

Analyses of the correlation of MRI determined hippocampal volume and scalp ictal EEG as well as inter-ictal scalp or depth-recorded spikes showed lower sensitivity and specificity of these EEG parameters to temporal lobe abnormalities, with values ranging from 41% to 59%. (See Table 1.)

DISCUSSION

Hippocampal atrophy established quantitatively by MRI was highly specific (66%) but not unique to patients with medial temporal lobe seizure onset as recorded by depth electrodes. Sensitivity of quantitative hippocampal MRI analysis to hippocampal seizure onset was also quite high (72%). These observations suggest that, at least in medial temporal lobe, MRI and EEG are better correlated than previously reported. The differences are probably due to our use of more uniformly sensitive measures of atrophy (quantitative MRI) and of electrographic

Table 1. Sensitivity and Specificity of MRI-Based Quantitative Hippocampal Atrophy for Temporal Lobe EEG Findings (by Various Methods)

EEG findings and methods	Sensitivity	Specificity
	(of MR based hippocampal atrophy)	
Scalp inter-ictal, predominantly unilateral temporal spikes	57%	41%
Scalp ictal, unilateral temporal seizure discharge	57%	53%
Intracranial interictal, predominantly unilateral medial temporal spikes	59%	47%
Intracranial ictal, unilateral medial temporal seizure onset	72%	66%

localisation (intracranial EEG). They also support the recently reported sensitivity and specificity of MRI hippocampal atrophy in predicting mesial temporal sclerosis, the underlying pathological diagnosis in most of these patients.

Hippocampal atrophy was much less sensitive or specific for temporal lobe electrographic localisation obtained by scalp ictal EEG or inter-ictal scalp or intracranial recordings; the reduced sensitivity of those EEG techniques themselves as evidence of focal epileptogenicity may be the primary reason for this observation. These results (for scalp and inter-ictal EEG) are predictably more consistent with previous studies showing poorer correlation of MRI and EEG localisation, because those studies also relied on scalp-recorded EEG (Boon et al., 1991; Dowd et al., 1991). Thus, Boon et al. found that EEG localisation of seizure onset was to the site of the lesion in only 23%, and to the side of the lesion in 56% of patients (Boon et al., 1991).

Quantitation of hippocampal atrophy by MRI is neither a completely specific nor a completely sensitive method for the diagnosis of epilepsy of medial temporal lobe origin. The technique is thus only one of many studies that should be used to localise the zone of epileptogenicity. Nevertheless, it offers a highly effective, non-invasive, localising criterion with a very substantial yield and accuracy for defining the epileptogenic zone. Further improvements in defining zones to be measured, normal values and absolute control volumes will probably improve the yield even more in the future.

Definition of significant absolute volumetric deviations from normal for medial temporal and other cerebral regions, including temporal neocortex, may enable further EEG/MRI correlations with improved predictive value for localisation. The application of signal changes to prediction of EEG localisation is also an area that is likely to be elucidated.

REFERENCES

Berkovic, S.F., Andermann, F., Olivier, A., et al.,, 1991, Hippocampal sclerosis in temporal lobe epilepsy demonstrated by magnetic resonance imaging, Ann Neurol. 29: 175–182.

Boon, P.A., Williamson, P.D., Fried, I., et al.,, 1991, Intracranial, intraaxial, space occupying lesions in patients with intractable partial seizures: An anatomo-clinical, neurophysiological and surgical correlation, Epilepsia 32: 467–476.

Cascino, G.D., Jack, C.R., Parisi, J.E., et al.,, 1991, Magnetic resonance imaging-based volume studies in temporal lobe epilepsy; pathological correlations, Ann Neurol. 30: 31–36.

Cascino, G.D., Jack, C.R., Parisi, J.E., et al., 1992, MRI in the presurgical evaluation of patients with frontal lobe epilepsy and children with temporal lobe epilepsy: pathologic correlation and prognostic importance, Epilepsy Res. 11: 51–59.

Diaz-Arrastia, R., Resor, S. and Silver, J., 1992, Clinical and electroencephalographic correlates of mesial temporal sclerosis (MTS) identified by magnetic resonance imaging, Neurology 42 (suppl 3): 206.

Dowd, C.F., Dillon, W.P., Barbaro, N.M., and Laxer, K.D., 1991, Magnetic resonance imaging of intractable complex partial seizures: pathologic and electroencephalographic correlation, Epilepsia 32: 454–459.

Jack, C.R., Jr., Sharbrough, F.W., Twomey, C.K., et al., 1990, Temporal lobe seizures: Lateralization with MR volume measurements of the hippocampal formation. Radiology 175: 423–429.

Lencz, T., McCarthy, G., Bronen, R., et al.,, 1992, Quantitative MRI of the hippocampus in temporal lobe epilepsy, Ann Neurol. 31: 629–637.

Rich, K.M., Goldring, S., and Gado, M., 1985, Computed tomography in chronic seizure disorder caused by glioma, Arch Neurol. 42: 26–7.

Spencer, D.D., Spencer, S.S., Williamson, P.D., and Mattson, R.H., 1984, Intracerebral masses in patients with refractory partial epilepsy, Neurology 34: 432–436.

Spencer, D.D., Spencer, S.S., and Fried, I., 1991, Presurgical localisation: Neurophysiological and neuroimaging studies, in: "Neurosurgical Aspects of Epilepsy," M. Apuzzo, ed., American Association of Neurological Surgeons, Park Ridge, 73–86.

Spencer, S.S., 1993, Temporal lobectomy: Selection of candidates, in: Wyllie, E., ed. "The Treatment of Epilepsy: Principles and Practice," E. Wyllie, ed., Lea and Febiger, Malvern, pp. 1062–1074.

PRINCIPLES OF STEREOTAXY APPLIED TO MRI AND EEG

L. Lemieux

Institute of Neurology
Queen Square
London, WC1N 3BG
United Kingdom

INTRODUCTION

Stereotaxy consists of techniques for the accurate localisation of structures within the body based on external means. From the early work of Bancaud to modern imaging-based techniques, stereotaxy has played an important role in functional neurosurgery, particularly for the implantation of depth electrodes. Whereas 'CT stereotaxy' has been based on the analysis of single slices, recent advances in computing have made possible the analysis and visualisation of entire volume data sets, as well as the development of new techniques for the correlation of data from various modalities (Levesque et al., 1990; Lemieux et al., 1992; Peters et al., 1992a).

Although the principles of CT stereotaxy can be applied to MRI, in general, the accuracy of MRI based stereotaxy is inferior due to field inhomogeneities, as demonstrated by phantom studies (Schad et al., 1987; Peters et al., 1992b). Accurate anatomical information contained in high-quality MRI data is playing an increasingly important role in the interpretation of electrophysiological data. Recent progress in imaging has also allowed the development of increasingly accurate head models for the purpose of EEG modelling (Meijs et al., 1988; Gevins et al., 1990); this also requires the accurate localisation of the electrodes relative to the anatomical structures underlying the electrical activity.

CURRENT RESEARCH

We have developed a computer program for stereotactic surgery planning, called TACT, which contains a special tool for depth electrode implantation (Figure 1), as well as other tools for the accurate registration of multimodality image data. A number of methods for the registration and visualisation of volume data, based both on conventional frames (such as in TACT) and frameless technology, are based on the determination of a single transformation matrix, called the volume transformation matrix (VTM). This transformation maps an entire

Magnetic Resonance Scanning and Epilepsy, Edited by S.D. Shorvon et al.,
Plenum Press, New York, 1994

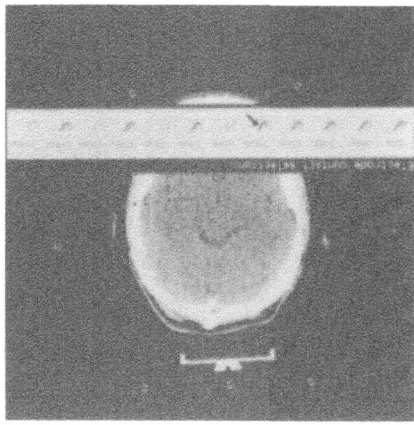

Figure 1. TACT's depth electrode implantation tool.

tomographic volume onto an external reference space. As illustrated in Figure 2, this can result in a certain loss of accuracy compared to conventional stereotaxy (Lemieux and Wootton, 1992). TACT also enables the comparison of post electrode implantation stereotactic radiographs and MRI, which can be used to assess the accuracy of MRI-based stereotaxy in human subjects (Figure 3). We are also currently developing a method for the accurate registration of tomographic data and radiography based on volume rendering (Figure 4).

DISCUSSION

Sophisticated image analysis techniques are providing new means of correlating image data from various modalities. The required level of registration accuracy depends on the type of application, for example, the correlation of electrode positions with image data for EEG modelling, it is reasonable to assume that the effect of (random) electrode localisation errors is relatively small for scalp measurements, due to the low fields involved (Stok, 1987). However, this may not be the case for intracranial measurements, where the generator may be located near the electrodes, and therefore requires anatomically accurate localisation of the

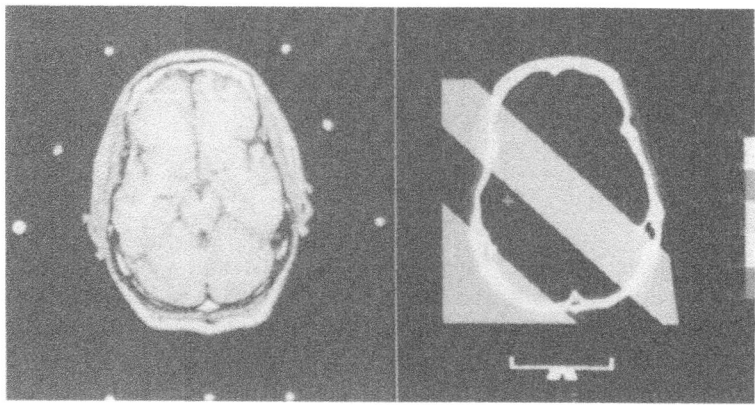

Figure 2. Stereotactic registration of CT and MRI using TACT, with VTM-related localisation error represented as superimposed colour map.

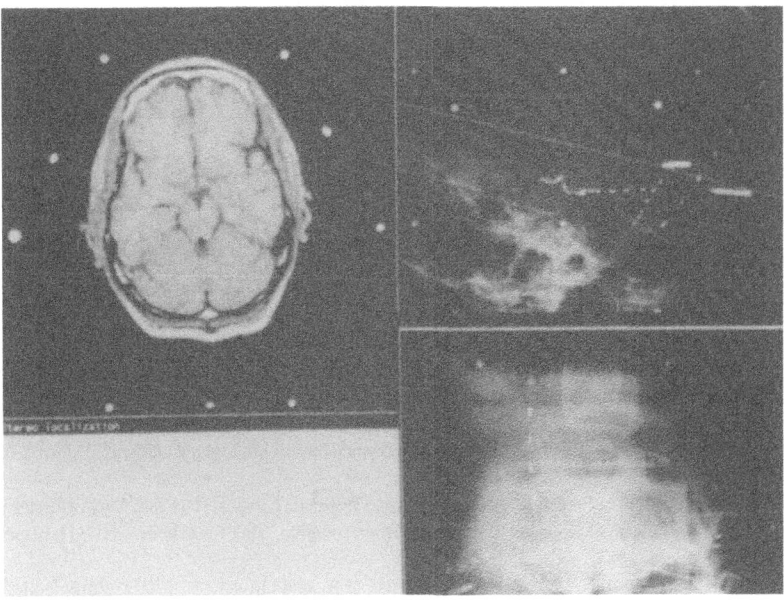

Figure 3. Localisation of intracranial electrodes from a pair of radiographs, and correlation with MRI.

electrodes. Although this can be achieved using the frame-based methods described above, a more flexible and potentially more accurate approach may be based on high quality visualisation of the anatomy combined with new image correlation methods.

PROBABLE DEVELOPMENT OVER THE NEXT FIVE YEARS

Stereotaxy is currently being redefined and is probably going to enter a phase of expansion into new fields of application. In parallel to this, better image acquisition and new analysis

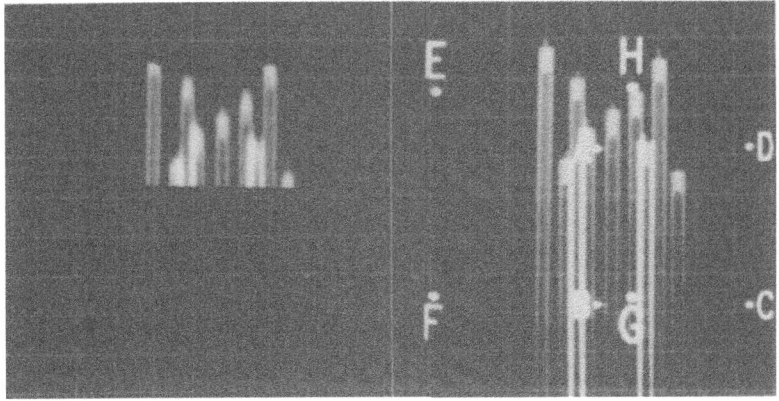

Figure 4. Registration of CT and radiographs of skull phantom based on a non-linear least-squares routine. The routine finds the VTM for which a measure of the similarity of the images is maximum.

techniques will provide more geometrically accurate MR images. The development of three-dimensional image analysis will provide new means of accurately correlating image data from various modalities, as well as with other forms of data. We anticipate that the future of conventional stereotaxy will be decided on the basis of its own record on accuracy as well as the levels of accuracy required for specific surgical procedures.

REFERENCES

Gevins, A., Brickett, P., Costales, B., Le, J., and Reutter, B., 1990, Beyond topographic mapping: functional-anatomical imaging with 124-channel EEGs and three-dimensional MRIs, Brain Topogr. 3: 53–64.

Lemieux, L., Lester, S., and Fish, D., 1992, Multimodality imaging and intracranial EEG display for stereotactic surgery planning in epilepsy, Electroenceph Clinical Neurophysiol. 82: 399–407.

Lemieux, L., and Wootton, R., 1992, The mathematics of stereotactic tomographic image display, in: "Image Directed Surgery of Brain Tumors," D.T. Thomas, ed., Churchill Livingstone, Edinburgh.

Levesque, M.F., Zhang, J., Wilson, C.L., Behnke, E.J., Harper, R.M., Lufkin, R.B., Engel, J., and Crandall, P.H., 1990, Stereotactic investigation of limbic epilepsy using a multimodal image analysis system, J Neurosurg. 73: 792–797.

Meijs, J.W.H., ten Voorde, B.J., Peters, M.J., Stok, C.J., and Lopes da Silva, F.H., 1988, The influence of various head models on EEGs and MEGs, in: "Functional Brain Imaging," G. Pfurtscheller and F.H. Lopes da Silva, ed., Huber, Toronto, 1988.

Peters, T.M., Henri, C.H., Collins, D.L., Lemieux, L., Pike, G.B., and Olivier, A., 1992a, Stereotactic Neurosurgery planning using integrated three-dimensional stereoscopic images, in: "Computers in Stereotactic Neurosurgery," P.J. Kelly and B.A. Kall, ed., Blackwell, Cambridge, MA.

Peters, T.M., Pike, G.B., and Clark, J.A., 1992b, A personal computer-based workstation for the planning of stereotactic neurosurgical procedures, in: "Computers in Stereotactic Neurosurgery," P.J. Kelly and B.A. Kall, eds, Blackwell, Cambridge, MA.

Schad, L., Lott, S., Schmitt, F., Sturm, V., and Lorenz, W.J., 1987, Correction of spatial distortion in MR imaging: a prerequisite for accurate stereotaxy, J Comp Assist Tomogr. 11: 499–505.

Stok, C.J., 1987, The influence of model parameters on EEG/MEG single dipole source estimation, IEEE Trans Biomed. 34: 289–296.

MRI STEREOTACTIC PLACEMENT OF INTRACRANIAL ELECTRODES

D.D. Spencer, G. McCarthy, M.L. Luby, and S.S. Spencer

Yale University School of Medicine
New Haven, Connecticut 06510

INTRODUCTION

Intracranial electrode evaluations in patients with medically intractable epilepsy are meant to define regions of epileptogenesis when this is not possible by non-invasive methods.

At Yale, the only patients who undergo direct resective surgery without invasive study are those with MRI volumetrically measured unilateral hippocampal atrophy or with a space-occupying mass in any cortical location and whose remaining evaluation is concordant with the MRI abnormality (Spencer and Pappas, 1992). If the non-invasive evaluation is not concordant (approximately 50% of our patients), intracranial study is required.

The questions to be asked of these invasive studies is quite individual but falls into the general categories of refining the epileptogenic region in presumptive unilateral temporal lobe epilepsy (TLE) or defining an extratemporal source.

There may also be a need to study the electrical characteristics of an MRI abnormality in relationship to surrounding cortex for the purposes of providing ictal and functional information.

CURRENT RESEARCH

Our present MRI stereotactic system in based on the CORITECH computer workstation which uses a 80486 processor and T134020 high-resolution graphics subsystem. The software was originally developed in 1987 on a micro Vax II used to support the BRW stereotactic frame of Radionics. As the workstation has changed with research and development, it now interfaces with the Radionics CRW and Leksell frames (McCarthy et al., 1991).

The 24 cm field of view (FOV) images are obtained with any of the fixed frame fiducial systems. Recent advances in fast MR provide protocols with spoiled gradient recall (SPGR) acquisition of contiguous 1–3 mm slices at a TR:TE of 24:7. The thin slices allow off-axis computation for fine tuning of trajectory and three-dimensional rendering. The fiducial rods in each image allow a target-centered cartesian system such

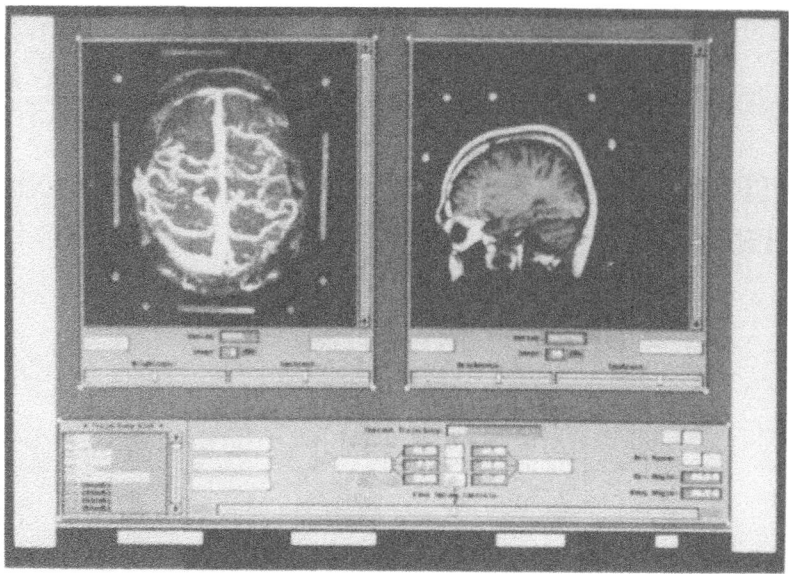

Figure 1. CORITECH workstation screen demonstrating three completed electrode trajectory plans. The right screen is a SPGR sagittal section with the proposed electrode tracts. The left screen is an axial MRA for viewing the superficial venous drainage. Image manipulation bars are noted alongside and beneath each viewing window.

as the Leksell to be used with maximum flexibility for the entire trajectory of an entry-target tract. Magnetic resonance angiography (MRA) in both the arterial and venous sequence is obtained following the SPGR views. Figure 1 shows the operator's display after six electrode paths have been planned. For representation purposes, two windows are displayed here but normally the screen shows one large window and two smaller ones such that all three axes can be viewed simultaneously. Images are stored in memory and clicking on the bar beside each picture allows the operator to drag quickly through the entire sequence. Images can be exchanged quickly and an electrode trajectory is created by simply clicking onto the entry and target point in any image. The horizontal bar at the base of the screen allows one to select the entry or the target and move the entire projected trajectory horizontally, vertically or laterally.

A typical hippocampal electrode placement is illustrated in Figures 2 and 3. Figure 2 demonstrates that the first step is to click on a target and entry point in the sagittal plane. The MRA is displayed in the second window such that any vessels in the proposed path are quickly identified. The operator moves to the coronals (Figure 3) and adjusts the electrode path such that it traverses the lateral third of the hippocampal formation. The MRA is again viewed simultaneously. The axial cuts are then brought up such that the electrode passage can be adjusted for the midbrain. The axial cuts are then thoroughly scrutinized for entry point surface veins and sulci through which the electrode may be passing. The MRA is rechecked in each axis and this pattern is repeated for each electrode.

For subdural electrode positioning, the entry and target points are noted and the curvilinear distance between is measured.

The following day, an MRI is obtained to verify electrode placement.

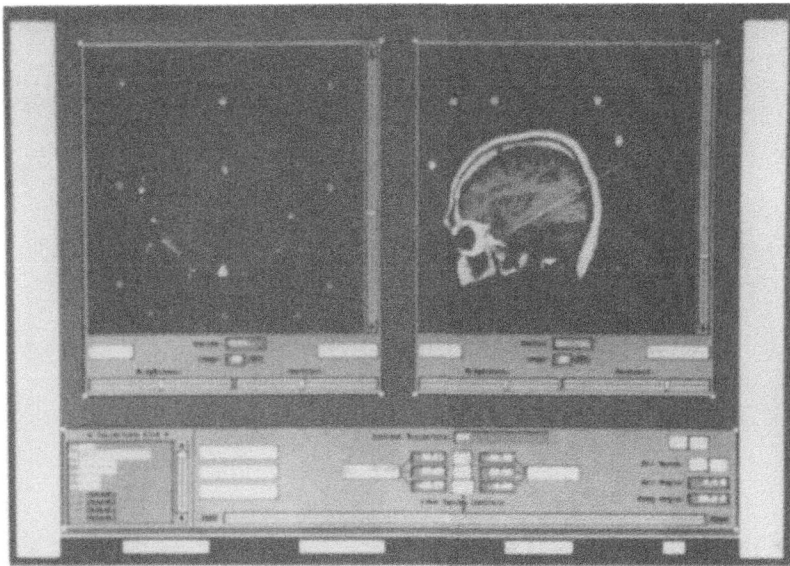

Figure 2. Electrode trajectory planning for the temporal lobe begins with identifying a target and entry point on a T1 sagittal cut through the hippocampus (right viewing window). The left viewing window demonstrates the MRA venous system at the entry point.

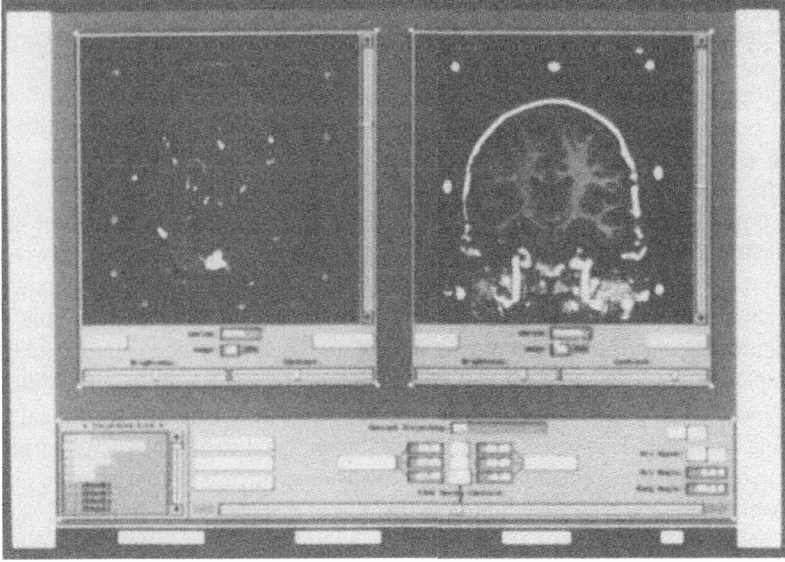

Figure 3. The next step in designing temporal lobe electrode trajectories is to bring up the coronal image set and adjust the electrode (right viewing window) to the lateral 1/3 of the hippocampus, avoiding the choroid plexus and sulci. The left viewing window illustrates the trajectory in relationship to the MRA reconstructed posterior cerebral artery.

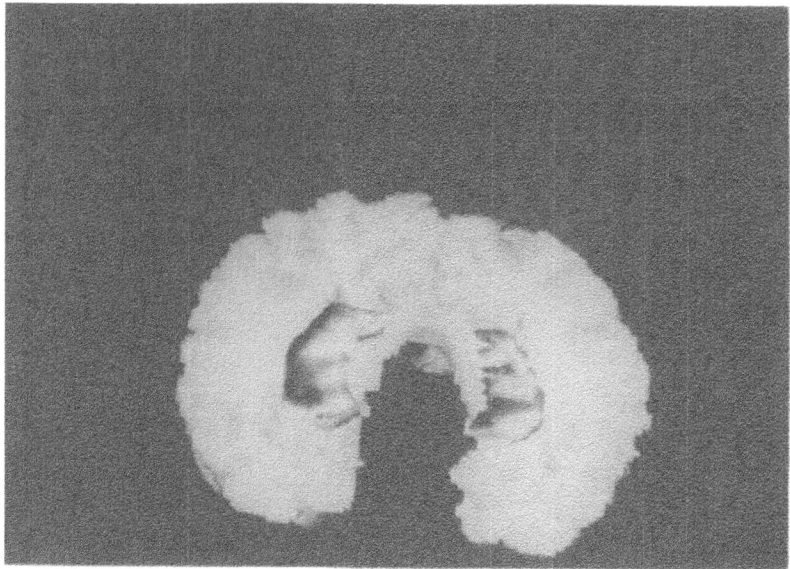

Figure 4. A Theraview volume reconstructed axial image paralleling the hippocampi. Note the left hippocampus is much smaller than the right. This volume difference can be easily quantitated.

DISCUSSION

The major changes in MRI stereotaxy in the past five years relate to fast MR sequences, MRA and speedier computer programs that allow multiple electrode trajectories to be created, reviewed and modified for cortical and vascular anatomy. Although not discussed in detail here, electrode contact material and shape has undergone revision to provide more accurate post placement data with less paramagnetic distortion.

FUTURE DEVELOPMENTS

Three major developments in MRI stereotaxy are immediately foreseeable; the use of three-dimensional anatomical reconstruction in trajectory planning and review; coupling contour cortical MRI maps for subdural strip and grid localisation; and the juxtaposition of three-dimensional volumes, contour mapping, and functional imaging. For example, Figure 4 is a three-dimensional volumetric representation of the hippocampi of a patient with unilateral hippocampal atrophy. The program for this modelling is performed on a Hewlett-Packard three-dimensional graphics workstation provided by Theraview, a three-dimensional biomedical imaging company. This workstation provides multiplanar two-dimensional reformations, contouring by edge discrimination for three-dimensional surface reconstruction and three-dimensional volumetric reconstruction. The first use of this program will be accurate surface contour rendering co-registered with post grid placement MRI images. Three-dimensional maps of ictal localisation, inter-ictal fields, evoked potentials, and functional localisation will be used for resective surgical strategies. This same three-dimensional program can be used to quantify volumetrics and to co-register with other dynamic imaging such as PET and SPECT. Ultimately, echo planar MR may be directly available in this three-dimensional format allowing the investigator to visualise motor, sensory, language and memory facets without invasive stimulation. The use of echo planar MR in this regard is the next quantum leap in revolutionising our understanding of normal brain function, its perturbation by disease, and our design of safer and more reliable medical and surgical therapies.

REFERENCES

McCarthy, G., Spencer, D.D., and Riker, R.J., 1991, The stereotaxic placement of depth electrodes in epilepsy, in: "Epilepsy Surgery," Luders, H., ed., Raven Press, New York.

Spencer, D.D., and Pappas, C.T.E., 1992, Surgical decisions regarding medically intractable epilepsy, in: "Clinical Neurosurgery," vol. 38, Selman, W., ed., Williams and Wilkins, Baltimore.

FRAMELESS STEREOTAXY

Technical Aspects

T.M. Peters, A.C. Evans, and A. Olivier

Montreal Neurological Institute
McGill University
Montreal, Quebec
Canada

INTRODUCTION

Until recently, stereotactic surgery has required that a stereotactic frame be fixed to the head of the patient during both imaging and surgery (Peters et al., 1989). However, with the stereotactic frame fixed to the patient in this manner, access to the surgical site is limited by the geometry of the frame, and some approaches are not possible. Removal of the frame from the operating room gives the operator complete freedom in the planning of the procedure. In addition, procedures that previously were performed using conventional techniques may take advantage of image guidance techniques developed for stereotaxy. The advent of sophisticated computer techniques has hastened the development of image-guided approaches to complement the surgical procedure (Kelly and Kall, 1992).

CURRENT RESEARCH

The objective of our work is to establish an environment that will remove the need for a stereotactic frame while preserving existing stereotactic functionality. Central to the project is the integration of the numerous stereotactic imaging modalities currently in use at our institute into a flexible imaging workstation that can be readily employed in the operating room by the surgical team. For a project such as this to be successful, and its fruits accepted by its eventual users, the user interface to the computer system is of utmost importance. Particular emphasis is being placed on the development of an intuitive system that enables the operator to manipulate the image as naturally as he would measure and dissect an anatomical specimen. We seek the following goals: (1) to establish and validate the methodology for frameless stereotaxy, using skin-mounted fiducial markers that are compatible with CT, MRI, digital subtraction argiography (DSA) and positron emission tomography (PET) as well as to investigate the use of natural surface anatomical landmarks for image correlation purposes; (2)

Magnetic Resonance Scanning and Epilepsy, Edited by S.D. Shorvon et al.,
Plenum Press, New York, 1994

to evaluate the use of computer-linked surgical-probe technology with existing surgery planning systems to determine its utility intra-operative use; (3) to integrate this methodology with multi-modality stereoscopic imaging (Henri et al., 1991); and (4) to integrate global and local volume-of-interest atlas information and segmented/classified MR datasets with the three-dimensional image volumes. Concurrent with the development of applications specific to frameless stereotaxy we are employing the ISG Allegro/Wand (ISG Technologies Inc., Mississauga, Canada) combination in the laboratory and operating room environment as an aid in both stereotactic and non-stereotactic surgery procedures. Such use is enabling us to evaluate the ultimate potential of three-dimensional interactive imaging workstations in the operating room, and is assisting us in specifying the functionality for future systems. The experience to date of the use of the prototype system in the operating room is the topic of Chapter 35.

INTERACTIVE SURGICAL PROBE

One of the critical elements in an intra-operative image-guided surgical system is the surgical probe. We are in the process of integrating such a rigid mechanical probe into our existing surgery planning systems to determine the accuracy with which landmarks on the patient surface may be correlated with the same points within three-dimensional image data sets. This methodology will then be integrated into the stereoscopic three-dimensional surgical workstation under development. The surgical probe is a critical component of this system because it provides the definitive link between the patient and the computer planning system. We have chosen a mechanical system consisting of articulated arms anchored to a base that is rigidly clamped to the patient head-clamp during surgery. The choice of the mechanical system was made on the basis of reliability and robustness. Other systems exist that use ultrasound (Reinhardt and Zweifel 1990), magnetic fields (Kato et al 1989, Pelizzari et al 1991) and optical tracking devices. The accuracy of ultrasonography and optical systems may be compromised when objects in the operating room interfere with the line of sight between transducers, whereas the magnetically operated systems are inaccurate in the presence of ferromagnetic objects, which are common in an operating room environment. Although these systems provide a greater degree of flexibility and manoeuvrability than mechanical devices, it is of utmost importance in a surgical situation that measurement accuracy be maintained at all times.

As the probe assembly is rigidly clamped to the head restraint, it provides a fixed reference with respect to the patient's skull, which is itself firmly immobilised (whether or not a stereotactic frame is being used in the procedure).

STEREOSCOPIC DISPLAY

We consider that an important feature of our proposed workstation will be its ability to display three-dimensional image information to the observer in a truly three-dimensional manner through the use of stereoscopy. Stereoscopic radiography has been used routinely for the past 50 years at the Montreal Neurological Institute. In the past 6 years it has also been adapted to a neurosurgical workstation, as well as digital fluoroscopy and angiography. The experience gained recently relating to the use of stereoscopic images in a clinical environment has been invaluable in designing the system that will be employed with the integrated surgical workstation that is currently under development.

There are two principal methods of displaying stereoscopic information to an observer via a TV screen. We have found that the approach using an active polarising shutter placed in front of the TV monitor, in conjunction with lightweight polarised glasses, has a high degree

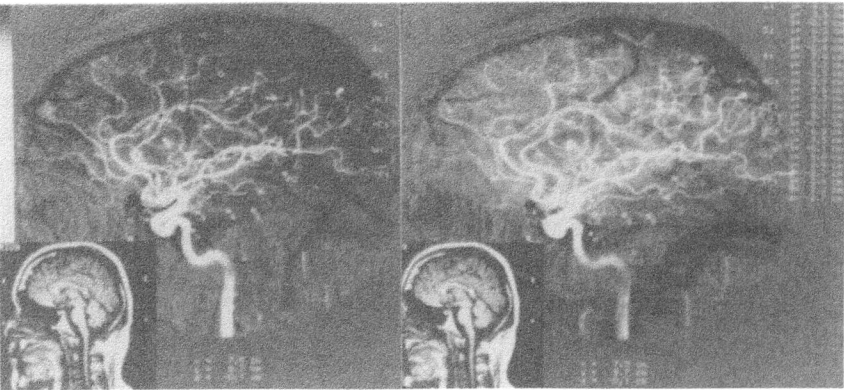

Figure 1. Stereoscopic DSA images with the positions of planned implanted depth electrodes shown within the volume. The three-dimensional cursor that is placed within vascular volume is reflected in the adjacent MR image. The image pair may be viewed stereoscopically using a crossed-eye technique.

of user acceptance. The alternative method employs electrically controlled shutters built into lightweight glasses worn by the observer, with no requirement for additional filters in front of the monitor screen. This system has increased its user acceptance recently as the weight of the active glasses has been reduced.

We have used a stereotactic image analysis workstation equipped with such a stereoscopic display during the surgical planning process routinely over the past 6 years, both during pre-surgical planning and during the operative procedure itself. The most common application of the system was to correlate the positions of cerebral vessels with MR or CT-based anatomy, during the implantation of depth electrodes used to localise seizure foci. A typical example of the use of stereoscopic images in this situation is shown in Figure 1, where the objective is to place multiple recording electrodes deep within the brain, while avoiding the intracerebral vessels. An added advantage of this approach is that the cortex of the brain, as defined by the cortical vessels, is also well appreciated in three dimensions. Note that the target points are also referenced to a sagittal MR slice from the same patient. Although in this example, the absolute stereotactic coordinates, and correlation with the anatomical image, were calculated on the basis of a stereotactic frame (Henri et al., 1991), these images demonstrate the value to be gained from stereotaxy in the more general situation of frameless stereotaxy, or image-guided neurosurgery.

For the integration of stereoscopic visualisation techniques into a more generalised three-dimensional neurosurgical workstation, there are a number of important issues that must be considered.

- Are there image-processing procedures that can be employed to improve the perception of the image by the observer (Cavanagh, 1987)?
- Is it necessary to include additional stereoscopic cues (perspective boxes etc.) within the image (Barham and McAllister, 1991)?
- What is the optimum nature of the three-dimensional cursor that is used for probing the three-dimensional stereoscopic space?
- What are the consequences of viewing the stereoscopic images with geometries that differ from that for which the reconstructed image was intended (variations in viewing distance, viewing angle etc.)?

Although we have already examined the geometrical aspects of this last question (Henri et al., 1991), we do not yet fully understand the effects of this phenomenon on the interpretation of the image. We have therefore begun to evaluate the qualitative effects of displaying images at sub-optimal geometries, a situation that occurs frequently in practice when the screen is observed by multiple operators, and/or being employed in an operating room where there is no fixed relationship between the screen and the observer. Fortunately, the quantitative aspects of this problem (when, for example, the operator is making measurements from a cursor placed in the stereoscopic volume) are independent of the viewing geometry and perceived image distortion.

PATIENT/IMAGE MATCHING

In the context of neurosurgical planning we employ the ISG Viewing-wand system to assist with image guidance during the surgical procedure. This system provides a hand-held probe that can be manipulated by the surgeon and at the same time be observed on the workstation monitor. To achieve this goal, it is necessary to register a three-dimensional image (derived from a set of CT or MR scans), to the patient surface itself. As the two-dimensional (original tomographic) images are intrinsically linked to the three-dimensional surface-rendered representation of the patient, the latter is employed to effect the registration.

As discussed by Oliver et al. (Chapter 35), the raw data are transformed into a three-dimensional image using ISG's "ALLEGRO" software, prior to being loaded into the "Viewing-wand" system. In order to perform the registration, the user points to easily visible landmarks on the patient's skin surface (tip of nose, corner of eyes, etc.) while simultaneously identifying the same points on the three-dimensional image with a mouse-driven cursor. The registration algorithm internal to the Viewing-wand system computes the best-fit between the two sets of three-dimensional coordinate pairs.

Early in clinical trials of this system it was observed that the correlated-points method was not sufficiently accurate when using normal pre-operative scans, because the visible landmarks used to register were too few and not sufficiently accurate to be delineated by a human observer. Errors of the order of 5 mm or more were common.

To improve these measurements, a second procedure, used to refine the previously calculated transformation, allows the operator to identify a sparse model of a patch of the patient's surface by touching with the probe a number of points randomly spaced over the skin, and sends to the computer at each point the real-world probe position. This then maps out a sparse model of the surface of the skin. Sufficient numbers of points define a shape which is a reasonably accurate description of the patient's surface in the area of interest. The computer then matches this shape to the shape of the three-dimensional surface model which was formerly reconstructed, to obtain a registration transform which is likely to be more accurate.

Accurate matching of the patient surface with the three-dimensional images is not without its problems. Poor scan quality or insufficient scan extent can lead to a poor fit. This is generally visually obvious, as the user can point the probe at known landmarks and touch the skin in several areas, to review the accuracy. Another problem is created by patient movement during the scan and in the operating room. High-quality imaging may be achieved using comfortable head restraints during the scanning procedure, and relative motion between the patient's head and the probe mount may be avoided by mounting it directly on the head clamp rather than the operating table.

We, along with others, have begun performing experiments to assess the accuracy of these systems. Initial experience indicates that it is generally possible to obtain accuracies on a par with stereotactic equipment, and Zinreich at al. (1993) have shown that an accuracy of registration in the order of 2–3 mm can be obtained throughout the volume when the initial data consist of a high-resolution CT data set derived from a high-contrast phantom. We caution that where the data are derived from MRI in a realistic patient situation, we cannot always expect to achieve this kind of accuracy, due to the factors mentioned above.

At present, the device is being employed as an image-guided adjunct to conventional neurosurgical approaches, including frame-based stereotaxy. In this manner we are accumulating the accuracy data to allow us to validate the use of this device for generalised frameless stereotactic neurosurgery. A typical example of the use of this system is demonstrated in Figure 2, where the hand-held probe is shown with respect to the MRA derived vessels seen within a "window" into the three-dimensional brain image.

DISCUSSION

We have found that a three-dimensional workstation coupled with a position sensor (Viewing-wand system) provides a valuable adjunct to neurosurgical procedures, and provides us with a level of accuracy that permits its effective use in image-guided neurosurgery. It has proved to be particularly useful in assessing probe trajectories, establishing lesion margins and determining optimal craniotomy strategies. The major difficulty with the use of such a device is the lack of on-line feedback between the image and the status of the brain at any time during the operation. Although the brain within the skull vault may well correspond with the three-dimensional image immediately prior to the procedure, this is not necessarily the case after a craniotomy or after tissue has been removed from the brain. Further work is required to assess the extent of this effect for the various procedures for which image-guided surgery is used, and where possible, to develop techniques (using ultrasound imaging and/or on-line video methods) to correct, or allow for this phenomenon.

PROBABLE DEVELOPMENTS OVER THE NEXT FIVE YEARS

The concept of image-guided surgery is likely to become a routine reality in all aspects of neurosurgery. Key developments will be (a) faster computer processing and increased interactivity with the image; (b) integration of on-line ultrasonography and video microscope imaging with the procedure (Roberts et al., 1992); (c) and increased accessibility within the

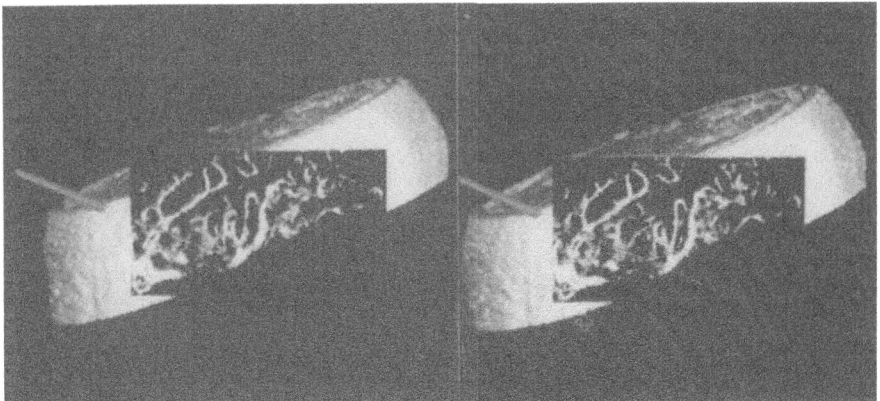

Figure 2. Three-dimensional rendered brain image showing position of probe with respect to the patient surface and internal vessels imaged with MR angiography. This image pair may be viewed stereoscopically using the crossed-eye technique.

three-dimensional imaging environment to multiple modality image information, both ana-tomical and functional. There is evidence that in a slightly longer-term time frame, virtual reality (Fuchs, 1990) may play an important part in operating room-based imaging systems.

REFERENCES

Barham, P.T., and McAllister, D.F., 1991, A comparison of stereoscopic cursors for the interactive manipulation of b-splines, in: "Symposium on electronic imaging and technology, SPIE/IS&T," 96.

Cavanah, P., 1987, Reconstructing the third dimension: interaction between colour, texture, motion, binocular disparity and shape, Comp Vision, Graphics, Image Proc. 37: 171–195.

Fuchs, H., 1990, Systems for display of three-dimensional medical data, in: "Three-dimensional Imaging in Medicine. Algorithms, Systems and Applications," K.H. Hoehner, H. Fuchs, S. Pizer, eds. Nato ASI series F Computers and System Sciences, Vol. 60. pp 315–331.

Henri, C.J., Collins, D.L., and Peters, T.M., 1991, Multi-modality image integration for stereotactic surgical planning, Med Phys. 18: 167–177.

Kato, A., Yoshimine, T., Hayakawa, T., et al., 1991, A frameless, armless navigational system for computer-assisted neurosurgery, J Neurosurg. 74: 845–849.

Kelly, P., and Kall, B., eds, 1992, "Computers in Stereotactic Neurosurgery," Blackwell, Oxford.

Pellizari, C., Chen, G.T.Y., Spelbring, D.R., et al., 1989, Accurate three-dimensional registration of CT, MR and PET images of the brain, J Comp Assist Tomogr. 13: 20–26.

Peters, T.M., Clark, J.A., Pike, G.B., et al., 1989, Stereotactic neurosurgery planning on a PC based workstation, J Digital Imag. 2: 1–7.

Reinhardt, H.F., and Zweifel, H.J., 1990, Interactive sonar-operated device for stereotactic and open surgery, Stereotactic and Functional Neurosurgery 54–55: 393–397.

Roberts, D.W., Pavlidis, J.D., Friets, E.M., et al., 1992, Computer image display during frameless stereotactic surgery, in: "Computers in Stereotactic Neurosurgery," P. Kelly and B. Kall, eds. Blackwell, Oxford, pp. 313–319.

Zinreich, J. et al., 1993, Frameless stereotactic integration of CT imaging data. Accuracy and initial application, Radiology 188: 735–742.

CORRELATION OF MRI AND MEG

K. Abraham-Fuchs,[1] H. Stefan,[2] P. Schueler,[2] J. Uebler,[1] S. Schneider,[1] and G. Naser[1]

[1] Siemens AG Medical Engineering Group
[2] Department of Neurology
University of Erlangen-Nuerenberg
Erlangen
Germany

INTRODUCTION

Biomagnetism provides information on electrophysiological function by three-dimensionally localising sources of electric activity within the human body from the non-invasively measured magnetic field, i.e. from the magnetoencephalogram (MEG).

Depending on the signal-to-noise ratio of the data, a localisation accuracy of a few millimetres can be achieved (Schneider et al., 1990). The 37-channel biomagnetic measurement system KRENIKON® is one of the systems which are installed in a hospital with the aim to explore the clinical potential of the method. The result of biomagnetic source localisation can then be combined with anatomical imaging such as MR or CT, in order to enhance the value for diagnosis and therapy.

For this purpose a common reference system of coordinates for the two instruments has to be established. An example from the evaluation of an inter-ictal epileptic spike is shown in Figure 1. Having established such a common reference system, it is then possible to quantify the correlation of the diagnostic result of MRI and MEG, for example by measuring the distance of the biomagnetically localised epileptogenic area to the border of a lesion.

CURRENT RESEARCH

Most image fusion techniques already known from the attempt to combine MRI, CT, PET and SPECT images (Evans, 1990) are applicable to biomagnetism with only slight modifications. The choice of the method depends on the accepted trade-off between accuracy, patient friendliness and reproducibility in different measurement sessions. The following techniques have been used in the combination of MRI and MEG so far: highest accuracy and reproducibility are achieved with stereotactic frames screwed into the skull, but this is only tolerable if a neurosurgical intervention is planned. A head mould, combined with a conventional Leksell

Magnetic Resonance Scanning and Epilepsy, Edited by S.D. Shorvon et al.,
Plenum Press, New York, 1994

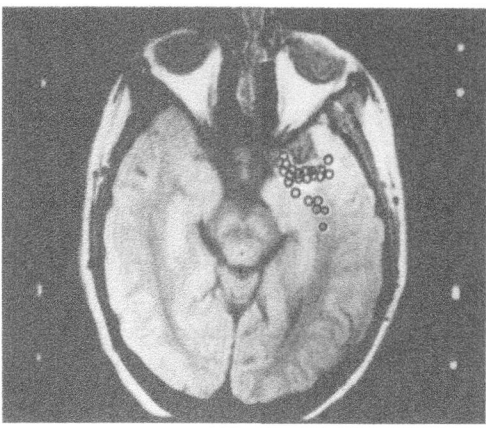

Figure 1. Example of biomagnetic dipole localisation fused with axial MR image. Each small black
circle marks a dipole localised during the time
course of an averaged spike-wave event, revealing
the border of a fronto-temporal lesion as the epileptogenic zone. (By courtesy of E. Hellstrand,
Karolinska Hospital, Sweden.)

frame, is used as a compromise during pre-surgical biomagnetic epilepsy diagnosis (Hellstrand
et al., 1990) (Figure 2). Less accuracy, but a more user friendly handling and a more flexible
system for recording sessions is offered by a dental frame, especially designed for use in
biomagnetism and MR head coils (Stefan et al., 1990) (Figure 3). These patient fixation systems
are connected with the biomagnetic and MRI measurement frame in a rigid, known way. A
variety of external markers attached to the patient are in use, (Orrison et al., 1990; Schneider
et al., 1990). The principle of these markers is that they use both an MR contrast agent and a
current source which can be localised from its magnetic field, mostly a circular current coil.
Easy to handle and with a sufficient accuracy for many applications, although less accurate
than the methods described above, is the use of anatomical landmarks, which can be identified
in the MR image. Electromagnetic transceiver devices are used most often to record the
three-dimensional coordinates of these landmarks in the biomagnetic measurement frame
(Crum et al., 1987). An alternative method uses the biomagnetic sensors also as receivers for
the magnetic field of a set of three orthogonal current coils (Ahlfors and Ilmoneimi, 1989) in
a stylus, used to scan the surface of the investigated object. The body surface contours so
yielded can be fitted to MR images, thereby establishing the common reference system of

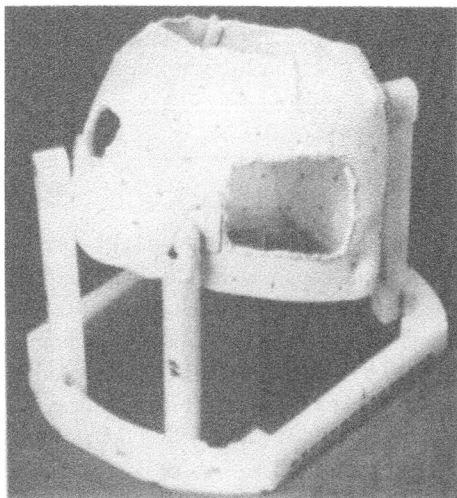

Figure 2. Head mould combined with a stereotactic
Leksell frame, used during pre-surgical epilepsy diagnosis (MR, CT, PET, biomagnetism) as well as during
radiosurgery by the gamma-knife technique. (By courtesy of E. Hellstrand, Karolinska Hospital, Sweden.)

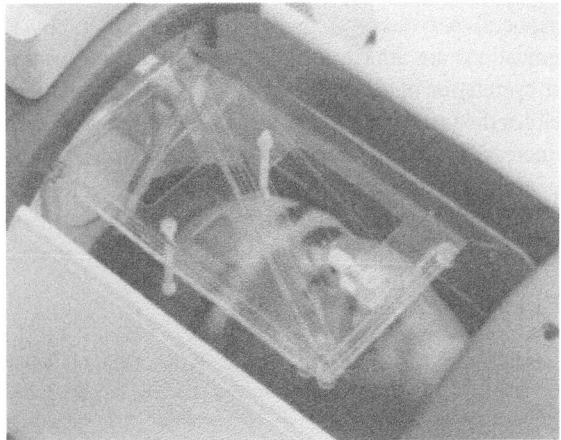

Figure 3. Dental frame for patient fixation, designed to fit in an MR head coil and in the biomagnetic measurement device KRENIKON®.

coordinates. This very recent development is of an accuracy nearly comparable to that of a stereotactic frame (Pelizzari et al., 1989; Abraham-Fuchs et al., 1991).

DISCUSSION

The method of choice is primarily determined by the clinical needs. By means of stereotactic frames or by surface contour fitting the accuracy achievable is determined by the MR image pixel size, being in the order of 1 mm. The accuracy with the head mould is estimated to be 2 mm–5 mm, depending on the head region.

The dental frame is capable of the same accuracy as the head mould but requires patient cooperation. This accuracy is sufficient for surgical interventions such as tailored resections or gamma-knife treatment (Hellstrand et al., 1990) in epilepsy therapy. Use of anatomical landmarks offers an accuracy of between 5 mm and 15 mm, which is often sufficient to differentiate the anatomical or functional structure that has been localised biomagnetically. A constraint which has to be observed in biomagnetism is that all patient-positioning devices have to be constructed avoiding ferromagnetic material, which in some cases made modifications of existing devices necessary.

In addition to the correlation of the biomagnetic localisations with the brain anatomy, a pilot study was carried through in eight epileptic patients in order to quantify the distance of a morphological lesion, visible in the MRI, and the MEG results (Stefan et al., 1991). The earliest activity at the onset of an epileptic spike which could be localised using the equivalent current dipole model was defined as the "primary epileptogenic area (PFA)". The distance of this biomagnetic localisation to the nearest border of the morphological lesion was then measured in the patient's MRI. In seven of eight patients, this distance was less than 10 mm, revealing a close correlation of morphological and electro-physiological pathology in the clear majority of the investigated patient group.

PROBABLE DEVELOPMENT OVER THE NEXT FIVE YEARS

Biomagnetism might be of use in the clinical diagnosis of epilepsy and in the pre-surgical functional mapping of the sensorimotor cortex. The number of multichannel systems in use is slowly increasing. The ongoing research work with these systems is expected to establish other clinical applications in the future, such as the diagnosis of brain ischaemias, transient ischaemic attacks and infarctions (Vieth, 1990). Another new field currently explored are disorders in the peripheral nervous system by magnetoneurography (Curio et al., 1991). Most of these applications are aimed at three-dimensional localisation of electro-physiological processes. The correlation of biomagnetism with imaging modalities such as MRI, CT or ultrasonography enables the visualisation of the electric activity with respect to morphology. Diagnostic value is increased hereby. The different fields of applications, as well as the differing demands on the accuracy, requires a variety of patient fixation systems and fiducial point strategies. Therefore an increase in research and development is expected in this field.

REFERENCES

Abraham-Fuchs, K., Lindner, T., Wegener, P., Nestel,F., and Schneider, S., 1991, Fusion of biomagnetism with MR or CT images by contour-fitting, Biomed. Technik 36 (suppl): 88–89.

Ahlfors, S., and Ilmoniemi, R., 1989, Magnetometer position indicator for multi-channel MEG, in: "Advances in Biomagnetism," S.J. Williamson, M. Hoke, G. Stroink, M. Kotani, eds, New York, p. 693.

Crum, D., Westley, R., Greenblatt, R., Toussaint, R., and Hirschkoff, E., 1987, Apparatus and method for making biomagnetic measurements, US Patent, April 1987.

Curio, G., Erne, S.N., Sandforth, J., Scheer, J., Stehr, R., and Trahms, L., 1991, Exploratory mapping of evoked neuromagnetic activity from human peripheral nerve, brachial plexus and spinal cord, Electroencephalogr Clin Neurophysiol 81:450–453.

Evans, N.T.S., 1990, Combining imaging techniques, Clin Phys Physiol Meas. 11a: 97–102.

Hellstrand, E., Abraham-Fuchs, K., Jernberg, B., Kihlstroem, L., Knutsson, E., Lindqvist, C., Schneider, S., and Wirth, A., 1993, MEG localisation of inter-ictal epileptic focal activity and concomitant stereotactic irradiation therapy. A new non-invasive approach for patients with focal epilepsy, Physiol Meas 14: 131–136.

Orrison, W.W., Davis, L.E., Sullivan, G.W., Mettler, F.A., and Flynn, E.R., 1990, Anatomic localisation of cerebral cortical function by magnetoencephalography combined with MR imaging and CT, AJNR 11: 713–716.

Pelizzari, C., Chen, G., Spelbring, D., Weichselbaum, R., and Chen, C., 1989, Accurate three-dimensional registration of CT, PET and/or MR images of the brain, J Comp Ass Tomogr. 13: 20–26.

Schneider, S., Hoenig, E., Reichenberger, H., Abraham-Fuchs, K., Daalmans, G., Moshage, W., Oppelt, A., Roehrlein, G., Stefan, H., Vieth, J., Weikl, A., and Wirth, A., 1990, Multichannel biomagnetic system for high-resolution functional studies of brain and heart, Radiology 176: 825–830.

Stefan, H., Schneider, S., Abraham-Fuchs, K., Bauer, J., Feistel, H., Pawlik, G., Neubauer, U., Roehrlein, G., and Huk, H.J., 1990, Magnetic source localisation in focal epilepsy: Multichannel magnetoencephalography correlated with magnetic resonance brain imaging, Brain 113: 1347–1359.

Stefan, H., Abraham-Fuchs, K., Schueler, P., and Schneider, S.,1991, Ictal and inter-ictal multichannel magnetic field recording of epileptiform activity, Proc.8th Int.Conf.on Biomagnetism, Muenster, 18–24 August 1991, 183–184.

Vieth, J., 1990, Magnetoencephalography in the study of stroke, in: "Advances in Neurology," Sato, S., ed., Raven Press, New York.

29

VOLUMETRIC MAGNETIC RESONANCE IMAGING

Impact on Neuropsychological Studies

M. Jones-Gotman

Montreal Neurological Institute
3801 University Street
Montreal, Quebec
Canada H3A 2B4

INTRODUCTION

In the past, the understanding of brain–behaviour relationships has made considerable advances through the study of epileptic patients who undergo focal surgical resection for seizure relief. Information about the site and size of resection was based upon estimates made by the surgeon at operation, and those measurements were used in conjunction with patients' performance on cognitive tests to infer the function of the brain region that had been excised. Reasoning that a given cognitive test was sensitive to dysfunction in a given area of brain, the information derived from postoperative testing was then applied to predict the site of brain dysfunction in patients prior to surgery. This approach has yielded a wealth of information over the years, but it is limited in several ways.

First, it has become very clear recently that there is a relatively high margin of error in the estimates of extent of removal that are made during surgery (Awad et al., 1989). This adds a considerable degree of uncertainty to postoperative lesion groupings made as a function of those estimates, especially when the groupings are based on small measurement differences. A second important limitation is that there has been no means of independent confirmation of conclusions drawn from preoperative cognitive test results. Thus, any fine distinctions one might attempt to draw about subregions within a brain area could neither be verified nor disproved.

A salient example of this problem is found in the study of the specific hippocampal contribution to learning and memory. Tests "sensitive to hippocampal dysfunction" (e.g. Jones-Gotman, 1991a,b) have been identified in postoperative studies, and, using those tests, conclusions regarding the function of hippocampus separately from that of temporal neocortex have been attempted for unoperated patients. In one such study that aimed to ascertain whether performance on a learning test could differentiate patients with from those without damage specifically in the hippocampus (Milner, 1978), patients were tested before surgery, and

Magnetic Resonance Scanning and Epilepsy, Edited by S.D. Shorvon et al.,
Plenum Press, New York, 1994

afterwards they were classified as having intact or damaged hippocampus using the surgeon's estimate of damage as determined by visual inspection during the operation. Another method, certainly more accurate but also more painstaking, has been to count cells in a resected hippocampus and to relate cell loss to preoperative memory scores (Rausch and Babb, 1987; Sass et al., 1990). In either method one has information only about the resected hippocampus and not about the contralateral one.

To progress more rapidly in our understanding of specific functions of subregions of the brain, it is clear that we need to be able to evaluate structural differences in the brain as a whole, and not just in small areas accessed or resected from patients who undergo surgery. To this end, the development of quantified MRI as a means to measure brain structures objectively is greeted with enthusiasm by cognitive neuroscientists.

CURRENT WORK

The quality and resolution of the images obtained through MRI have improved vastly over the space of a few years, and with this improved resolution has come the possibility to quantify the volume of separate structures and regions. That the measurements are meaningful has been shown in studies comparing preoperative volume estimates from MRI scans with postoperative cell counts from resected tissue (Cascino et al., 1991; Lencz et al., 1992). In those studies, the severity of cell loss was shown to correlate significantly with hippocampal volume measurements, such that the more atrophic hippocampi (small measured volumes) showed the greatest histopathologic changes. Also, volume measurements appear to be reliable: comparison of measurements made twice by the same rater and of measurements made independently by two different raters yield highly similar results (Cendes et al., 1992).

If we accept that the volumetric MRI measurements yield meaningful information, those measurements can be used to study performance on cognitive tests. Data from such studies are just beginning to appear, and the usefulness of the high-resolution MRI for the study of patients whose lesions are not otherwise verifiable is abundantly clear. Thus, Press et al., (1989) have reported hippocampal atrophy in three amnesic patients, confirming in living patients the pathology that until now has been possible to document only in the rare case that comes to post mortem examination. Studies of language disorders will surely benefit in a similar manner. It will be possible to relate the deficits in speech and language, which have been examined in minute detail for many years without confirmation of the underlying cerebral abnormalities, to anatomical findings revealed by MRI. Indeed a preliminary study has been reported recently for three patients with verbal auditory agnosia (Filipek et al., 1987). Similarly, MRI allows the cognitive findings in patients who undergo callosotomy to be analysed as a function of more precise information about the extent and placement of the callosal section performed (Bogen et al., 1988; Risse et al., 1989).

Initial reports have begun to appear on the application of MRI measurements to verify the site of cerebral abnormality predicted by performance on cognitive tests in patients with temporal-lobe epilepsy. Thus, a recent study by Lencz et al. (1992) showed that left hippocampal atrophy, as assessed by MRI volumetric measurement, was related to deficient verbal memory (assessed by a paragraph memory test), and that a small left temporal lobe was related to deficient performance on a word learning test. Furthermore, postoperative pathology confirmed the MRI findings: the hippocampal atrophy inferred from the MRI measurements correlated with a reduced neuronal density in the hippocampal CA fields and dentate gyrus, as observed in cell counts carried out on the excised hippocampus.

The same group examined neuronal density in hippocampal subfields in conjunction with performance on memory tests during an intracarotid sodium amobarbital (ISA) procedure, again by postoperative cell counts in the excised tissue (Sass et al., 1991). Their results showed significant cell loss specifically from CA3 in patients who had failed the amobarbital procedure memory tests when injection had been made into the hemisphere opposite the seizure focus. An earlier study by Rausch and Babb (1989) had also shown a significant incidence of failure on ISA memory tests in patients with marked hippocampal cell loss, but they found a less systematic relationship between ISA memory performance and degree of cell loss when hippocampal damage was moderate. Quantified MRI should contribute to clarifying the circumstances that lead to ISA memory failures. We are currently pursuing this line of enquiry using MRI measurements that give separate values for amygdala and hippocampus (Watson et al., 1992) in patients with unilateral versus bilateral temporal lobe abnormality according to EEG.

Frontal lobe function has intrigued neuroscientists since the mid-1800s, when Phineas Gage received a crow-bar through the frontal lobes and lived to tell the tale. Our store of knowledge about specific functions that are lost as a result of damage to the frontal lobes is increasing steadily, but much more can be learned with the aid of neuroimaging. For example, Anderson et al., (1991) recently raised a note of caution against overinterpretation of the Wisconsin Card Sorting test, which is widely used to assess frontal lobe function: those authors failed to discriminate frontal from nonfrontal cases in 91 patients whose lesions were delineated using CT and MRI scans. The present and future high-resolution MRI scans should allow further exploration of specific deficits in conjunction with well-defined areas of damage within the expanse of frontal lobe cortex.

PROBABLE DEVELOPMENTS OVER THE NEXT FIVE YEARS

The hippocampus is believed to play an important role in learning and memory, but it is largely unknown what specific contribution is made by the hippocampus and what by the amygdala or other medial temporal structures (parahippocampal gyrus, entorhinal cortex, perirhinal cortex). Studies of the separate roles of these structures in different aspects of learning and memory can be carried out relatively easily in experimental animals, but has seldom been attempted in human subjects. It is now possible to measure MRI volume in the amygdala separately from hippocampus, allowing exploration of this issue in patients. Preoperatively, one can explore the effect of reduced volume in amygdala versus reduction in the hippocampus, in patients in whom such reduction in these structures occurs independently.

After operation, verification of the extent of resection separately for amygdala and hippocampus is important. For example, in an experiment investigating odour memory in patients with focal surgical resection, it was found that a "small hippocampal resection" resulted in a greater deficit than did a "large hippocampal resection" (Jones-Gotman and Zatorre, 1993). The finding was interpreted as possibly owing to a more extensive amygdala resection in the cases with "small hippocampal removal", an interpretation based on the observation that a more complete removal of amygdala was attempted in the patients in whom hippocampus would be spared. That intriguing notion can be substantiated or refuted only by careful MRI measurement of the structures in question.

An important clinical issue in evaluation of memory in patients with temporal lobe epilepsy is prediction of postoperative memory loss. There is some evidence indicating that patients with better preoperative memory function tend to show the greatest postoperative memory losses. This suggests that excision of a healthy hippocampus interrupts memory, whereas excision of a damaged hippocampus does not. Future studies relating memory performance to hippocampal volume should shed light on this question.

In studies of auditory function, knowledge about the integrity of Heschl's gyrus is of prime importance. In the future, this area will be studied more precisely with volumetric measurements. Study of the contributions of subcortical regions to cognitive functions will also become more prominent. As mentioned above, knowledge of frontal lobe function is particularly difficult to obtain: frontal cortex is vast, the site of lesions within frontal cortex varies considerably, and patients with surgical excision from a frontal lobe are less numerous than those with temporal lobe resection. Precise MRI measurements of different areas of the frontal lobe will allow one to relate function to these different regions.

Quantification of structure volumes in brain images is still in its infancy. Although validation studies have been carried out, more confirmation will be necessary before volumetric MRI findings can be considered definitive. Should they prove to be as reliable as they seem, they will revolutionise the study of brain-behaviour relationships.

REFERENCES

Anderson, S.W., Damasio, H., Jones, R.D., and Tranel, D., 1991, Wisconsin Card Sorting Test performance as a measure of frontal lobe damage, J Clin Exp Neuropsychol. 13: 909–922.

Awad, I.A., Katz, A., Hahn, J.F., Kong, A.K., Ahl, J., and Lüders, H., 1989, Extent of resection in temporal lobectomy for epilepsy, I. Interobserver analysis and correlation with seizure outcome, Epilepsia 30:756–762.

Bogen, J.E., Schultz, D.H., and Vogel, P.J., 1988, Completeness of callosotomy shown by magnetic resonance imaging in the long term, Arch Neurol. 45: 1203–1205.

Cascino, G.D., Jack, C.R., Parisi, J.E., Sharbrough, F.W., Hirschorn, K.A., Meyer, F.B., Marsh, W.R., and O'Brien, P.C., 1991, Magnetic resonance imaging-based volume studies in temporal lobe epilepsy: pathological correlations, Ann Neurol. 30: 31–36.

Cendes, F., Andermann, F., Watson, C., Evans, A., Gloor, P., Jones-Gotman, M., Melanson, D., Olivier, A., Leroux, G., and Peters, T., 1992, MRI volumetric measurements of amygdaloid body and hippocampal formation: Intra- and inter-rater differences, Can J Neurol Sci. 19: 285.

Filipek, P.A., Kennedy, D.N., Caviness, V.S., Klein, S., and Rapin, I., 1987, In vivo MRI-based volumetric brain analysis in subjects with verbal auditory agnosia, Ann Neurol. 22: 410.

Jones-Gotman, M., 1991a, Localization of lesions by neuropsychological testing. Epilepsia 32 (suppl 5): S41-S52.

Jones-Gotman, M., 1991b, Presurgical neuropsychological evaluation for localization and lateralization of seizure focus, in: "Epilepsy Surgery," H. Lüders, ed., Raven Press, New York.

Jones-Gotman, M., and Zatorre, R.J., 1993, Odor recognition memory in humans: Role of right temporal and orbitofrontal regions, Brain Cogni. 22: 182–198.

Lencz, T., McCarthy, G., Bronen, R.A., Scott, T.M., Inserni, J.A., Sass, K.J., Novelly, R.A., Kim, J.H., and Spencer, D.D., 1992, Quantitative magnetic resonance imaging in temporal lobe epilepsy: Relationship to neuropathology and neuropsychological function, Ann Neurol. 31: 629–637.

Milner, B., 1978, Clues to the cerebral organization of memory, in: "Cerebral Correlates of Conscious Experience," INSERM Symposium No. 6, P. Buser and A. Rougeul-Buser, eds, Elsevier, Amsterdam,

Press, G.A., Amaral, D.G., and Squire, L.R., 1989, Hippocampal abnormalities in amnesic patients revealed by high-resolution magnetic resonance imaging, Nature 341: 54–57.

Rausch, R., and Babb, T.L., 1987, Evidence for memory specialization within the mesial temporal lobe in man, in: "Fundamental Mechanisms of Human Brain Function," J. Engel, G. Ojemann, H. Lüders, and P. Williamson, eds, Raven Press, New York.

Rausch, R., Babb, T.L., Engel, J., and Crandall, P.H., 1989, Memory following intracarotid amobarbital injection contralateral to hippocampal damage, Arch Neurol. 46: 783–788.

Risse, G.L., Gates, J. Lund, G., Maxwell, R., and Rubens, A., 1989, Interhemispheric transfer in patients with incomplete section of the corpus callosum: Anatomic verification with magnetic resonance imaging, Arch Neurol. 46: 437–443.

Sass, K.J., Spencer, D.D., Kim, J.H., Westerveld, M., Novelly, R.A., and Lencz, T., 1990, Verbal memory impairment correlates with hippocampal pyramidal cell density, Neurology 40: 1694–1697.

Sass, K.J., Lencz, T., Westerveld, M., Novelly, R.A., Spencer, D.D., and Kim, J.H., 1991, The neural substrate of memory impairment demonstrated by the intracarotid amobarbital procedure, Arch Neurol. 48: 48–52.

Watson, C., Andermann, F., Gloor, P., Jones-Gotman, M., Peters, T., Evans, A., Olivier, A., Melanson, D., and Leroux, G., 1992, Anatomic basis of amygdaloid and hippocampal volume measurement by magnetic resonance imaging, Neurology 42: 1743–1750.

MRI AND INTELLECTUAL DECLINE IN EPILEPSY

M.R. Sperling

Comprehensive Epilepsy Center
Graduate Hospital
University of Pennsylvania School of Medicine
Philadelphia, Pennsylvania

INTRODUCTION

Two categories of cognitive impairment are described in epilepsy, static cognitive impairment and progressive cognitive decline. Static impairments are common in children and adults with epilepsy, especially in the acquired epilepsies. Cognitive decline is less well understood and controversial. Recurrent seizures might cause progressive decline in intellectual and cognitive abilities. A small number of investigators have serially evaluated cognition in epilepsy patients with a matched control population, and have suggested that some children with refractory epilepsy do experience progressive mental decline (Bourgeois et al., 1983; Rodin et al., 1986). Other factors influencing cognitive function include the age at onset of epilepsy, seizure type, seizure frequency, number of medications, drug levels, and socioeconomic status. The age at which seizures first appear may be particularly critical as shown in some animal models and human studies (seizures arising beyond a certain age may be far less harmful than if they had surfaced earlier) (Dikmen et al., 1977; Bourgeois et al., 1983). Holmes and colleagues (1990) demonstrated deleterious effects of seizures on memory, learning, behaviour, and activity levels in genetically epilepsy-prone rats.

MRI and CT have been used to study the size of various brain structures in health and disease. Morphometric changes, chiefly diminishing cortical volume and increasing CSF volume, accompany the normal ageing process (Jernigan et al., 1990). MRI and CT have been correlated with mental ability in other neurological diseases. Cognitive deficits were reported in multiple sclerosis patients with clinically isolated demyelinating plaques (Callanan et al., 1989). Hippocampal atrophy is found in Alzheimer's disease (Jack et al., 1992), and Kesslak and colleagues (1991) found that a reduction in hippocampal and parahippocampal volume correlated with decline in the Mini-mental Status score. A CT study in Down's syndrome demonstrated progressive cerebral atrophy which was more marked in demented patients compared with non-demented patients (Schapiro et al., 1989).

Magnetic Resonance Scanning and Epilepsy, Edited by S.D. Shorvon et al.,
Plenum Press, New York, 1994

CURRENT RESEARCH

Hippocampal atrophy is commonly present in patients with temporal lobe epilepsy (Jackson et al., 1990). The amount of atrophy correlates with the degree of cell loss (Cascino et al., 1991). Moreover, the degree of memory impairment correlates with hippocampal pyramidal cell density and may be specific for only some subfields (Sass et al., 1990; O'Rourke et al., 1992). Long-term studies are currently under way to evaluate cognitive abilities serially in epilepsy surgery patients with parallel control populations.

DISCUSSION

The studies cited above either provide a limited static view of cognition and lack longitudinal follow-up, or evaluate a highly selected subpopulation who have undergone a therapeutic intervention that altered the natural history of epilepsy. Nevertheless, preliminary data in subjects with several neurological diseases suggest that MRI-derived volumetric studies provide insights regarding the function of specific brain structures.

PROBABLE DEVELOPMENT OVER THE NEXT FIVE YEARS

Detailed comparisons of cognitive abilities, histopathological abnormalities, and MRI volumetric studies in surgical specimens should provide useful data. It may be possible to predict neuropsychological outcome after resective surgery by correlating pre-operative MRI anatomy with post-operative cognitive changes. Studies must be carried out to define more carefully cognitive and intellectual changes over time in epilepsy. Careful control of variables, especially age, medication, and seizure type and frequency will be required. Serial MRI scans (with particular attention to limbic cortex) can be performed in conjunction with repeated neuropsychological assessments, to determine if volume changes occur and if they correlate with cognitive changes. Because of the normal ageing process and practice effects, a normal control population will be needed for purposes of comparison.

Additionally, MR techniques for imaging blood flow can be applied to study active mental processes. Specific cognitive tasks can be devised and patterns of brain activation studied. It may be possible to then study cognitive reorganisation in people with epilepsy for understanding of fundamental mechanisms of brain response to injury and prediction of clinical outcome.

REFERENCES

Bourgeois, B.F.D., Prensky, A.L., Palkes, H.S., Talent, B.K., and Busch, S.G., 1983, Intelligence in epilepsy: A prospective study in children, Ann Neurol. 14: 438–444.

Callanan, M.M., Logsdail, S.J., Ron, M.A., and Warrington, E.K., 1989, Cognitive impairment in patients with clinically isolated lesions of the type seen in multiple sclerosis: A psychometric and MRI study, Brain 112: 361–374.

Cascino, G.D., Jack, C.R., Parisi, J.E., Sharbrough, F.W., Hirschorn, K.A., Meyer, F.B., Marsh, W.R., and O'Brien, P.C., 1991, Magnetic resonance imaging based volume studies in temporal lobe epilepsy: pathologic correlations, Ann Neurol. 30: 31–36.

Dikmen, S., Mathews, S.G., and Harley, J.P., 1977, Effect of early versus late onset of major motor epilepsy on cognitive-intellectual performance: further considerations, Epilepsia 18: 31–36.

Holmes, G.L., Thompson, J.L., Marchi, T.A., Gabriel, P.S., Hogan, M.A., Carl, F.G., and Feldman, D.S., 1990, Effects of seizures on learning, memory, and behavior in the genetically epilepsy-prone rat, Ann Neurol. 27: 24–32.

Jack, C.R., Peterson, R.C., O'Brien, P.C., and Tangalos, E.G., 1992, MR-based hippocampal volumetry in the diagnosis of Alzheimer's disease, Neurology 42: 183–188.

Jackson, G.D., Berkovic, S.F., Tress, B.M., Kalnins, R.M., Fabinyi, G.C.A., and Bladin, P.F., 1990, Hippocampal sclerosis can be reliably detected by magnetic resonance imaging, Neurology 40: 1869–1875.

Jernigan, T.L., Press, G.A., and Hesselink, J.R., 1990, Methods for measuring brain morphologic features on magnetic resonance images: Validation and normal aging, Arch Neurol. 47: 27–32.

Kesslak, J.P., Nalcioglu, O., and Cotman, C.W., 1991, Quantification of magnetic resonance scans for hippocampal and parahippocampal atrophy in Alzheimer's disease, Neurology 41: 54–54.

O'Rourke, D.M., Saykin, A.J., Gilhool, J.J., Harley, R., O'Connor, M.J., and Sperling, M.R., 1993, Unilateral hemispheric memory and hippocampal neuronal density in temporal lobe epilepsy. Neurosurgery 32: 574–581.

Rodin, E.A., Schmaltz, S., and Twitty, G., 1986, Intellectual functions of patients with childhood-onset epilepsy, Dev Med Child Neurol. 28: 25–33.

Sass, K.J., Spencer, D.D., Kim, J.H., Westerveld, M., Novelly, R.A., and Lencz, T., 1990, Verbal memory impairment correlates with hippocampal pyramidal cell density, Neurology 40: 1694–1697.

Schapiro, M.B., Luxenberg, J.S., Kaye, J.A., Haxby, J.V., Friedland, R.P., and Rapoport, S.I., 1989, Serial quantitative CT analysis of brain morphometrics in adult Down's syndrome at different ages, Neurology 39: 1349–1353.

MRI AND SPECT IN EPILEPSY SURGERY

C.R. Jack, Jr., F.W. Sharbrough, and G.D. Cascino

Mayo Clinic
Rochester, Minnesota 55905

INTRODUCTION

It is axiomatic in epilepsy surgery that the epileptogenic focus must be resected in order to achieve a good result. Imaging modalities which are directed toward this localisation can be divided into two major categories: anatomical and functional. MR has superseded CT for anatomic imaging in epilepsy (Kuzniecky et al., 1987; Jack et al., 1990a; Jackson et al., 1990; Ashtari et al., 1991; Berkovic et al., 1991; Bronen et al., 1991; Cook et al., 1992; Lencz et al., 1992). PET, SPECT, MR spectroscopy, and MR perfusion/diffusion imaging fall into the category of functional imaging. Further discussion of functional imaging here will be limited to SPECT which can be performed inter-ictally or peri-ictally (Stefan et al., 1987; Lee et al., 1988; Rowe et al., 1989; Tatum et al., 1990; Rowe et al., 1991).

Precise figures are not known but reasonable estimates of the accuracy of MRI in identifying the major pathological substrates of chronic epilepsy are: structural lesions (tumour, arteriovenous malfunction, migration anomalies)—100%; mesial temporal sclerosis—90%; non-specific neocortical gliosis or no pathological abnormality—0% (Kuzniecky et al., 1987; Jack et al., 1990a; Jackson et al., 1990; Berkovic et al., 1991; Bronen et al., 1991; Lencz et al., 1992). Virtually all patients undergo MRI imaging prior to epilepsy surgery in order to identify structural lesions which must be resected if a good result is to be achieved. However, additional useful information beyond simple lesion localisation on cross-sectional images can be extracted from MRI. Specifically, surface renderings of the cortex can be generated from an appropriately designed three-dimensional volumetric MR pulse sequence using off-line image processing algorithms. With these views, the relationship of surface lesions to key anatomical surface landmarks (such as the sensory motor cortex) can be identified pre-operatively. This information can be useful in selecting patients for surgery, identifying the most appropriate type of surgery, and identifying the most appropriate surgical approach (Jack et al., 1990b).

As outlined above, MRI is quite accurate in localising most pathological substrates of chronic epilepsy. However, at least 15–20% of patients in most epilepsy surgery series will have negative, or unrevealing, histology upon examination of the tissue specimen. The MRI likewise is usually unrevealing in these cases. It is particularly in

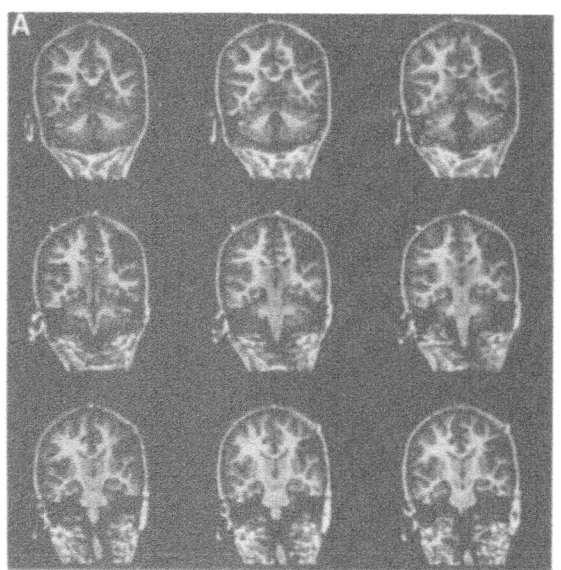

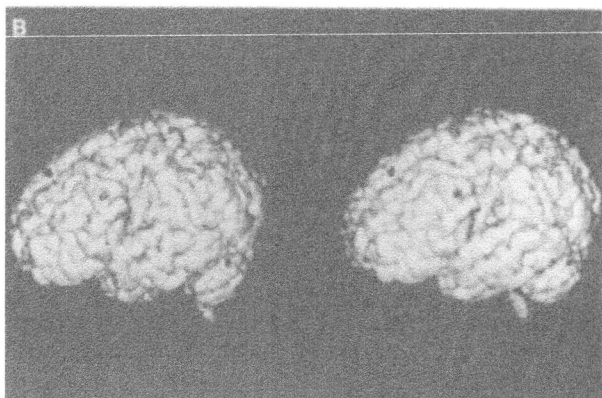

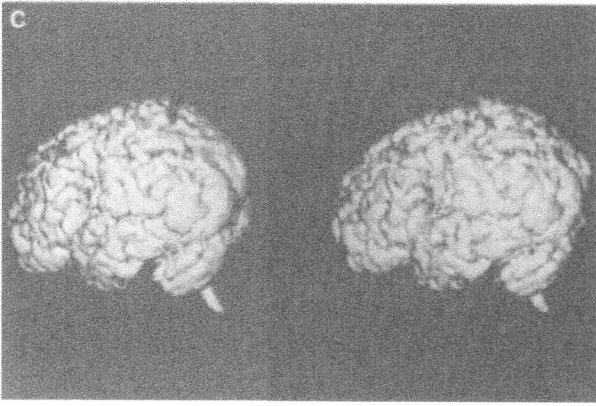

Figure 1. Adolescent female who suffered a left hemisphere stroke in early life. She suffered from intractable seizures for a number of years, the right arm was paretic, but motor function in the right leg as well as speech were intact. (A) Series of cross-sectional coronal MR images through the zone of infarction. From these images it was difficult to identify the precise extent of the infarcted area with respect to surrounding topographic landmarks. Specifically, it was unclear that a complete resection of the encephalomalacic lesion could be accomplished without damage to the normally functioning sensorimotor cortex and speech area. Initially a focal cortical resection was not planned, rather a palliative corpus callosotomy was planned. (B,C) Three-dimensional surface rendering which are progressively rotated from the viewer's perspective. These views clearly demonstrated the position of the infarcted cortex relative to the sensorimotor strip. It is seen from these images that the zone of infarction in fact is quite narrow in its anteroposterior extent. A clearly definable margin is seen between the lesion and the leg portion of the anatomic sensorimotor homunculus as well as the expected location of Broca's area. Accordingly, a focal cortical resection of this area was carried out, and the patient has been seizure-free postoperatively.

these cases that functional imaging studies, such as PET or SPECT, could provide localising information. However, the largest, and most carefully done, interictal SPECT studies (Rowe et al., 1989, 1991) have reported a disappointing sensitivity rate for localisation of the epileptogenic zone. Therefore, techniques to improve the sensitivity of SPECT in epilepsy seem to be a worthwhile goal.

CURRENT RESEARCH

Recent research at our institution into the question of the optimal use of MR and SPECT in surgical epilepsy has taken two forms: clinical application of MRI-based surface rendering and efforts to improve SPECT imaging.

MRI-based Surface Rendering of the Brain

Views of the brain surface can be generated from an appropriately designed three-dimensional volumetric MRI data set. These views can be generated by either of two general techniques: surface rendering or volume rendering. With either of these techniques, the relationship between abnormal surface topography (i.e. a lesion or lesions presumably responsible for seizures) and key anatomical landmarks can be displayed. These displays can be rotated to any desired viewer perspective, and are quite useful for surgical planning. An example of such a case is seen in Figure 1.

Improved SPECT Imaging

The second category in which we have been conducting research is that of improving the ability of SPECT to identify the epileptogenic focus. We have investigated two means of improving SPECT in epilepsy:

(1) Integration of inter-ictal SPECT and MR images (Erickson and Jack, 1993). A problem inherent to SPECT imaging is its poor spatial resolution. Volume averaging of metabolically inert CSF spaces on inter-ictal SPECT studies can mimic zones of tissue hypoperfusion which are the hallmark of the epileptogenic zone. This diagnostic ambiguity inherent in inter-ictal SPECT imaging is one correctable problem which may decrease its accuracy. The solution to this problem is integrating MR with SPECT. Two general approaches have been used: (a) point-to-point transformation of one data set to the reference framework of the other, and (b) surface-to-surface matching. We have developed a point-to-point iterative minimisation technique using externally fixed fiducial markers. Recently completed validation studies have demonstrated that registration can be performed to greater accuracy than that of the lower resolution image (SPECT) (Erickson and Jack, 1993). We have also begun working with a surface-to-surface matching algorithm. Advantages of the point-to-point method include greater speed and potentially greater accuracy. The surface-to-surface method, however, carries a formidable advantage over the point-to-point techniques in that no surface markers need be attached, and therefore image registration may be done retrospectively.

(2) A second problem SPECT imaging has is the inherently low sensitivity of regional hypoperfusion (inter-ictal imaging) as a marker for the epileptogenic focus. Studies by Rowe et al. (1989, 1991) have indicated that imaging peri-ictal hyperfusion may provide strikingly greater sensitivity. When ictal SPECT imaging is registered with

MRI, the potential exists for precise registration of the peri-ictal flow abnormality on a highly detailed MRI generated anatomical map of the cerebral cortex (Jack et al., 1990b; Erickson and Jack,1993) (Figure 2).

DISCUSSION/FUTURE DEVELOPMENTS

(1) In the future it is likely that payers will not reimburse medical care providers for every test in every patient and will demand verification of the utility of each test employed in the pre-operative evaluation of surgical epilepsy patients. The result for pre-operative imaging in surgical epilepsy will be the development of a paradigm(s) outlining when MRI imaging alone is sufficient and when SPECT or other imaging studies are indicated.

(2) It is likely that all SPECT imaging will be interpreted after having been integrated with an MRI-generated anatomic template via surface-to-surface matching algorithms.

(3) MRI based surface renderings of the brain will play an increasingly important role in the selection and planning of surgical cases in epilepsy.

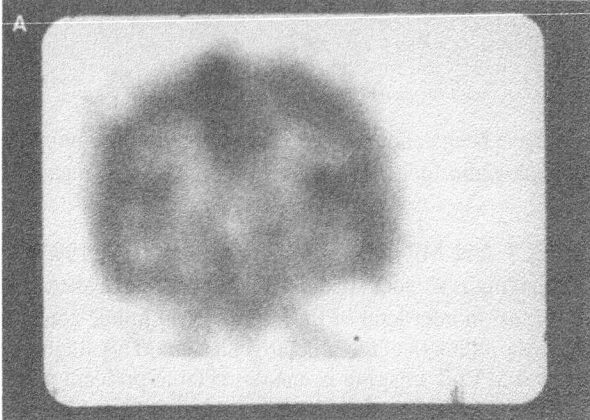
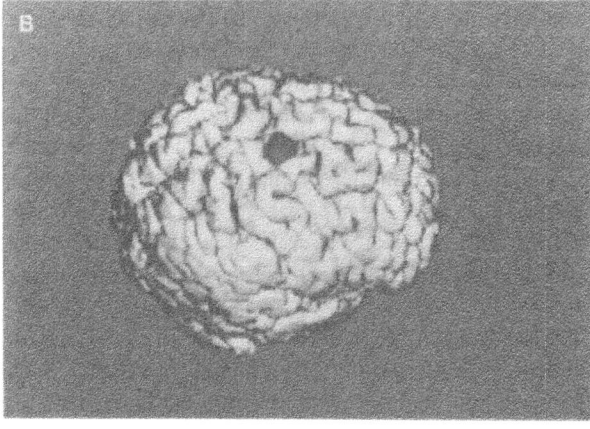

Figure 2. A male in his late forties with reflex simple partial motor seizures involving the left leg. The patient could induce left leg seizures by tensing the muscles of his lower extremity. An ictal SPECT study was performed by injecting the isotope during the planned ictal event. (A) A coronal ictal SPECT study, which demonstrates a focal area of increased uptake in the right parasagittal cortex. Whereas this abnormality could be demonstrated on the SPECT study, it could not be precisely localised relative to cortical anatomy because of the poor spatial resolution of SPECT. (B) Three-dimensional surface rendering of the brain MR images. The MR and SPECT data sets have been fused, and the "hot spot" of the SPECT scan is projected onto the three-dimensional surface rendering. This technique of integrating MR and ictal SPECT imaging data enables precise placement of the ictal cerebral perfusion abnormality on an MR-generated surface map of the brain. The ictal perfusion abnormality correlates well with the patients clinical seizure activity as it is located in the leg portion of the anatomic motor strip homunculus, and also in the pre-motor area on the right.

REFERENCES

Ashtari, M., Barr, W., Schaul, N., and Bogerts, B., 1991, Three-dimensional flash imaging and computerised volume measurements of the hippocampus in patients with chronic epilepsy of the temporal lobe, AJNR 12: 941–947.

Berkovic, S.F., Andermann, F., Olivier, A., Ethier, R., et al., 1991, Hippocampal sclerosis in temporal lobe epilepsy demonstrated by magnetic resonance imaging, Ann Neurol. 29: 175–182.

Bronen, R.A., Cheung, G., Charles, J.T., Kim J.H. et al., 1991, Imaging findings in hippocampal sclerosis: correlation with pathology, AJNR 12: 933–940.

Cook, M., Fish, D., Shorvon, S., and Stevens, J., 1992, Distribution of hippocampal atrophy in temporal lobe epilepsy: volumetric MRI assessment, Neurology 42 (suppl 3): 205.

Erickson, B.J., and Jack, C.R., Jr, 1993, A method for image correlation with validation studies, AJNR 14: 713–720.

Jack, C.R., Jr., Sharbrough, F.W., Twomey, C.K., et al., 1990a, Temporal lobe seizures: lateralisation with MR volume measurements of hippocampal formation, Radiology 175: 423–429.

Jack, C.D., Jr., Marsh, W.R., Hirschorn, K.A., et al., 1990b, EEG scalp electrode projection onto three-dimensional surface rendered images of the brain, Radiology 176: 413–418.

Jackson, G.D., Berkovic, S.F., Tress, B.M., Kalnins, R.M., Fabinyi, G.C.A., and Bladin, P.F., 1990, Hippocampal sclerosis can be reliably detected by magnetic resonance imaging, Neurology 40: 1869–1875.

Kuzniecky, R., De la Sayette, V., Ethier, R., et al., 1987, Magnetic resonance imaging in temporal lobe epilepsy: pathological correlations, Ann Neurol. 22: 341–347.

Lee, B.I., Markand, O.N., Wellman, H.N., et al., 1988, HIPDM-SPECT in patients with medically intractable complex partial seizures, Arch Neurol. 45: 397–402.

Lencz, T., McCarthy, G., Bronon, R., et al., 1992, Quantitative MRI and the hippocampus in temporal lobe epilepsy, Ann Neurol. 31: 629–637

Rowe, C.C., Berkovic, S.F., Sia, S.T.B., et al., 1989, Localisation of epileptic foci with postictal single photon emission computed tomography, Ann Neurol.. 26: 660–668.

Rowe, C.C., Berkovic, S.F., Austin, M.C., McKay, W.J., and Bladin, P.F., 1991, Patterns of postictal cerebral blood flow in temporal lobe epilepsy: qualitative and quantitative analysis, Neurology 42: 1096–1103.

Stefan, H., Pawlik, G., Bocher-Schwarz, H.G., et al., 1987, Functional and morphological abnormalities in temporal lobe epilepsy: a comparison of inter-ictal and ictal EEG, CT, MRI, SPECT and PET, J Neurol. 234: 377–384.

Tatum, W.O., Sperling, M.R., O'Connor, M.J., and Jacobstein, J.G., 1990, Inter-ictal SPECT in the pre-surgical evaluation of intractable partial epilepsy, Epilepsia 31: 670.

MR-DIRECTED STEREOTACTIC RESECTIONS AND PER-OPERATIVE SCREENING USING LOW-FIELD MRI

D.G.T. Thomas and G.P. Kratimenos

National Hospital for Neurology and Neurosurgery
Queen Square
London, WC1N 3BG
United Kingdom

INTRODUCTION

Precision resection of stereotactically defined volume presents one of the current applications of "volumetric stereotaxis". Computer-assisted reconstruction of serial outlines of the volume for resection obtained with modern computerised neuroimaging methods defines the spatial coordinates of that volume and allows its interpolation in a three-dimensional matrix (Kelly et al., 1984). Information derived from stereotactically performed computerised imaging allows the suspension of the given volume into a stereotactic three-dimensional space and its precise resection using a stereotactic technique. Experience with CT-directed volumetric resections indicates that the method is satisfactory. The ability of magnetic resonance imaging (MRI) to define the boundaries of most intracranial structures more accurately and its superior diagnostic image sensitivity make its use in stereotactic volumetric resections highly desirable. The use of MRI, however, in computerised volumetric stereotactic surgery presents considerable difficulties. Problems concerning the construction of stereotactic hardware materials such as fiducials, frame and stabilising devises have now been successfully addressed. Computer software compatible with current imaging and stereotactic hardware has also been developed and used in clinical practice and although the problem of linear distortion still remains, especially in the periphery of the image, it is now possible to use MRI-derived information in volumetric stereotactic resections either indirectly by registration of the stereotactic coordinates or directly through specially developed software (Kelly et al., 1987).

CURRENT RESEARCH

CT-directed stereotactic volumetric resections of non-tumorous cerebral volumes have been clinically tried in cases of medically refractory epilepsy where a stereotactic volumetric amygdalo-hippocampectomy was thought the best form of treatment (Kelly et al., 1987;

Magnetic Resonance Scanning and Epilepsy, Edited by S.D. Shorvon et al.,
Plenum Press, New York, 1994

Kratimenos et al., 1992). Six patients (three male and three female patients with a mean age of 23 years) underwent selective-directed volumetric amygdalo-hippocampectomy using the Kelly-Goerss-Kall "COMPASS" stereotactic system. Patients with tumours identified on CT or MRI scanning were excluded from this series and in this respect these patients belong in a larger series of patients undergoing stereotactic volumetric excisions. All patients have had medically intractable complex partial seizures for an average length of 14 years (range: 11–19). Four patients had a unilateral mesial temporal focus identified on video telemetric EEG recordings; one patient had bilateral mesial temporal foci on EEG telemetry (but with clinical and neuropsychological localisation to the left, MRI findings supportive of more advanced left-sided atrophy and electro-physiological predominance of a ratio of 7 to 1 to the left). Finally one patient had a large unilateral temporal epileptogenic area defined with imaging and recording studies. Four patients underwent a left and two patients a right craniotomy with removal of the amygdalo-hippocampal complex. The patient with the large epileptogenic area had a supplementary excision of the ipsilateral temporal pole in addition to the selective amygdalo-hippocampectomy. Three patients remained seizure free since the operation and three had a considerable reduction in seizure frequency. All patients stayed on anti-epileptic medication. Three of the patients with unilateral mesial foci have been seizure free post-operatively. The patient with bilateral temporal foci has had a reduction in seizure frequency from 3–4 attacks per day to 2 per week whereas the patient with the larger temporal epileptogenic focus has also had a marked reduction in seizure frequency but is still having occasional absence attacks. Histopathological examination of the resected specimens showed medial hippocampal sclerosis in five patients, whereas the patient with the large epileptogenic region was found to harbour a medial temporal, completely excised, cryptic angioma. Post-operative MRI was performed in all patients and in some cases indicated the possibility of achieving a larger and potentially more beneficial resection; this will be possible when direct MRI guidance becomes available at the time of surgery. This was especially true in the cases where the number of the epileptic seizures of the patients were decreased post-operatively but not totally controlled.

DISCUSSION AND PROBABLE DEVELOPMENT OVER THE NEXT FIVE YEARS

There is no doubt that MR imaging has greater diagnostic sensitivity and is more accurate than CT in outlining intracerebral structures. This makes its use highly desirable in intra-parenchymal stereotactic volumetric surgery. The peripheral linear distortion of MR images, however, combined with the poor imaging of bony structures excludes its sole uses at present in skull base stereotactic surgery. Intra-operative MRI guidance would potentially offer higher precision in stereotactic resections and would allow the complementary use of multiple computerised imaging modalities. Cross-registration of stereotactic points and volumes could be done in real time and verified continuously during the resection. Interactive image displays depicting the progress of the resection as it happens could also make volumetric resections more precise and safe. There are, however, numerous problems to be addressed before intra-operative MRI screening could offer effective guidance in stereotactic operations. Planning of operation units with non-ferromagnetic instruments and appropriate surgical equipment would be an essential step permitting the installation of an MRI suite in operating rooms. Appropriate operation table tops permitting imaging with the patient in situ and open imaging units combined with low field MRI or other shielded system would also be required. Finally control units adjacent or placed inside the operating rooms and housing the appropriate computing and imaging hardware would be required to allow for stereotactic image manipulation and continuous real time information feedback.

REFERENCES

Kelly, P.J., Kall, B.A., and Goerss, S. J., 1984, Transposition of volumetric information derived from computed tomographic scanning into stereotactic space, Surgi Neurol. 21: 465–471.

Kelly, P.J., Sharbrough, F.W., Kall, B.A., et al., 1987, Magnetic resonance imaging-based computer assisted stereotactic resection of the hippocampus and amygdala in patients with temporal lobe epilepsy, May Clin Proc. 62: 103–108.

Kratimenos, G.P., Pell, M.F., Thomas, D.G.T., Shorvon, S.D., Fish, D.R., and Smith, S.J.N., 1992, Open stereotactic selective amygdalo-hippocampectomy for drug resistant epilepsy, Acta Neurochirurg (Wien). 116: 150–154.

Section 5

MR and Lesional Epilepsy Syndrome

NON-MALIGNANT TUMOURAL LESIONS

G.D. Cascino, C.R. Jack, Jr., F.W. Sharbrough, and P.J. Kelly

Mayo Clinic and Mayo Foundation
Rochester, Minnesota 55905

INTRODUCTION

Magnetic resonance imaging (MRI) is the most sensitive and specific structural imaging technique available to demonstrate non-malignant or low-grade tumours in patients with epilepsy (Lee et al., 1985; Bergen et al., 1989). The low-grade neoplasms associated with chronic seizure disorders include gangliogliomas, gliomas and dysembryoplastic neuroepithelial tumours (Cascino, 1990) (Figures 1–3).

The most common tumours in these patients are low-grade astrocytomas (Cascino, 1990). MRI is a non-invasive study that has no known biological toxicity and may indicate the aetiology of the seizure disorder and assist in localising the epileptogenic region or zone, i.e. the site of seizure onset (Bergen et al., 1989; Brooks et al., 1990). MRI may identify a focal intracranial lesion in patients with intractable partial epilepsy being evaluated for epilepsy surgery (Jabbari et al., 1986; Brooks et al., 1990). Seizures are the most common presenting symptom in patients with low-grade intracranial neoplasms (Penfield et al., 1940). The tumour histology is related to the epileptogenic potential of the lesion (Le Blanc and Rasmussen, 1974). Approximately 10–20% of patients with intractable partial epilepsy have a tumoural lesion revealed at the time of epilepsy surgery (Penfield et al., 1940; Le Blanc and Rasmussen, 1974; Babb and Brown, 1987). The foreign-tissue abnormalities may be imaged by MRI without producing X-ray computed tomography (CT) alterations (Laster et al., 1985).

CURRENT RESEARCH

The sensitivity of long repetition time/echo time pulse sequences (predominantly T2-weighted images) using a high-field strength magnet (1.5 T) in detecting alterations associated with non-malignant tumoural lesions in patients with partial epilepsy has been confirmed (Bergin et al., 1989; Brooks et al., 1990). Tumours characteristically produce a prominent increase in T1 and T2 relaxation times of tissue (Jabbari et al., 1986; Bergen et al., 1989; Brooks et al., 1990) (Figures 1–3). T2-weighted images are more sensitive in revealing the foreign-tissue pathology (Figure 2). A focal T2-weighted signal intensity alteration is most commonly observed in patients with mass lesions and partial epilepsy (Figures 1–3). Gadolinium-DTPA-

Magnetic Resonance Scanning and Epilepsy, Edited by S.D. Shorvon et al.,
Plenum Press, New York, 1994

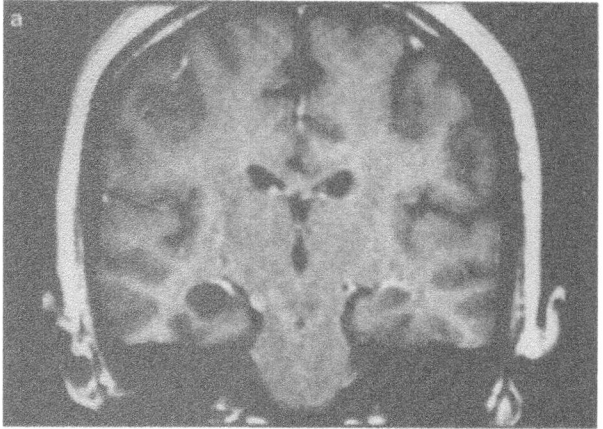

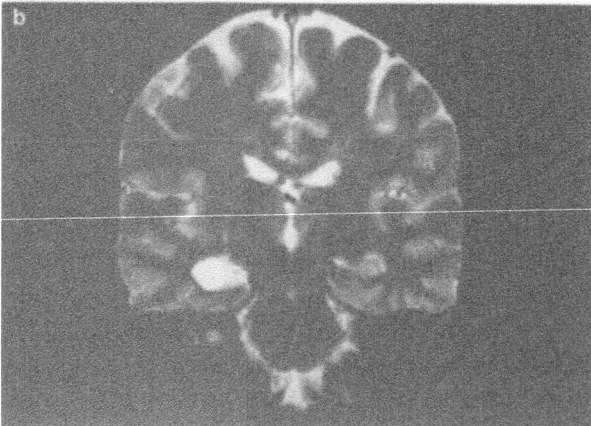

Figure 1. Grade I-II mixed oli-godendroglioma-astrocytoma. (a) A gadolinium-DTPA-enhanced MRI using a short repetition/echo time pulse sequence revealing a right temporal lobe abnormality associated with an increase in T1 signal. No pathological enhancement was noted. (b) A focal T2-weighted signal intensity abnormality identified on the long repetition time/echo time pulse sequence

enhanced MRI may be useful in patients with lesional pathology to indicate the pathological process and differentiate the tumour from oedema (Cascino et al., 1989). Gadolinium produces a prominent T1 shortening effect and is employed with a T1-weighted image sequence. The enhanced images have not proved useful in patients with cortical gliosis and mesial temporal sclerosis. MRI has been demonstrated to be more sensitive and specific than CT in patients with foreign-tissue pathology and intractable partial epilepsy (Laster et al., 1985).

MRI identified lesional pathology has been shown to be a favourable prognostic indicator of surgical outcome in patients with intractable partial epilepsy who undergo epilepsy surgery (Cascino et al., 1992a). Results of MRI in the pre-surgical evaluation directly affect patient selection for surgery and may alter the operative technique. Patients with MRI-identified epileptogenic lesions should be considered favourable candidates for surgery and not exposed to unnecessary anti-epileptic medication trials. Surgical strategies that do not include excision of tumoural lesions are usually unsuccessful in significantly reducing the seizure tendency (Awad et al., 1991; Fish et al., 1991). Focal cortical resections of epileptogenic cortex in patients with posterior temporal or extra-temporal lesions has been associated with a less favourable outcome (Fish et al., 1991). The extent of resection of the foreign-tissue pathology is the most important predictor of surgical outcome in patients with lesional epilepsy (Awad et al., 1991; Palmini et al., 1991). Surgical techniques designed to resect the lesion and not the epileptogenic cortex—lesionectomy—may significantly reduce seizure activity in 74%

of patients during long-term follow-up (Cascino et al., 1992b). Selected patients have been rendered seizure-free after lesionectomy and successfully withdrawn from anti-epileptic drug medication (Cascino et al., 1992b). The duration of epilepsy, seizure-type, anatomical local-isation of scalp-recorded inter-ictal and ictal epileptiform activity, and age at seizure onset have not been shown to be significant factors in predicting seizure outcome after lesionectomy (Cascino et al., 1992b). Post-operative EEG recordings have correlated with the operative outcome. Patients who have not benefited from the procedure, i.e. continue to have seizures, are more likely to have inter-ictal epileptiform discharges in extracranial EEG studies per-formed after lesionectomy. Comparative studies have suggested that the most effective procedure in patients with lesion epilepsy for reducing seizure activity is excision of the mass lesion with resection of the epileptic brain tissue (Awad et al., 1991). Potentially, lesionectomy may be associated with a reduced operative morbidity compared to focal corticectomy (Cascino et al., 1992b). MRI has made possible the development of stereotactic lesionectomy which allows selective excision of tumoural lesions from eloquent cortex with a low morbidity (Cascino et al., 1992b). Stereotactic lesionectomy has been useful for histopathological confirmation of intracranial structural abnormalities, and resecting epileptogenic lesions in patients with partial epilepsy. Post-operative MRI studies are performed to indicate the extent of lesion resection. Patients who fail lesionectomy may subsequently be a candidate for a focal corticectomy to resect the epileptogenic cortex (Cascino et al., 1992b).

PROBABLE DEVELOPMENT OVER THE NEXT FIVE YEARS

MRI-based hippocampal volumetry has been shown to be a reliable indicator of mesial temporal sclerosis in patients with partial epilepsy (Jack et al., 1990; Cook et al., 1992a). Hippocampal formation volume studies may be useful to evaluate patients with temporal lobe extra-hippocampal lesions and medically refractory seizures (Cascino et al., 1993a). There is conflicting evidence regarding the results of hippocampal volume studies in patients with

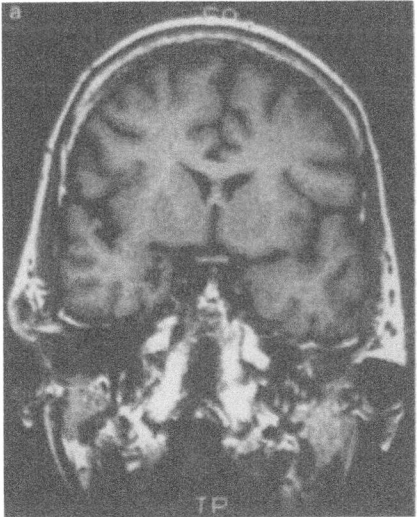 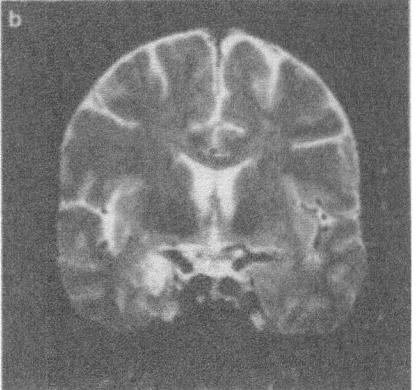

Figure 2. Ganglioglioma. (a) MRI performed in the coronal plane using a short repetition time/echo time pulse sequence revealing a subtle abnormality in the right anterior mesial temporal region. (b) The long repetition time/echo pulse sequence showing an increase T2 signal alteration.

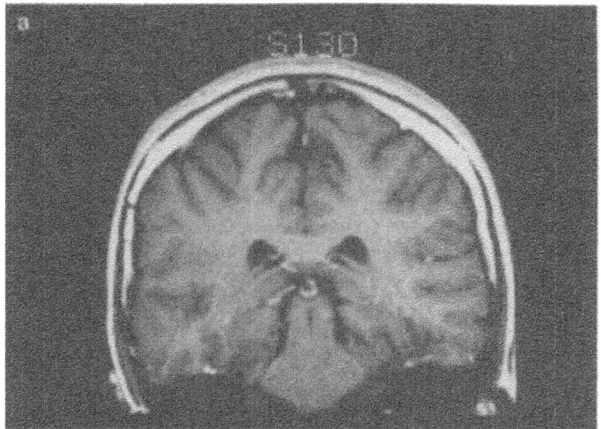

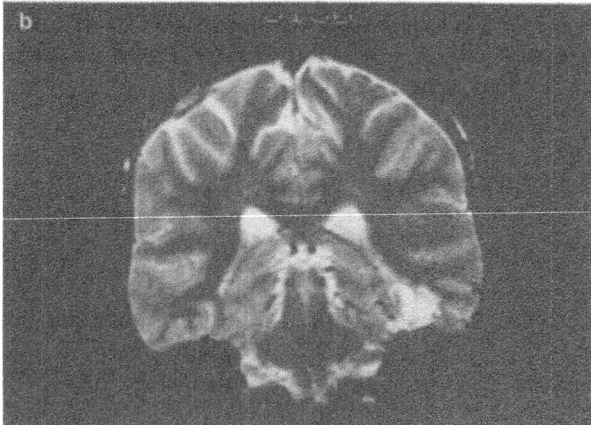

Figure 3. Dysembroplastic neuro-epithelial tumour. (a) An MRI using a short repetition time/echo time pulse sequence revealing a left posterior temporal lobe lesion associated with an increase in the T1 signal. (b) The long repetition time/echo time pulse sequence indicating a focal area of increased T2 signal.

temporal lobe lesions (Cook et al., 1992b; Cascino et al., 1993a). A Mayo Clinic study indicated that MRI may reveal ipsilateral medial temporal atrophy in patients with temporal lobe foreign-tissue lesions, i.e. MRI-identified dural pathology (Cook et al., 1992b; Cascino et al., 1993a). The reason for the different results in the volumetric studies in patients with extra-hippocampal temporal lobe lesions may be the relatively rare occurrence of atrophy in these patients (Cook et al., 1992b; Cascino et al., 1993a). Lesionectomy has been shown to be ineffective in patients with intractable partial epilepsy and temporal lobe dual pathology (Cascino et al., 1993a). Subsequent anterior temporal corticectomy in a small series of patients was associated with a favourable seizure outcome (Cascino et al., 1993a). The surgically excised hippocampi revealed mesial temporal atrophy, and extra-hippocampal non-malignant tumours may prove to be candidates for lesionectomy without requiring resection of the hippocampus.

A final issue that remains to be settled concerns the pre-operative evaluation in patients with tumoural lesions and intractable partial epilepsy (Cascino et al., 1993b). Should all patients be submitted to long-term EEG monitoring, and when if ever should chronic intracranial EEG recordings be performed? Should patients with MRI-identified foreign-tissue lesions be "denied" surgery if the electrophysiological evaluation cannot determine the site of seizure onset? Patients at the Mayo Clinic with low-grade tumours and medically refractory seizures almost invariably undergo surgery without chronic intracranial EEG monitoring. The latter electrophysiologial studies in selected patients may be inaccurate and misleading in determining the site of seizure onset in patients with foreign-tissue lesions (Williamson et al., 1992). Subdural electrodes, however, may be used for functional mapping and during electro-corticography. Ultimately, the surgical strategy in patients with intractable partial epilepsy related to tumoural lesions should include excision of the intracranial mass regardless of the pre-operative electrophysiological studies (Fish et al., 1991).

REFERENCES

Awad, I., Rosenfeld, J., Ahl, H., Hahn, J.F., and Luders, H., 1991, Intractable epilepsy and structural lesions of the brain: mapping, resection strategies, and seizure outcome, Epilepsia 32: 179–186.

Babb, T.L., and Brown, W.J., 1987, Pathological findings in epilepsy, in: "Surgical Treatment of the Epilepsies," Engel, J., Jr, ed., Raven Press, New York

Bergen, D., Bleck, T., Ramsey, R., Clasen, R., Ristanovic, R., Smith, M., and Whistler, W., 1989, Magnetic resonance imaging as a sensitive and specific predictor of neoplasms removed for intractable epilepsy, Epilepsia 30: 3 18–321.

Brooks, B.S., King, D.W., El Gammal, T., Meador, K., Yaghami, F., Gay, J.N., Smith, J.R., and Flanigin, H.F., 1990, MR imaging in patients with intractable partial epileptic seizures. AJNR, 11: 93–99.

Cascino, G.D., Hirschorn, K.A., Jack, C.R., Jr, and Sharbrough, F.W., 1989, Gadolinium-DTPA enhanced magnetic resonance imaging in intractable partial epilepsy, Neurology 39: 1115–1118.

Cascino, G.D., 1990, Epilepsy and brain tumours: implications for treatment, Epilepsia 31 (suppl 3) S37-S44.

Cascino, G.D., Jack, C.R., Jr, Parisi, J.E., Marsh, W.R., Kelly, P.J., Sharbrough, F.W., Hirschorn, W.A., and Trenerry, M.R., 1992a, MRI in the presurgical evaluation of patients with frontal lobe epilepsy and children with temporal lobe epilepsy: pathologic correlation and prognostic importance, Epilepsy Res. 11: 51–59.

Cascino, G.D., Kelly, P.J., Sharbrough, F.W., Hilihan, J.F., Hirschorn, K.A., and Trenerry, M.R., 1992b, Long-term follow-up of stereotactic lesionectomy in partial epilepsy: predictive factors and electroencephalographic results, Epilepsia 33: 639–644.

Cascino, G.D., Jack, C.R., Jr, Parisi, J.E., Sharbrough, F.W., Schreiber, C.P., Kelly, P.J., and Trenerry, M.R., 1993a Operative strategy in patients with MRI-identified dual pathology and temporal lobe epilepsy, Epilepsy Res. in press.

Cascino G.D., Boon, P.A., and Fish, D.R., 1993b Lesional epilepsy, in: "Surgical Treatment of the Epilepsies," Engel, J., Jr, ed., Raven Press, New York, in press.

Cook, M.J., Fish, D.R., Shorvon, S.D., Straughan, K., and Stevens, J.M., 1992a, Hippocampal volumetric and morphometric studies in frontal and temporal lobe epilepsy, Brain 115: 1001–1015.

Cook, M.J., Cendes, F., Andermann, F., Free, S.L., Fish, D.R., Shorvon, S.D., and Stevens, J.M., 1992b, Hippocampal volumetric studies in extratemporal epilepsies: 50 cases, Epilepsia 33 (suppl 3): 72.

Fish, D.R., Andermann, F., and Olivier, A., 1991, Complex partial seizures and small posterior temporal or extratemporal structural lesions: surgical management, Neurology 41: 1781–1784.

Jabbari, B., Gunderson, C.H., Wippold, F., Citrin, C., Sherman, J., Bartoszek, D., Daigh, J.D., and Mitchell, M.H., 1986, Magnetic resonance in partial complex epilepsy, Arch Neurol. 43: 869–872.

Jack, Jr, C.R., Sharbrough, F.W., Twomey, C.K., Cascino, G.D., Hirschorn, K.A., Marsh, W.R., Zinsmeister, A.R., and Scheithauer, B., 1990, Temporal lobe seizures: lateralisation with MR volume measurements of the hippocampal formation, Radiology 40: 423–429.

Laster, D.W., Penry, J.K., Moody, D.M., Ball, M.R., Witcofski, R.L., and Riela, A.R., 1985, Chronic seizure disorders: contribution of MR imaging when CT is normal, AJNR 6: 177–180.

Le Blanc, F.E., and Rasmussen, T., 1974, Cerebral seizures and brain tumours, in: "Handbook of Clinical Neurology," Vinken, P.J., and Bruyn, G.W., eds, North- Holland, Amsterdam.

Lee, B.C.P., Kneeland, J.B., Cahill, P.T., and Deck, M.D.F., 1985, MR recognition of supraentorial tumours, AJNR 6: 871–878..

Palmini, A., Andermann, F., Olivier, A., et al., 1991, Focal neuronal migrational disorders and intractable partial epilepsy: results of surgical treatment, Ann Neurol. 30: 750–757.

Penfield, W., Erickson, T.C., and Tarlov, I., 1940, Relation of intracranial tumours and symptomatic epilepsy, Arch Neurol Psychol. 44: 300–315.

Williamson, P.D., Boon, P.A., Thadani, V.M., Darcey, T.M., Spencer, D.D., Spencer, S.S., Novelly, R.A., and Mattson, R.H., 1992, Parietal lobe epilepsy: diagnostic considerations and results of surgery, Ann Neurol. 31: 193–201.

VASCULAR ANOMALIES IN EPILEPSY

MRI Contribution

M. Bracchi,[1] M. Casazza,[2] G.B. Bradac,[1] G. Avanzini,[2] G. Broggi,[3] and
M. Grisoli[4]

[1] Department of Neuroradiology
  University of Turin, Turin
[2] Department of Neurophysiology
[3] Department of Neurosurgery
[4] Department of Neuroradiology
  National Neurological Institute
  Milan
  Italy

INTRODUCTION

Vascular anomalies are responsible for about 5% of cases of secondary partial epilepsy. The term "anomalies" covers a spectrum of different forms, from the true "malformation" to the "anatomical variant" (Rao and Lee, 1988 Lasjaunias et al., 1991). Even if arteriovenous malformations (AVMs) are the most well-known vascular anomalies, "occult" vascular malformations (cavernomas, capillary telangiectasias and "venous angiomas") are in reality more frequent in pathological studies, and they also represent the most important group of vascular lesions found in patients with partial epilepsy. With CT, and especially MRI, all the different types of "vascular anomalies" are detectable in vivo, and have a similar prevalence and frequency to that found in pathological studies (Robinson et al., 1991). Sturge-Weber syndrome, giant aneurysm, and dural fistula are other rarer examples of vascular lesions responsible for epilepsy.

As many of these "lesions" may be totally asymptomatic during a whole lifespan, it is important to establish a significant relationship between the "anomaly" and the presence of a seizure focus in patients with partial epilepsy. This is largely the province of neurophysiological studies; however, it can be useful to try also to define morphological criteria of "epileptogenicity" using MRI (Trussart et al., 1989).

This is a particular problem with small cavernomas and venous angiomas, which are now easily detected by MRI, both in patients with epilepsy and as incidental findings in asymptomatic subjects, because cavernomas are susceptible to surgical therapy in many cases.

Magnetic Resonance Scanning and Epilepsy, Edited by S.D. Shorvon et al.,
Plenum Press, New York, 1994

CURRENT RESEARCH

MRI diagnoses of occult vascular malformations performed in two neuroradiological centres (University of Turin and Istituto Nazionale Neurologico of Milan) have been reviewed. We selected a group of 23 patients with repeated seizures, operated on for cavernomas in the last 4 years at the Istituto Nazionale Neurologico of Milan and followed with clinical and MRI studies. In 13 cases seizures lasted for more than 5 years. The diameter of the lesions ranged between 0.8 and 3 cm, in all except one case (6 × 4 cm). The location was purely cortical in 10 cases, cortico-subcortical in 11, and subcortical in 2. Most of the lesions (11) were in the temporal lobe. Five patients had other smaller cavernomas. The semiology of seizures was concordant with the lesion location in 18 cases, contralateral in 1 case, and did not fit completely in 4 more cases. Scalp EEG showed slow and/or epileptiform abnormalities on the same side and site in 13 cases, on the same side in 3 cases, on the contralateral hemisphere in 1 case, and was normal, even after sleep deprivation, in 6 cases.

All these patients were operated on with a microsurgical technique. Post-surgical MRI was performed in 15 cases and showed complete removal of the lesion, with persistence in 5 cases of minimal portions of the peripheral ring of hypointensity on T2-weighted images due to haemosiderin deposits.

Sixteen patients became seizure free, in two cases after antiepileptic drug withdrawal; five patients have experienced single or sporadic seizures; two patients presented again with seizures one month after surgery.

DISCUSSION

Surgery has a double goal in cavernomas: to prevent haemorrhages and to relieve seizures. The risk of severe bleeding of a cavernoma is low (Del Curling et al., 1991). However, in our group, three patients with previous epileptic symptoms, had subsequent large, symptomatic haematomas. Post-surgical seizure control rate is good in our series as in others in the literature (Robinson et al., 1991). Nevertheless, precise criteria for surgical resection of cavernomas have not yet been established for either haemorrhage prevention or seizure control. Pre- and post-surgical MRI studies can refine these criteria. The removal of the surrounding glial scar and haemosiderin-laden tissue has been recommended in order to guarantee seizure control (Del Curling et al., 1991). In our series, although the surgical procedure was limited to excision of the cavernoma, only small remnants of the hypointense rim due to haemosiderin deposits were discovered at MRI, indicating that these deposits rarely exceed the border of the lesion.

Regarding the criteria of "epileptogenicity", the size and the location are important factors (Trussart et al., 1989). The multiplanar studies of MRI can assess them precisely.

Peri-lesional high-intensity signal on T2-weighted images is another important finding commonly seen in vascular malformations, and may be due to oedema, gliosis or chronic ischaemia. In our experience it is rare for cavernomas presenting with seizures to have a peri-lesional hyperintensity on T2-weighted images; this is most frequent when there has been sudden bleeding. Exceptionally the peri-lesional hyperintensity is attributable to functional changes following prolonged epileptic activity. Clinical–MRI correlation may help to distinguish these possibilities (Trussart et al., 1989).

MRI diagnosis of cavernoma cannot be specific, because several other forms with the same haemorrhagic pathophysiological properties may have the same appearance (Imakita et al., 1989; Rapacki et al., 1990). The differentiation of the various types of "occult" vascular malformations (Sigal et al., 1990) might be of value, as may the identification of evolving lesions with serial studies.

PROBABLE DEVELOPMENT OVER THE NEXT FIVE YEARS

Another interesting lesion is the so-called "venous angioma", which is the most frequent "vascular anomaly" (about 60%, Garner et al., 1991), and is usually an incidental finding in pathological studies. Indeed, the term "venous angioma" is misleading, because it is usually not a pathological process, but a variation of the venous drainage. The term "developmental venous anomaly" (DVA) seems more appropriate (Lasjaunias et al., 1991). DVAs have a broad range of expression, from a single vein through the white matter, to a complete reorganisation of the veins of one hemisphere. Bleeding of DVAs is extremely rare. They may be associated with cavernomas (Sasaki et al., 1991). DVAs are often incidental findings, but the association with epilepsy has been proposed and the exact relationship needs to be better defined (Garner et al., 1991). The application of the above mentioned criteria for the identification of "epileptogenicity characters" to large series of MRI studies in DVAs will offer a better understanding of this problem.

REFERENCES

Del Curling, O., Kelly, D.L., Elster, A.D., and Craven, T.E., 1991, An analysis of the natural history of cavernous angiomas, J Neurosurg. 75: 702–708.

Garner, T.B., Del Curling, O., Kelly, D.L., and Laster, D.W., 1991, The natural history of intracranial venous angiomas, J Neurosurg. 75: 715–722.

Imakita, S., Nishimura, T., Yamada, N., Naito, H., Takamiya, M., Yamada, Y., Kikuchi, H.,Yonekawa, Y., Sawada, T., and Yamaguchi, T., 1989, Cerebral vascular malformations: applications of magnetic resonance imaging to differential diagnosis, Neuroradiology 31: 320–325.

Lasjaunias, P., Piske, R., and Alvarez, H., 1991, The venous system from the anomaly to the malformation, in: "First Refresher Course of the ESNR," P.Lasjaunias and M.Leonardi Eds, Del Centauro, Udine, Italy, 7–20.

Rao, K.C.V.G., and Lee, S.H., 1988, Cerebrovascular anomalies, in: "Magnetic Resonance Imaging," D.D.Stark and W.G.Bradley eds, The C.V. Mosby Company, St Louis, 473–505.

Rapacki, T.F.X., Brantley M.J., Furlow, T.W., Geyer, C.A., Toro, V.E., and George E.D., 1990, Heterogenicity of cerebral cavernous hemangiomas diagnosed by MR imaging, J Comput Assist Tomogr. 14: 18–25.

Robinson, J.R., Awad, I.A., and Little, J.R., 1991, Natural history of the cavernous angioma, J Neurosurg. 75: 709–714.

Sasaki, O., Tanaka, R., Koike, T., Koide, A., Koizumi, T., and Ogawa, H., 1991, Excision of cavernous angioma with preservation of coexisting venous angioma, J Neurosurg.75: 461–464.

Sigal, R., Krief, O., Houtteville, J.P., Halioni, P., Doyon, D., and Pariente, D, 1990, Occult cerebrovascular malformations: follow-up with MR imaging, Radiology 176: 815–819.

Trussart, V., Berry, I., Manelfe, C., Arrue, P., and Castan, P., 1989, Epileptogenic cerebral vascular malformations and MRI, J Neuroradiol. 16: 273–284.

MAGNETIC RESONANCE AND NEOCORTICAL EPILEPSY ATROPHIES

B. Oliver and A. Russi

Instituto de Neurologia y Neurocirugia
Barcelona
Spain

INTRODUCTION

Focal cerebral atrophies are more likely to be surgically treatable than diffuse cerebral atrophies.

In 1954, Penfield and Jasper classified surgically treatable epileptogenic lesions into expanding and atrophic lesions. In the last group, three main types of lesions were included: (1) meningocerebral cicatrix (focal atrophy and scar), atrophy secondary to penetrating head injuries, infectious brain diseases; (2) simple atrophic lesions, secondary to brain vascular diseases, closed head injuries; and (3) lesions of birth and infancy; cerebral hemiatrophies, acquired porencephalies, temporal lobe and incisural sclerosis, and "local microgyria" (small and closely placed gyri or gyrus, in an otherwise normal hemisphere, which have failed to grow due to an early brain insult).

Moderate and large atrophic lesions of the neocortex are easily diagnosed by MRI, with a better anatomical definition than by CT, so avoiding invasive diagnostic procedures. The detection of small areas of atrophic or gliotic gyri and/or subtle reduction of regional brain volumes is difficult but is of great importance in the pre-surgical evaluation of epileptic patients.

CURRENT RESEARCH

At present, most patients evaluated for epilepsy surgery have mesial temporal sclerosis and the number of patients with neocortical epilepsy is small. Most surgical cases have grey matter heterotopias and mass lesions. A limiting factor prior to MRI was the inability in imaging methods to identify these lesions, and therefore systematic studies of atrophic lesions in neocortical epilepsies are few. MRI provides new opportunities in this field.

Focal atrophies detected by MRI have been reported in 2% of all cases of epilepsy (Convers et al., 1990). MRI abnormalities in frontal epilepsies were previously not detected

(Convers et al., 1990) but are increasingly reported in studies (Robitaille et al., 1992). Hyperintense signals on T2-weighted images are the most frequently reported positive findings in cryptogenic neocortical epilepsies. These high signals have diverse morphological correlates (Rougier et al., 1988) and occasionally transient MRI phenomena may occur during frequent seizures (Kramer et al., 1987).

We studied retrospectively 100 patients evaluated for epilepsy surgery between 1989 and 1992, of whom 68 patients were surgically treated. MRI examinations were performed with a 0.5 or 1.5 T unit. All patients had a 32-channel video-telemetry long-term monitoring, and 15% an additional intracranial EEG study. Significant MRI abnormalities were detected in 75 patients and in 45 the findings were classified as atrophic lesions. Patients with neocortical involvement in their epileptogenic area had atrophic changes in 32%. In our MRI findings the following were considered insignificant: irrelevant occipital white matter hyperintensities and some parenchymal and choroidal fissure cysts. Some cortical dysplasias were associated with focal or diffuse atrophies. The correlation between the atrophic lesion detected by MRI and the seizure-onset zone was good in cases with temporal lobe atrophy and discrete extra-temporal lesions, except in one case of parieto-occipital porencephaly which became seizure free after anterior temporal resection. The patients with more widespread cortical involvement were not seizure free or were not operated on, indicating the difficulties in delineating the seizure-onset zone.

PROBABLE DEVELOPMENT OVER THE NEXT 5 YEARS

In the future, the following developments are likely:

(1) The introduction of quantitative MRI measurements in neocortical epilepsies.
(2) The establishment of a data-bank for volumes of various cerebral structures (e.g. temporal, frontal, occipital lobes, corpus callosum, total or regional grey and white matter) correlated to age, sex and handedness.
(3) The use of relative values or normalised volumes to allow comparison among subjects, and the definition of normal ranges and physiological asymmetries.
(4) The exploration of the significance, in clinical practice, of the deviations from the normal range.
(5) Possibly new MRI techniques will prove helpful in defining functional epileptogenic areas in relation to the anatomical and/or MRI signal abnormalities.

REFERENCES

Convers, P., Bierme, T., Ryvlin, P., et al., 1990, Apport de l'imagerie par resonance magnetique dans 100 cas d'epilepsie partielle rebelle a scanner X normal, Rev Neurol (Paris). 146: 330–337.
Kramer, R.E., Lüders, H., Lesser, R.P., et al., 1987, Transient focal abnormalities of neuroimaging studies during focal status epilepticus, Epilepsia 28: 528–532.
Robitaille, Y., Rasmussen, T., Dubeau, F., et al., 1992, Histopathology of non- neoplastic lesions in frontal lobe epilepsy. Review of 180 cases with recent MRI and PET correlations, Adv Neurol. 57: 499–513.
Rougier, A., Biset, J.M., Kien , P., et al., 1988, I.R.M. et chirurgie de l'épilepsie. Neurochirurgie 33: 188–193.

Section 6

MR Spectroscopy in Epilepsy

APPLICATION OF SPECTROSCOPY TO EPILEPSY

K.D. Laxer, J.W. Hugg, G.B. Matson, and M.W. Weiner

University of California
San Francisco, California

INTRODUCTION

A variety of imaging techniques have been used to characterise the ictal and inter-ictal metabolic abnormalities associated with focal epilepsy. Position emission tomography (PET) and SPECT scanning have demonstrated the inter-ictal focus to be hypoperfused and hypometabolic. Magnetic resonance spectroscopy (MRS) allows the non-invasive measuring of chemicals within the body and can be performed on many conventional MRI systems. MRS exploits the principle that every chemically distinct nucleus in a compound resonates at a slightly different frequency. Nuclear magnetic resonance (NMR) signals from many compounds can be detected simultaneously in one MRS experiment and magnetic resonance spectroscopic imaging (MRSI) with phase encoding has the ability to obtain MRS signals from multiple regions simultaneously. ^{1}H MRS detects N-acetylaspartate (NAA), lactate, choline, creatine/phosphocreatine, and amino acids including glutamate, glutamine, aspartate and taurine. ^{31}P MRS detects phosphocreatine (PCr), ATP, inorganic phosphate (Pi), pH (from the chemical shift of Pi), free Mg^{2+} (from the chemical shift of ATP), phosphomonoesters (PME), and phosphodiesters (PDE) . PCr, ATP, Pi, pH and lactate provide information concerning bioenergetics. PDE, PME and choline provide information regarding lipid metabolism (Matson and Weiner, 1992). MRS studies in animals and in human neonates during seizures have confirmed previously reported alterations in energy metabolism including the depletion of PCr, ATP, and increased Pi, lactate and H^{+} (Young et al., 1985; Younkin et al., 1986). With the recognised metabolic abnormalities detected by PET and SPECT scanning inter-ictally, we questioned whether or not ^{1}H and ^{31}P MRS could document focal metabolic changes localised to the seizure focus which led to the following pilot studies.

CURRENT RESEARCH

Using a ^{31}P ISIS technique, we studied the temporal lobes in eight patients with medically refractory complex partial seizures (CPS) arising from the medial temporal lobes (Laxer et al., 1992). The ^{31}P MRS spectra were obtained in vivo prior to temporal lobectomy. All the patients have been seizure free since surgery. Electro-corticography, gross surgical findings and the microscopic pathology were all consistent with mesial temporal sclerosis. The ^{31}P spectra were obtained at 2.0 T on the Phillips Gyroscan System using ISIS for spatial localisation. The person performing and processing the MRS was "blind" to the side of the seizure focus. Volumes of interest (84–105 ml) in the right and left anterior temporal lobes were studied. No significant difference was found between ipsilateral and contralateral temporal lobe concentrations for ATP, PCr or PDE. The temporal lobe with the epileptic focus had increased pH and Pi compared to the non-epileptic side. Seven of the eight patients had an asymmetry of pH with the side of the epileptic focus being more alkaline; the seven patients with the ipsilateral temporal lobe alkalosis also had a greater Pi on the side of the focus. There was a trend for PME to be decreased ipsilaterally as well.

The results described above were obtained using pre-selected volumes. Using whole brain ^{31}P MRSI, we studied an additional population of patients with medically refractory CPS. MRSI simultaneously obtained spectra from multiple regions throughout the field of view and, from these spectra, metabolite images can be constructed. The advantage of this technique is that the hippocampus or any other region can be selected post-acquisition. Using this technique, a double-blind ^{31}P MRSI study of eight patients with medically refractory CPS was performed (Hugg et al., 1992). The spectra were obtained inter-ictally and again revealed the seizure focus to be more alkaline ($7.17 + 0.03$ vs $7.06 + 0.02$, $P < 0.01$), have increased Pi ($1.2 + 0.2$ mmol/l vs $0.6 + 0.1$ mmol/l, $P < 0.01$), and decreased PME ($2.1 + 0.03$ mmol/l vs $3.3 + 0.5$ mmol/l, $P < 0.01$). No asymmetry between the hemispheres was found for any phosphorus metabolite or pH in a normal control population. The ^{31}P MRSI correctly lateralised the seizure focus in all of the cases including a patient with a medial frontal focus.

Using a technique similar to the ^{31}P MRSI, we have performed proton spectroscopic imaging in a group of patients with medically refractory CPS arising from the medial temporal lobe. ^{1}H MRSI demonstrated a 78% decrease in the concentration of NAA in the epileptogenic hippocampus as compared to the contralateral side (Hugg et al., 1993).

From these studies, the epileptogenic focus can be defined by increased pH and Pi, decreased PME and NAA.

DISCUSSION

In patients being evaluated for seizure surgery, the ictal EEG recordings are the "gold standard" for cortical localisation; however, a variety of ancillary tests has been developed to provide supportive evidence, which, in some patients, allows the surgery to be performed without the use of intracranial electrodes. Patients in whom there is concordance of these ancillary tests have improved prognosis for seizure control. In a review of our patients with refractory temporal lobe epilepsy (TLE), patients with high-resolution MRIs demonstrating hippocampal atrophy or increased hippocampal T2 signal ipsilateral to the ictal EEG focus, 95% will become seizure free after operation, whereas patients with normal MRIs or discordant MRIs have only a 50% or 30% probability of becoming seizure free, respectively. Unfortunately, MRI scanning is normal or discordant in up to 50% of the patients with TLE and is rarely abnormal in non-lesional, neocortical epilepsy. Eighty per cent of patients with TLE and normal MRI scans have hypometabolism on PET scanning, whereas it is uncommon for PET to be abnormal in non-TLE patients without a focal neocortical abnormality on MRI (Ryvlin et al., 1992). Although these are only preliminary findings, it appears that MRSI will afford an accurate and sensitive adjunctive test in the evaluation of patients with epilepsy.

The aetiology of these metabolic changes is not clear. The alkalosis may represent a compensation for the intermittent ictal acidosis, perhaps through an up-regulation of the Na^+-H^+ anti-port system. It is equally possible that the inter-ictal alkalosis is causative to the epilepsy, because it is well established that increased pH can activate epileptogenic activity.

PROBABLE DEVELOPMENT OVER THE NEXT FIVE YEARS

It is expected that the explosion in technical developments of MR will continue during the next five years with machines that have higher and faster gradients without eddy currents, improving the signal-to-noise ratio and spatial resolution. These developments will allow better understanding of the underlying mechanisms and pathogenesis of seizures. MRS may be able to document metabolic signatures for each seizure type and will perhaps allow the better classification of seizure disorders based upon this metabolic characterisation. With the ability to measure more accurately and localise these metabolites including glutamate and gamma-aminobutyric acid (GABA), it may become possible to characterise those patients who will have the best response to each class of anti-convulsant. The increased spatial resolution will allow better definition of the seizure focus, enhancing the pre-operative work-up and increasing the post-operative prognosis for seizure control.

REFERENCES

Hugg, J.W., Laxer, K.D., Matson, G.B., Maudsley, A.A., Husted, C.A., and Weiner, M.W., 1992, Lateralisation of human focal epilepsy by ^{31}P magnetic resonance spectroscopic imaging, Neurology 42: 2011–2018.

Hugg, J.W., Laxer, K.D., Matson, G.B., Maudsley, A.A., and Weiner, M.W., 1993, Neuron loss localizes human temporal lobe epilepsy by in-vivo proton magnetic resonance, Ann Neurol. 34: 788–794

Laxer, K.D., Hubesch, B., Sappey-Marinier, D. and Weiner, M.W., 1992, Increased pH and inorganic phosphate in temporal seizure foci, demonstrated by ^{31}P MRS, Epilepsia 33: 618–623.

Matson, G.B., and Weiner, M.W., 1992, Spectroscopy, in: "MRI," D.D. Stark, and W.G. Bradley, eds, C.V. Mosby Yearbook, St. Louis.

Ryvlin, P., Philippon, B., Cinotti, L., Froment, J.C., Le Bars, D., and Mauguiere, F., 1992, Functional neuroimaging strategy in temporal lobe epilepsy: a comparative study of [18]FDG-PET and ^{99m}Tc-HMPAO-SPECT, Ann Neurol. 31: 650–656.

Young, R.S., Osbakken, M.D., Briggs, R.W., Yagel, S.K., and Rice, D.W., 1985, ^{31}P NMR study of cerebral metabolism during prolonged seizures in the neonatal dog, Ann Neurol. 18: 14–20.

Younkin, D.P., Delivoria-Papadopoulos, M., Maris, J., Donlon, E., Clancy, R., and Chance, B., 1986, Cerebral metabolic effects of neonatal seizures measured with in vivo ^{31}P NMR spectroscopy, Ann Neurol. 20: 513–519.

PROTON MR SPECTROSCOPIC IMAGING IN THE INVESTIGATION OF PATIENTS WITH TEMPORAL LOBE EPILEPSY

F. Cendes, F. Andermann, and D. L. Arnold

Montreal Neurological Institute and Hospital
McGill University
3801 University Street
Montreal, Quebec
Canada H3A 2B4

INTRODUCTION

MR spectroscopy (MRS) is a non-invasive technique that allows direct identification and quantitation of certain cerebral metabolites in vivo without the injection of radionuclides. Initial studies on small numbers of patients using phosphorus MRS demonstrated a relative alkalosis and an increase in inorganic phosphate in the temporal lobe responsible for temporal lobe epilepsy (TLE) (Kuzniecky et al., 1992; Laxer et al., 1992). Proton MRS has the advantage of much greater signal-to-noise ratio and, therefore, greater spatial resolution compared to phosphorus spectroscopy. Proton MRS studies reported to date have revealed a reduced N-acetylaspartate (NAA) relative resonance intensity in the temporal lobes of patients with TLE (Cendes et al., 1994; Matthews et al., 1990; Laxer et al., 1992).

Multiple lines of evidence indicate that a reduced signal from NAA reflects focal neuronal loss or damage (Moffet et al., 1991; Simmons et al., 1991; Tallen, 1957; Hanstock et al., 1988; Birken and Oldendorf 1989; Bruhn et al., 1989; Coyle et al., 1989; Gill et al., 1989; Petroff et al., 1989; Fenstermacher and Narayana, 1990; Menon et al., 1990; Arnold et al., 1992(b); Duijn et al., 1992; Graham et al., 1992; Slopis et al., 1992). The experience of the London group based on spectra from a single voxel, including the posterior temporal lobe of patients with TLE, as well as data obtained from patients with other disorders, such as multiple sclerosis (Matthews et al., 1991; Arnold et al., 1992), suggest that axonal loss or damage is an important contributor to the observed reduction in NAA signal intensity from white matter, and that such axonal and neuronal damage is more prevalent than generally appreciated.

The studies reported to date have been limited by two factors. First, the lateralisation of the TLE was not always known (Gill et al., 1989), so that agreement between the spectroscopic data and clinical-EEG lateralisation could not be determined. Second, the spectra were obtained

Magnetic Resonance Scanning and Epilepsy, Edited by S.D. Shorvon et al.,
Plenum Press, New York, 1994

from single volumes, the location of which was predetermined from the MRI prior to acquisition of the spectra. Thus, one could not determine whether the spectra were acquired from regions of maximal abnormality, i.e. whether the studies were optimised. This uncertainty can be resolved by MR spectroscopic imaging, which allows reconstruction of metabolic images, e.g. based on NAA resonance intensity, from which one can localise areas of maximal abnormality. The ability to analyse the regional distribution of the metabolic abnormality and to select the volume of maximal abnormality after data acquisition should confer an advantage to MRSI over single-voxel MR spectroscopy techniques (Cendes et al., 1994).

We recently studied 10 patients with intractable TLE and 5 normal controls using two-dimensional MRSI in a 1.5 T combined imaging and spectroscopic system (Philips Medical Systems, The Netherlands) (Cendes et al., 1994).

The normalised measure of asymmetry for NAA/Cr, i.e., [(right − left) / ((right + left) / 2)], for TLE patients as a group was significantly different from normal controls for all regions studied. The asymmetry was greater in the posterior temporal region than in the mid-temporal region, and was greater still when based on the region of maximal metabolic abnormality on MRSI, rather than the above anatomically defined regions of the temporal lobe.

NAA/Cr was low in the mid and posterior temporal regions in 7 of the 10 patients, and in the posterior temporal region only in the remaining 3. These foci of reduced NAA/Cr were ipsilateral to the predominant inter-ictal and ictal EEG abnormalities in every patient. Two patients had a widespread reduction in NAA/Cr in both temporal lobes, but the region of maximal reduction of NAA/Cr was ipsilateral to the side of the more active EEG abnormalities.

Lateralisation based on NAA/Cr correlated with atrophy of amygdala and hippocampus on MRI volumetric measurements in nine patients and with an increased signal from mesial temporal structures in T2-weighted MR images in two patients.

The spectroscopic images of NAA and NAA/Cr revealed regional asymmetries in the relative signal intensities of NAA and NAA/Cr in all patients. When these regions were used for quantitation of side to side differences, the magnitude of the asymmetries was greater than

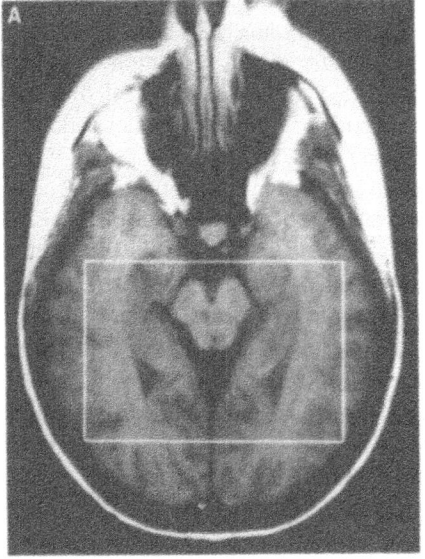
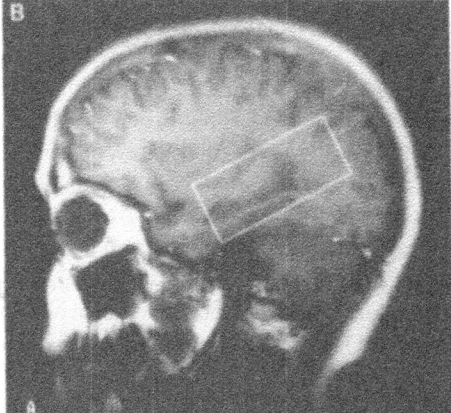

Figure 1. Region of interest (ROI) including both temporal lobes and excluding bone defined on axial (A) and sagittal (B) planes (multislice spin echo MRI, TR = 2000, TE = 30).

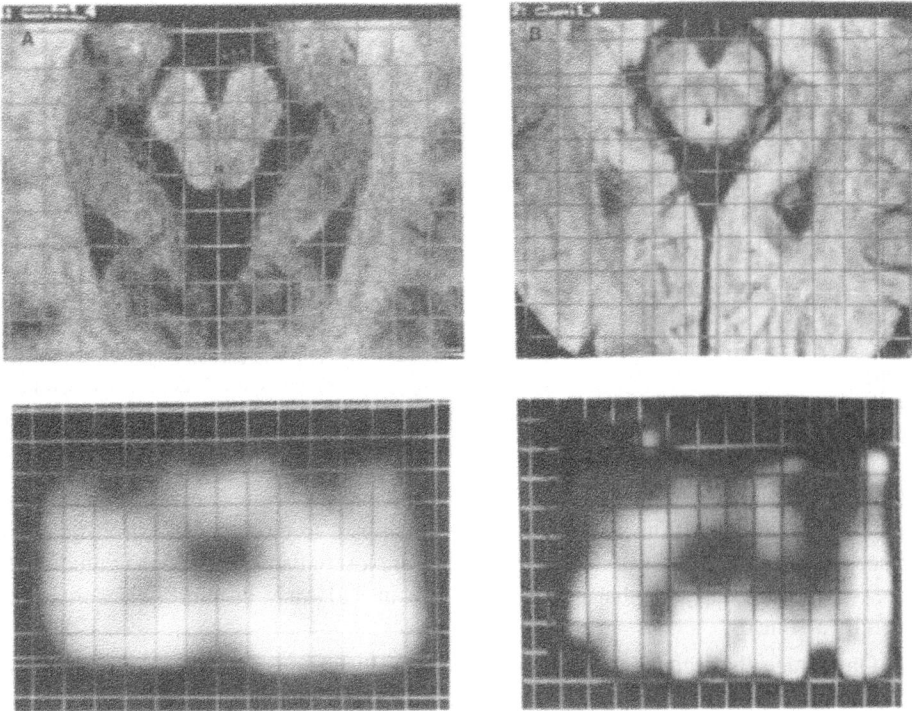

Figure 2. MRI and MRSI from a normal volunteer (a) and a patient with left TLE (b). The images on top show one slice of the conventional (water-based) MRI through the temporal lobes. The images on the bottom are generated from the resonance intensity ratio of NAA/Cr. The spectroscopic images have been smoothed for presentation. The VOI for the spectroscopic image and the original phase-encoding grid are shown superimposed on the images.

that for different other regions of the temporal lobes defined anatomically on the MRI. The foci of reduced NAA/Cr were ipsilateral to the predominant inter-ictal and ictal EEG abnormalities in all patients.

Eight patients underwent either selective amygdalo-hippocampectomy or anterior temporal lobe resection. All are seizure free since the operation (mean follow up 8 months, range 4–12 months).

Quantitative comparison of the side-to-side asymmetry in amygdala and hippocampal volumes with side to side asymmetry of NAA/Cr resonance intensities, suggests a good correlation, although the sample size is small. One patient with left temporal lobe seizures, who did not have any atrophy of amygdala or hippocampus on MRI volumetric measurements, and no abnormal signal in T2-weighted MRI images, showed a significant decrease of NAA/Cr within the left mid-posterior temporal lobe. This patient underwent a selective amygdalo-hippocampectomy and histopathological investigation showed mild mesial temporal sclerosis.

These results indicate that MRSI shows promise as a new means of lateralising TLE. Lateralisation by MRSI based on a reduced NAA/Cr resonance intensity ratio agreed with the side of ictal EEG onset in all patients. Lateralisation by MRSI also agreed with lateralisation by conventional, water-based MRI when significant atrophy was present on MRI volumetric studies or when abnormal signal was present on T2-weighted MR images. The fact that one patient with a normal MRI had reduced NAA/Cr ipsilateral to the EEG focus, and mild mesial sclerosis in this temporal lobe on post-operative histopathology, suggests that MRSI may be

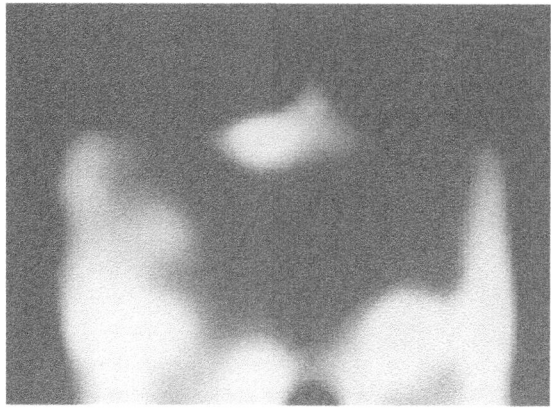

Figure 3. MRSI generated from the resonance intensity ratio of NAA/Cr from another patient with left TLE, without superimposition of the VOI and the original phase-encoding grid. Note the asymmetry with a decreased resonance intensity of NAA/Cr on the left side.

able to detect regional neuronal and/or axonal loss or damage with greater sensitivity than MRI can detect volume loss. This may be due, at least in part, to the fact that astrocytic gliosis replaces some of the volume of neurons when they are lost or damaged. The magnitude of the decrease in NAA suggests that neuronal damage in TLE may be more widespread than generally assumed.

On average, the decrease in NAA resonance intensity was greater in the posterior temporal lobes, rather than more anteriorly. This implies that the source of the decrease in NAA/Cr resonance intensity is in the axons which make up the white matter outflow tracts of the temporal lobe. This may explain the success of single-voxel examinations in which the volume of interest is chosen based on anatomical location (Gill et al., 1989; Kuzniecky et al., 1992; Laxer et al., 1992).

The regional distribution of maximal decrease in NAA varied in different patients. The ability to analyse the regional distribution of the metabolic abnormality and select the volume of maximal abnormality confers a distinct advantage on MRSI over single-voxel techniques.

Although the number of patients studied is small, it seems that the spatial extent and degree of reduction of NAA/Cr does not correlate with the frequency of inter-ictal EEG abnormalities or with the frequency of seizures over the year preceding the MRSI examination. This finding is in agreement with the volumetric studies and, as in the case of the volumetric studies, suggests that the abnormality measured is the cause rather than the result of the seizures.

The relative importance of ictal electrical phenomena versus associated structural and metabolic abnormalities in lateralising the epileptogenic area pre-operatively remains to be determined. The primary importance of the electrophysiological abnormality is axiomatic. However, the fact that seizures may begin on both sides, coupled with the fact that it may be not be feasible to record very many seizures means that there is a statistical likelihood of error in lateralisation when studying patients with bitemporal epilepsy. The structural and, presumably, the metabolic abnormality in TLE seem to reflect the pathological substrate of seizure genesis (Babb and Brown, 1987; Meencke and Veith, 1991; Bruton, 1988; Gloor, 1991). This may bear a sufficiently consistent relationship to the origin and severity of seizures that this determination may be as reliable or even more reliable than recording a few seizures in predicting the side from which most seizures originate. If this is confirmed in a larger series of patients, MRSI lateralisation could reduce the need for costly and prolonged hospitalisations and invasive EEG investigations now required for the pre-surgical assessment of TLE.

REFERENCES

Arnold, D.L., 1992, Reversible reduction of N-acetylaspartate after acute central nervous system damage, Proc Soc Magn Reson Med. 11:643 (abstract).

Arnold, D.L., Matthews, P.M., Francis, G.S., O'Connor, J., and Antel, J.P., 1992, Proton Magnetic resonance spectroscopic imaging for metabolic characterization of demyelinating plaques, Ann Neurol. 31: 235–241.

Babb, T.L., and Brown, W.J., 1987, Pathological findings in epilepsy, in: "Surgical treatment of the epilepsies, " Engel J, Jr, ed., Raven Press, New York..

Birken, D.L., and Oldendorf, W.H., 1989, N-Acetyl-L-aspartic acid: a literature review of a compound prominent in 1H-NMR spectroscopic studies of brain, Neurosci Biobehav Rev. 13: 23–31.

Bruhn, H., Frahm, J., Gyngell, M.L., Merboldt, K.D., Hanicke, W., and Sauter, R., 1989, Cerebral metabolism in man after acute stroke: new observations using localised proton NMR spectroscopy, Magn Reson Med. 9: 126–131.

Bruton, C.J., 1988, "The Neuropathology of Temporal Lobe Epilepsy," Oxford University Press, New York.

Cendes, F., Andermann, F., Preul, M., and Arnold, D.L., 1994, Focal metabolic abnormalities in temporal lobe epilepsy demonstrated by proton MR spectroscopic imaging Ann Neurol. 35:211–216.

Coyle, J.T., Robinson, M.B., Blakely, R.D., and Forloni, G-L., 1989, The neurobiology of N-acetyl-aspartyl-glutamate, in: "Allosteric modulation of amino acid receptors: therapeutic implications," E.A. Barnard and E. Costa, eds, Raven Press, New York.

Duijn, J.H., Matson, G.B., Maudsley, A.A., Hugg, J.W., and Weiner, M.W., 1992, Human brain infarction: proton MR spectroscopy, Radiology 183: 711–718.

Fenstermacher, M.J., and Narayana, P.A., 1990, Serial proton magnetic resonance spectroscopy of ischemic brain injury in humans, Invest Radiol. 25: 1034–1039.

Gill, S.S., Small, R.K., Thomas, D.G., et al., 1989, Brain metabolites as 1H NMR markers of neuronal and glial disorders, NMR Biomed. 2: 196–200.

Gloor, P., 1991, Mesial temporal sclerosis: historical background and an overview from a modern perspective, in:"Epilepsy Surgery," H. Luders, ed., Raven Press, New York.

Graham, G.D., Blamire, A.M., Howseman, A.M., et al., 1992, Proton magnetic resonance spectroscopy of cerebral lactate and other metabolites in stroke patients, Stroke 23: 333–340.

Hanstock, C.C., Rothman, D.L., Prichard, J.W., Jue, T., and Shulman, R.G., 1988, Spatially localised 1H NMR spectra of metabolites in the human brain, Proc Natl Acad Sci USA 85: 1821–1825.

Kuzniecky, R., Elgavish, G.A., Hetherington, H.P., Evanochko, W.T., and Pohost, G.M., 1992, In vivo 31P nuclear magnetic resonance spectroscopy of human temporal lobe epilepsy, Neurology 42: 1586–1590.

Laxer, K.D., Hubesch, B., Sappey-Marinier, D., and Weiner, M.W., 1992, Increased pH and inorganic phosphate in temporal seizure foci demonstrated by 31P MRS, Epilepsia 33: 618–623.

Matthews, P.M., Andermann, F., and Arnold, D.L., 1990, A proton magnetic resonance spectroscopy study of focal epilepsy in humans, Neurology 40:9 85–989.

Matthews, P.M., Francis, G.S., Antel, J., and Arnold, D.L., 1991, Proton magnetic resonance spectroscopy for metabolic characterization of plaques in multiple sclerosis, Neurology 41: 1251–1256.

Meencke, H.J., and Veith, G., 1991, Hippocampal sclerosis in epilepsy, in: "Epilepsy Surgery," H. Luders, ed., Raven Press, New York.

Menon, D.K., Sargentoni, J., Peden, C.J., et al., 1990, Proton MR spectroscopy in herpes simplex encephalitis: assessment of neuronal loss, J Comput Assist Tomogr. 14: 449–452.

Moffet, J.R., Namboodiri, M.A.A., Cangro, C.B., and Neale, J.H., 1991, Immunohistochemical localization of N-acetylaspartate in rat brain, NeuroReport 2:131–134.

Petroff, O.A.C., Spencer, D.D., Alger, J.R., and Prichard, J.W., 1989, High-field proton magnetic resonance spectroscopy of human cerebrum obtained during surgery for epilepsy, Neurology 39: 1197–1202.

Simmons, M.L., Frondoza, C.G., and Coyle, J.T., 1991, Immunocytochemical localization of N-acetyl-aspartate with monoclonal antibodies, Neuroscience 45:37–45.

Slopis, J.M., Lin, S., Butler, J.M., and Caprioli, R., 1992, Selective Corelease of N-Acetylaspartylglutamate and N-Acetyl-Aspartate from rat hypothalamus in vivo. Ann Neurol. 32(3):445–446 (abstract).

Tallen, H.H., 1957, Studies on the distribution of N-acetyl-L-aspartic acid in brain, J Biol Chem. 224:41–45.

PROTON MR SPECTROSCOPY IN THE EVALUATION OF MESIAL TEMPORAL SCLEROSIS

F. Triulzi, A. Falini, and G. Scotti

Department of Neuroradiology
Scientific Institute H.S. Raffaele
Milan
Italy

INTRODUCTION

Mesial temporal sclerosis (MTS) can be identified on MRI with a high degree of sensitivity and good specificity (Jackson et al., 1990). However, a further improvement in both MRI sensitivity and specificity should be of major clinical importance, in particular in patients with intractable temporal lobe epilepsy selected for surgical treatment. A potential improvement of the overall MRI accuracy could be obtained with the direct in vivo evaluation of some brain metabolites by means of localised proton MR spectroscopy (^{1}HMRS). With this technique the spectra are collected from a volume of interest of $2 \times 2 \times 2$ cm which can be directly selected on the basis of MR imaging. The number of metabolites currently available with clinical ^{1}HMRS (with echo time of 270 or 135 ms) are, however, limited to N-acetylaspartate(NAA), creatine(CR) and choline(CHO) and the evaluation of mesial temporal structures is affected by some technical limitations such as artefacts from carotid pulsatility and middle fossa bone, and relatively large volume of interest which cause a global decrease of the signal-to-noise ratio.

CURRENT RESEARCH

Different ^{1}HMRS data concerning the in vivo evaluation of the epileptogenic foci in patients with intractable partial epilepsy were recently reported (Matthews et al., 1990; Allard et al., 1992; Breiter et al., 1992; Connelly et al., 1992; Kato et al., 1992). The main finding of the ^{1}HMRS spectra collected in the epileptogenic focus was a relative decrease in NAA peak with regard to normal controls. The decrease of NAA concentration was reported in a percentage of epileptic patients ranging from 100% (Matthews et al., 1990; only two patients) to 21%. A variation of glutamatephis glutamine peak was also reported in some cases in comparison with normal volunteers. The presence of a low NAA peak and low NAA/Cho + Cr ratio in the epileptogenic lesions is concordant with the most recent in vitro ^{1}HMRS data

Magnetic Resonance Scanning and Epilepsy, Edited by S.D. Shorvon et al.,
Plenum Press, New York, 1994

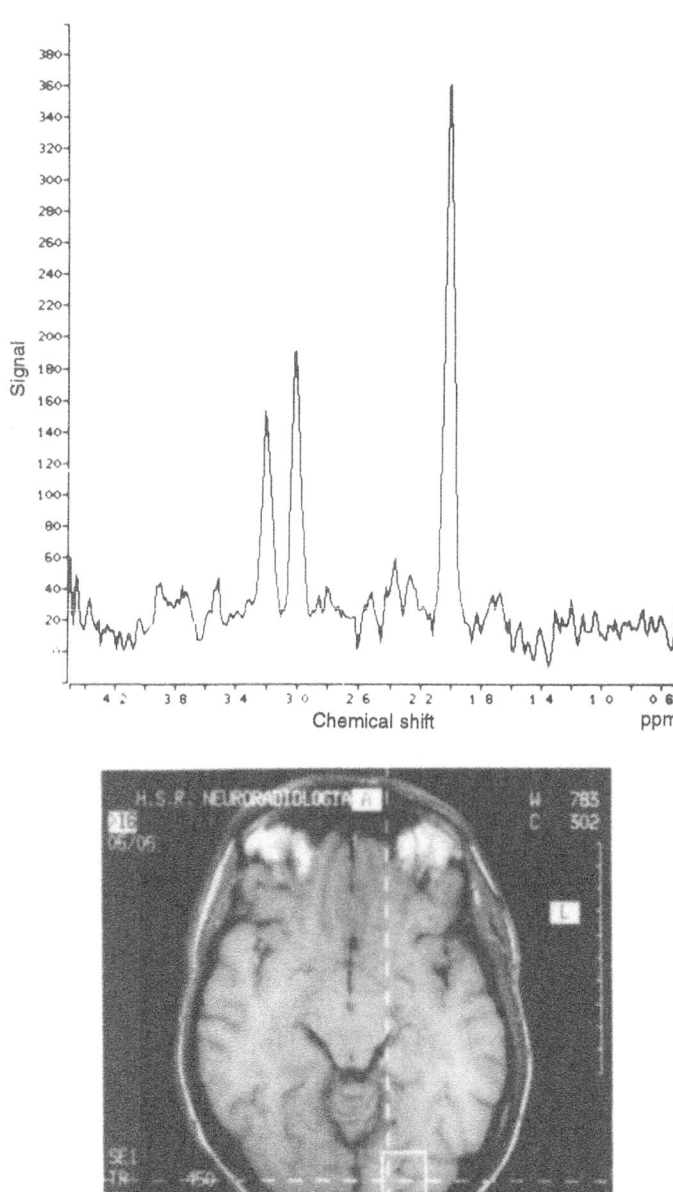

Figure 1. Normal volunteer, SE sequence with TE = 135 ms ^{1}H spectrum from the left occipital lobe shows a relatively high peak of NAA (2.00 p.p.m.) in comparison with choline (3.20 p.p.m.) and creatine (3.00 p.p.m.) peaks.

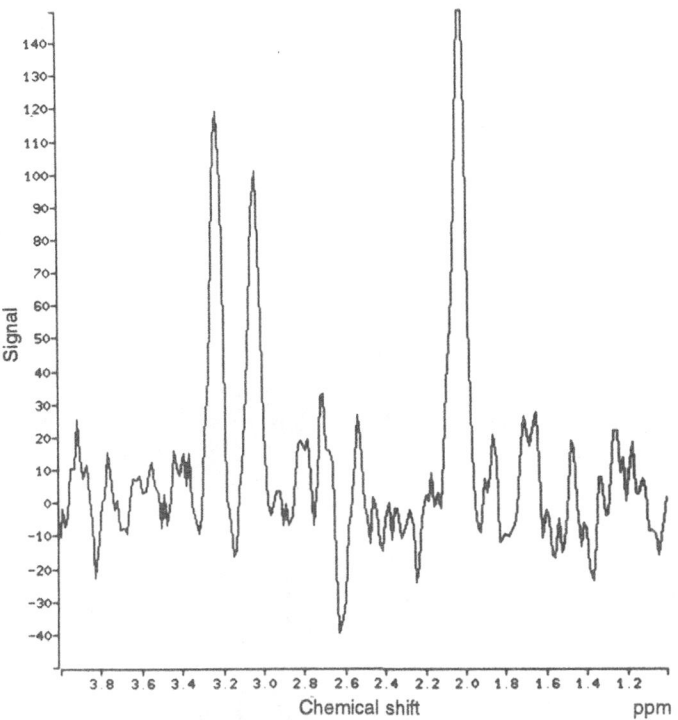

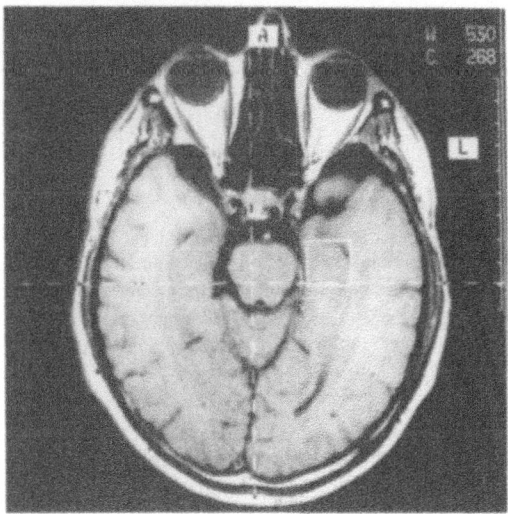

Figure 2. Normal volunteer, SE sequence with TE = 135 ms ^{1}H spectrum from the left hippocampal region shows a relative decrease of NAA peak with respect to choline and creatine peaks, with a reduction of NAA/Cho + Cr ratio.

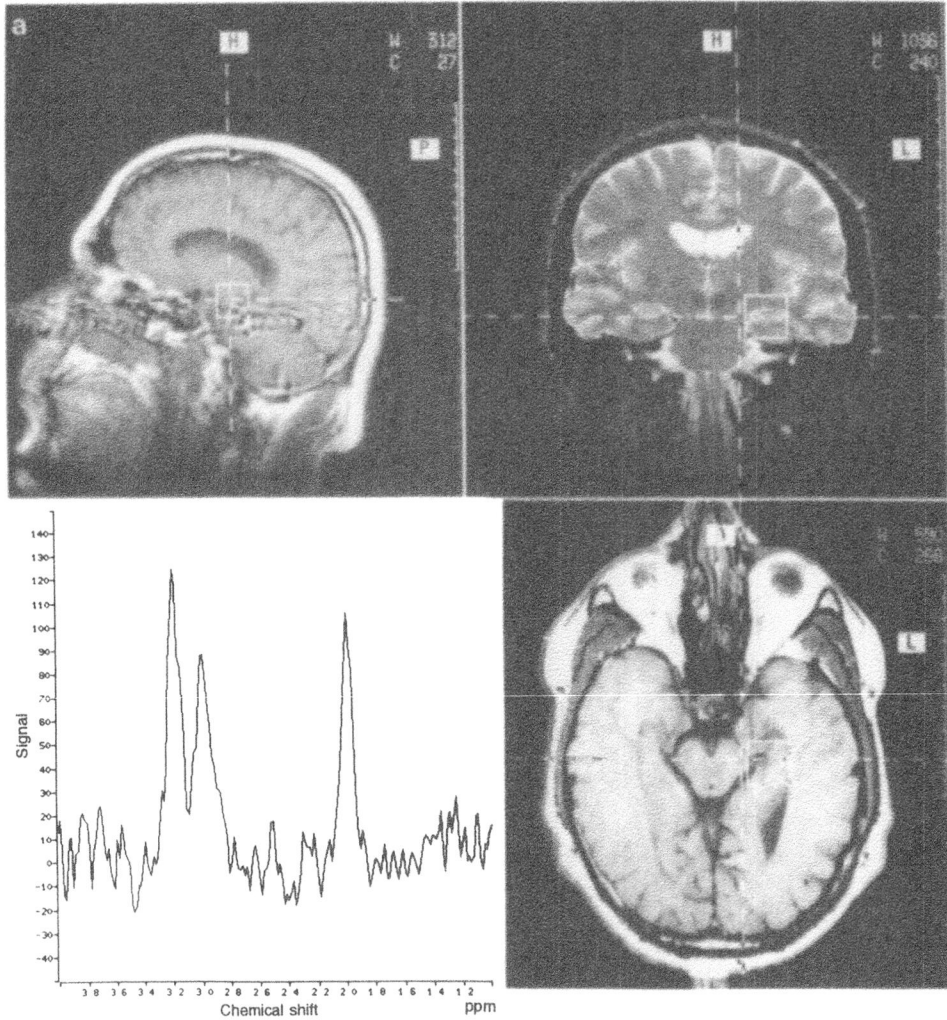

Figure 3. Patient with long-standing TLE and electrophysiological and MRI indicating (reduction in size of left hippocampus in comparison with the contralateral) left lateralisation of epileptogenic focus, SE sequence with TE = 135 ms. The spectrum of left hippocampus (a) shows a further decrease of NAA/Cho + Cr ratio in comparison with normal subjects; however, the NAA/Cho + Cr ratio of left hippocampus was higher than the NAA/Cho + Cr ratio of right hippocampus (b). The signal-to-noise ratio was reduced in both spectra, but the noise is particularly high in the right one.

which reported a striking decrease of NAA concentration in sclerotic hippocampus in comparison with normal hippocampus (Sutherland and Peeling, 1992). The reduction of NAA concentration could be reasonably due to the neuronal loss of the sclerotic regions, but a reduction of NAA concentration was reported by the same authors also in normal hippocampus with regard to the normal neocortex suggesting a normal regional variation of NAA between neo- and archicortex. Our personal experience carried out with a Magnetom Siemens SP 63, spin echo (SE) sequence, with TE (echo time) = 135, TR (relaxation time) = 1600 and 8 cm^3 VOIs, confirmed a regional variation of peak ratios in normal subjects, with a relative reduction of NAA in hippocampal regions (Figures 1 and 2).

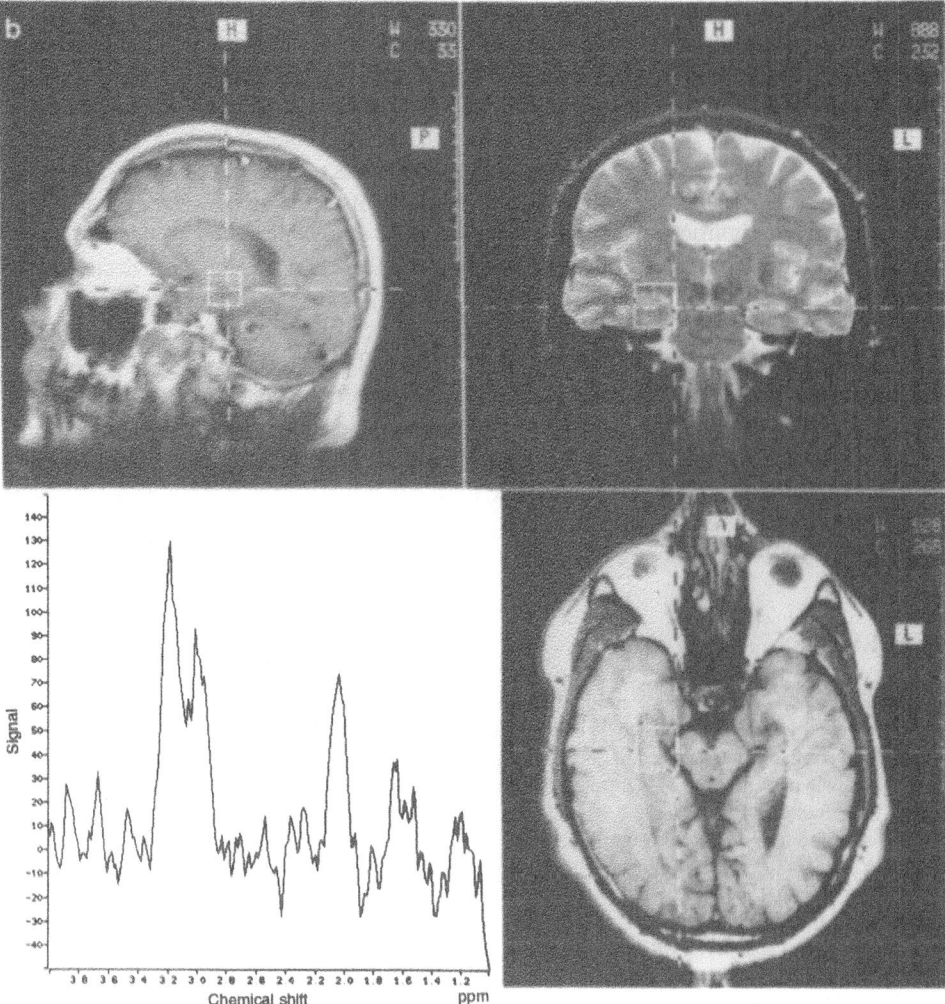

Due to the technical limitations previously reported the spectra collected in the temporo-mesial region showed an overall decrease of the signal-to-noise ratio and an increase in the normal inter-individual variation. The same difficulties were encountered in the evaluation of patients with temporal lobe epilepsy. Unlike the current literature we studied patients with long-standing, but relatively well controlled, TLE in which a previous lateralisation of the epileptogenic focus was obtained with routine MRI evaluation (Triulzi et al., 1988). In the four patients studied so far, the NAA/Cho and NAA/Cho + Cr ratios showed mainly a reduction in comparison with the normal data, but the reduction involved both sides with contradictory results with respect to the lateralisation of the focus achieved with electrophysiological and MRI techniques (Figure 3). If the sensitivity of the state-of-the-art localised ^{1}H-MRS technique did not appear to be superior to MRI, the specificity was not investigated at all, but it is well known from the literature that different types of primitive brain tumours, such as an infiltrating astrocytoma or an ependymoma, showed a "gliotic" spectral pattern, with a relative reduction of NAA (Alger et al., 1990).

PROBABLE DEVELOPMENT OVER THE NEXT FIVE YEARS

The localised ^{1}H-MRS technology clinically available today (TE values of 135 or 270 ms) does not show any clear advantage in the evaluation of ^{1}H-MRS in TLE patients in comparison with the traditional MRI evaluation or with the functional in vivo analysis of SPECT and PET. However, the recent development of new acquisition techniques could probably reduce some of the practical limitations. A promising technique in which the conventional TE of 135 or 270 ms was reduced to 20 ms was recently proposed (Frahm et al., 1991). Using a short echo time sequence, the reduction of the delay between excitation and detection causes a significant increase in signal-to-noise ratio which allows a decrease in the size of the volume of interest up to 4 ml. Secondly the reduction of delay time decreases the influence of the artefacts related to vessel pulsatility. Another interesting development in ^{1}H-MRS acquisition techniques, relatively close to clinical application, is the chemical shift imaging (CSI) technique (Sauter et al., 1991). With the CSI technique, spectra can be collected simultaneously from different volumes covering an entire brain section. CSI could be extremely useful in the direct comparison of the epileptogenic zone to the contralateral normal brain and in the evaluation of the extent of the epileptogenic lesion. Preliminary data concerning the CSI evaluation of patient with intractable focal epilepsy are encouraging; in all the cases the lateralisation of the epileptogenic focus was correctly predicted by CSI (Comair et al., 1992; Hugg et al., 1992; Miller-Lisse et al., 1992)

REFERENCES

Alger, J.R., Frank, J.A., Bizzi, A., et al., 1990, Metabolism of human gliomas: assessment with H-1 MR spectroscopy and F-18 fluorodeoxyglucose PET, Radiology, 177: 633–41.

Allard, M., Portais, J.C., Franconi, J.M., et al., 1992, In vivo proton magnetic resonance spectroscopy of focal epilepsy in humans, SMRM '92, Book of Abstracts, p. 1717.

Breiter, S.N., Barker, P.B., Mathews, V.P., et al., 1992, Proton magnetic resonance spectroscopy in patients with seizure disorders, SMRM '92, abstract p. 644.

Comair, Y.G., Ng, T.C., Xue, M., et al., 1992, Proton chemical shift imaging/ spectroscopy of epilepsy, SMRM '92, abstract p. 1945.

Connelly, A., Gadian, D.G., Jackson, G.D., et al., 1992, 1H spectroscopy in the investigation of intractable temporal lobe epilepsy, SMRM '92, abstract p 234.

Frahm, J., Bruhn, H., Hanicke, W., et al., 1991, Localised proton NMR spectroscopy from brain tumours using short-echo time STEAM sequences, J Comput Assist Tomogr. 15: 915–922.

Hugg, J.W., Laxer, K.D., Matson, G.B., et al., 1992, 1H MR spectroscopic imaging detects neuron loss more sensitively than MRI in focal epilepsy, SMRM '92, abstract p. 1913.

Jackson, G.D., Berkovic, S.F., Tress, B.M., et al., 1990, Hippocampal sclerosis can be reliably detected by magnetic resonance imaging, Neurology 40: 1869–1875.

Kato, T., Mikami, I., Takashima, S., et al., 1992, Proton MR spectroscopy of the pediatric brain with focal epilepsy, SMRM '92, abstract p. 2006.

Matthews, P.M., Andermann, F., and Arnold, D.L., 1990, A proton magnetic resonance spectroscopy study of focal epilepsy in humans, Neurology 40: 985–989.

Miller-Lisse, U., Truber, F., Layer, G., et al., 1992, Proton MR spectroscopic imaging (MRSI) in the pre-surgical diagnosis of temporal lobe epilepsy, SMRM '92, abstract p. 1946.

Sauter, R., Schneider, M., Wiclow, K., and Kolem, H., 1991, Localised 1H MRS of the human brain: single-voxel versus CSI techniques, J Magn Res Imag. 1, abstract 241.

Sutherland, G.R., and Peeling, J., 1992, 1H magnetic resonance spectroscopy of extracts of epileptic neocortex and hippocampus, SMRM '92, abstract p. 1914.

Triulzi, F., Franceschi, M., Fazio, F., and Del Maschio, A., 1988, MRI (1.5 T) in patients with non-refractory temporal lobe epilepsy, Radiology 166:181–185.

THE POTENTIAL OF PROTON MR SPECTROSCOPY FOR MONITORING

Pathological Alterations of Human Cerebral Metabolism In Vivo

H. Bruhn, K.D. Merboldt, W. Hänicke, and J. Frahm

Max-Planck-Institut für biophysikalische Chemie
Postfach 2841
37018 Göttingen
Germany

INTRODUCTION

Recent progress in image-controlled, localised proton MR spectroscopy (MRS) offers a non-invasive tool to gain metabolic information about pathologies of the human central nervous system (CNS) in vivo. Study protocols that are suitable for clinical examinations combine T1- and T2-weighted MR imaging based on fast-scan gradient echo sequences and proton MRS of multiple regions-of-interest within total investigational times of about one hour.

CURRENT RESEARCH

Insights into brain biochemistry by proton MRS rely on the identification (and quantification) of cerebral metabolites in localised spectral acquisitions. So far, more than a dozen compounds have been identified with the use of the short echo time STEAM localisation method (TE = 20 ms) (Frahm et al., 1990).

Proton MR spectra of healthy brain exhibit resonances from N-acetylaspartate (NAA) and N-acetyl-aspartyl-glutamate (both neuronal in origin), choline-containing compounds (Cho, predominantly phosphocholine, glycerophosphorylcholine and plasmalogen), creatines (Cr, creatine and phosphocreatine), glutamate (Glu), myo-inositol [(Ins) probably only in glial cells], scyllo-inositol, glucose (Glc) and lactate (Lac) (Frahm et al., 1991a; Merboldt et al., 1992; Michaelis et al., 1991, 1993a,b).

Figure 1 shows a typical proton MR spectrum of cerebral white matter obtained at 2.0 T (Siemens Magnetom). Spectral differences are observed for different brain regions. They have been quantified and attributed to variable levels of pertinent metabolites. For example, for a repetition time of TR=3 s, the Cho/Cr signal ratio is about 0.5–0.6 in cortical grey matter and

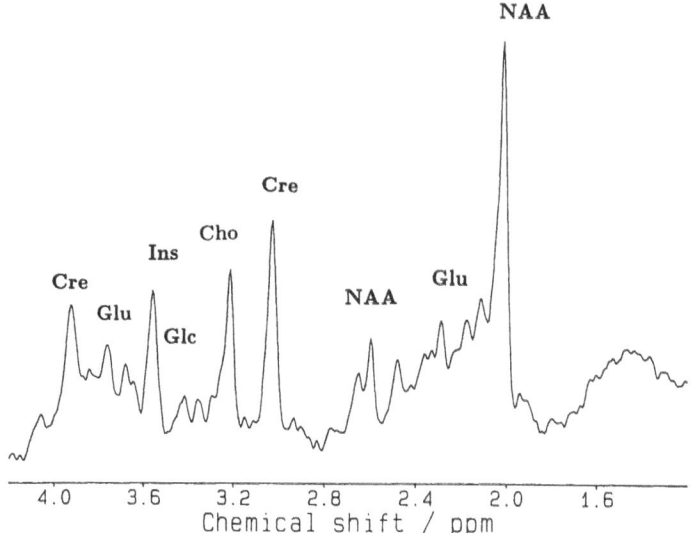

Figure 1. Proton magnetic resonance spectrum of a 4-year-old male in vivo (parietal white matter: 8 ml volume-of-interest, TR 3000/TE 20/128 scans). See text for abbreviations of resonance assignments.

0.9–1.0 in parietal white matter. Absolute metabolite concentrations may be determined by taking fully relaxed acquisitions (TR = 6 s) at a mild penalty in signal-to-noise per measuring time (Michaelis et al., 1991). The study of healthy subjects also reveals a dependence of the detectable metabolite pattern on age. Although the greatest changes occur during brain maturation in the first 6 months of life, e.g. a marked decrease of Cho and Ins and an increase of NAA (Bruhn et al., 1992a) more subtle changes such as a slow decrease in the NAA/Cr ratio proceed throughout ageing (Bruhn et al., 1992b).

The clinical use of proton MRS is still in its infancy. A large number of applications are currently being explored. So far, our studies aim at two major goals: (i) direct use for diagnostic purposes and therapy control, and (ii) a pathophysiological elucidation of disease to develop new diagnostic and therapeutic strategies. Although first applications dealt with focal brain lesions such as infarcts (Bruhn et al., 1989a), tumours (Bruhn et al., 1989b; Frahm et al., 1991b) and multiple sclerosis, (Bruhn et al., 1992c), various general affections of the CNS such as metabolic diseases of childhood and neurodegenerative diseases in adults are now being investigated (Bruhn et al., 1991a,b, 1992a,b). In most cases, proton MRS of brain pathologies reveals striking variations of the metabolite concentrations found in normal brain parenchyma. Moreover, the occurrence of resonances from elevated levels of, e.g. alanine, GABA, glutamine, glycine and mobile fatty acids yield valuable additional information on specific metabolic deficiencies. Exciting prospects have been demonstrated by the ability of proton MRS to monitor pathological alterations of the CNS that are caused by malfunction of internal organs, e.g. increased brain glucose in diabetes mellitus (Bruhn et al., 1991c) and increased brain glutamine in liver disease (Bruhn et al., 1991d, 1992a).

DISCUSSION

In general, MRS of cerebral metabolites adds a biochemical dimension to a modality well established for imaging anatomy at high spatial resolution and with excellent soft tissue contrast. However, the interpretation of spectral results is not always straightforward and detailed studies have to pave the way for a translation into clear-cut biochemical conclusions or medical decisions. Although pathologies may clearly demonstrate an abnormal metabolic behaviour by marked spectral alterations, the observations often lack an easy understanding and raise new questions rather than provide definite answers.

A typical example is shown in Figure 2 where the proton MR spectrum of a child with alternating hemiplegia reveals a relatively high Cho/Cr ratio and a low level of myo-inositol. How can these findings be related to the cerebrovascular malfunction as the putative cause of this disease? Speculative interpretations such as a preferential involvement of the glial cell population without affection of the neuronal cells may unravel previously unrecognised pathogenic clues to a specific but not well-understood disease; however, they do not necessarily solve any problem for the individual patient.

At this stage, general concepts for the interpretation of proton MR spectra from cerebral pathologies centre around only a few MR-sensitive "marker" substances that can be assigned to specific cell populations and/or linked to specific metabolic disturbances. Being both prominent and easy to detect, NAA is exclusively neuronal in origin and therefore could provide an objective in vivo assessment or "indicator function" for neuronal damage or loss. Further compounds include choline and myo-inositol (not in neurons?) for their biochemical role as intermediaries of phopholipids involved in membrane synthesis (cell proliferation) as well as lactate and alanine for their role in increased glycolysis and impaired mitochondrial respiration indicating vital cerebral tissue to be in jeopardy.

FUTURE PROSPECTS

Although further improvements in hardware technology will continue to improve the technical reliability of localised MRS data, software developments will be concerned with more automatised set-ups of MRS studies as well as with a user-independent and quantitative evaluation of spectral data. However, even the present development of localisation strategies, in addition to their practical implementation and technical handling, have reached a level suitable for more expanded use in clinical research. Experience and confidence based on an increasing number of applications will lead to clinical indications for proton MRS including

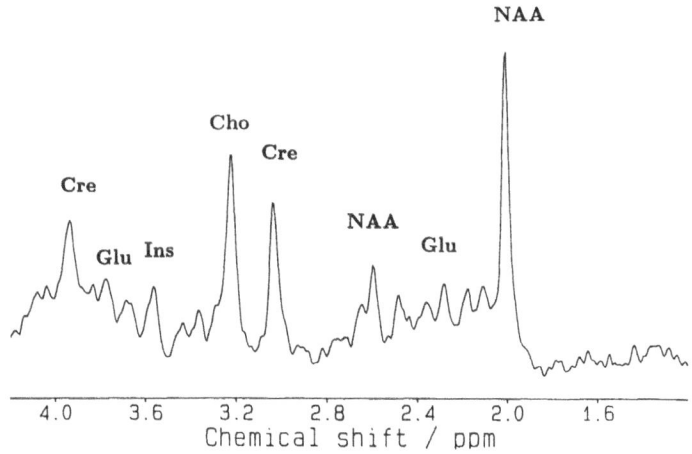

Figure 2. Proton MR spectrum (parietal white matter: volume-of-interest 8 ml, TR 3000/TE 20/128 scans) of a 4-year-old girl with alternating hemiplegia showing a decreased level of myo-inositol and an elevated ratio of Cho/Cr.

the elucidation of epileptic foci, e.g. in temporal lobe epilepsies. In the foreseeable future, the combination of metabolite spectroscopy with oxygenation-sensitive functional MR imaging (Frahm et al., 1992) looms at the horizon of epilepsy research.

REFERENCES

Bruhn,H., Frahm, J., Gyngell, M.L., Hänicke, W., and Sauter, R., 1989a, Cerebral metabolism in man after acute stroke. New observations using localised proton NMR spectroscopy, Magn Reson Med. 9: 126–131.

Bruhn, H., Frahm, J., Gyngell, M.L., Merboldt, K.D., Hänicke, W., Sauter, R., and Hamburger, C., 1989b, Noninvasive differentiation of tumours with use of localised H-1 MR spectroscopy in vivo: initial experience in patients with cerebral tumours, Radiology 172: 541–548.

Bruhn, H., Wilichowski, E., Hanefeld, F., Merboldt, K.D., Michaelis, T., and Frahm., J., 1991a, Cerebral findings in children with mitochondrial disorders. Metabolic disturbances detected by localised proton MRS, in: "SMRM Book of Abstracts," p. 192, Society of Magnetic Resonance in Medicine, Berkeley, CA.

Bruhn, H., Weber, T., Thorwirth, V., and Frahm, J., 1991b, In vivo monitoring of neuronal loss in Creutzfeldt-Jakob disease by proton MRS, Lancet 337: 1610–1611.

Bruhn, H., Michaelis, T., Merboldt, K.D., Hänicke, W., Gyngell, M.L., and Frahm, J., 1991c, Monitoring cerebral glucose in diabetics by proton MRS, Lancet 337: 745–746.

Bruhn, H., Merboldt, K.D., Michaelis, T., et al., 1991d, Proton MRS of metabolic disturbances in the brain of patients with liver cirrhosis and subclinical hepatic encephalopathy, in: "SMRM Book of Abstracts," p. 400, Society of Magnetic Resonance in Medicine, Berkeley, CA.

Bruhn, H., Kruse, B., Korenke, G.C., Hanefeld, F., Hänicke, W., Merboldt, K.D, and Frahm, J., 1992a, Proton NMR spectroscopy of cerebral metabolic alterations in infantile peroxisomal disorders, J. Comput Assist Tomogr. 16: 335–344.

Bruhn, H., Stoppe, G., Merboldt, K.D., Michaelis, T., Hänicke, W., and Frahm, J., 1992b, Cerebral metabolic alterations in normal aging and Alzheimer's dementia detected by localised proton magnetic resonance spectroscopy, in: "SMRM Book of Abstracts," p. 752, Society of Magnetic Resonance in Medicine, Berkeley, CA.

Bruhn, H., Frahm, J., Merboldt, K.D., Hänicke, W., Hanefeld, F., Christen, H.J., Kruse, B., and Bauer, H.J., 1992c, Multiple sclerosis in children: cerebral metabolic alterations monitored by localised proton magnetic resonance spectroscopy in vivo, Ann Neurol. 32: 140–150.

Frahm, J., Michaelis, T., Merboldt, K.D., Bruhn, H., Gyngell, M.L., Hänicke, W., 1990, Improvements in localised proton NMR spectroscopy of human brain. Water suppression, short echo times, and 1 ml resolution, J Magn Reson. 90: 464–473.

Frahm, J., Michaelis, T., Merboldt, K.D., and Hänicke, W., Gyngell, M.L. and Bruhn, H., 1991a, On the N-acetyl methyl resonance in localised proton NMR spectra of human brain in vivo, NMR Biomed. 4: 201–204.

Frahm, J., Bruhn, H., Hänicke, W., Merboldt, K.D., Mursch, K., Markakis, E., 1991b, Localised proton NMR spectroscopy of brain tumours using short echo-time STEAM sequences, J Comput Assist Tomogr. 15: 915–922.

Frahm, J., Bruhn, H., Merboldt, K.D., and Hänicke, K.D., 1992, Dynamic MRI of Human Brain Oxygenation During Rest and Photic Stimulation, J Magn Reson Imag. 2.

Merboldt, K.D., Bruhn, H., Hänicke, W., Michaelis, T., and Frahm, J., 1992, Decrease of glucose in the human visual cortex during photic stimulation, Magn Reson Med. 25: 187–194.

Michaelis, T., Merboldt, K.D., Hänicke, W., Gyngell, M.L., Bruhn, H., and Frahm, J., 1991, On the identification of cerebral metabolites in localised proton NMR spectra of human brain in vivo, NMR Biomed. 4: 90–98.

Michaelis, T., Helms, G., Merboldt, K.D., Hänicke, W., Bruhn, H., and Frahm, J., 1993a, Identification of scyllo-inositol in proton NMR spectra of human brain in vivo, NMR Biomed in press.

Michaelis, T., Bruhn, H., Gyngell, M.L., Hänicke, W., Merboldt, K.D., and Frahm, J., 1993b, Quantification of cerebral metabolites in man. Results using short-echo time localised proton MRS, in: "SMRM Book of Abstracts," p. 387, Society of Magnetic Resonance in Medicine, Berkeley, CA.

QUANTITATIVE PROTON MR SPECTROSCOPY OF THE HUMAN BRAIN

O. Henriksen, P. Christiansen, H.B.W. Larsson, and M. Stubgaard

Danish Research Center of Magnetic Resonance
Hvidovre Hospital
Hvidovre
Denmark

INTRODUCTION

Proton magnetic resonance spectroscopy (^{1}H-MRS) of the human brain has developed rapidly during the recent years. The techniques currently used include measurements in a single volume of interest or position-encoded spectroscopy (chemical shift imaging, CSI). The pulse sequences are based on stimulated echo techniques, (STEAM) (Frahm et al., 1989) or double spin echo techniques (compare Luyten et al., 1991) preceeded by water signal suppression pulses.

The metabolites which can be detected include N-acetylaspartate (NAA), creatine and phospocreatine (Cr + PCr), choline containing compounds (Cho), inositols (Ino) and glutamine/glutamate (Glu/Glu).

Quantification of metabolite concentrations of the human brain is associated with a number of experimental difficulties related to the MR equipment as well as to the biological systems. Among factors related to the MR equipment are variations in flip angles due to B_1 field inhomogeneities, inter-individual variation in receiver efficiency due to variation in coil loading etc. Biological factors include T1 and T2 relaxation processes, and nuclear coupling phenomena i.e. J-coupling. MR visibility also has to be considered. A thorough presentation of different approaches for quantification of metabolite concentration has been given by Tofts and Wray (1988). By including external standards (samples with known solutions) the problems of coil loading are solved. Still supplementary studies for B_1 inhomogeneities and spatial variations in receiver coil sensitivity are needed. The use of internal standards may be more attractive because all the problems related to the MR equipment mentioned above can be solved. The concentration of the internal standard has to be known and to remain constant during the different physiological and pathophysiological conditions.

We propose the use of the unsaturated water signal as internal standard for the following reasons: the water signal can be obtained with a high signal-to-noise ratio in one acquisition, and the total water content of brain tissue varies very little (probably less than 10% in most

Magnetic Resonance Scanning and Epilepsy, Edited by S.D. Shorvon et al.,
Plenum Press, New York, 1994

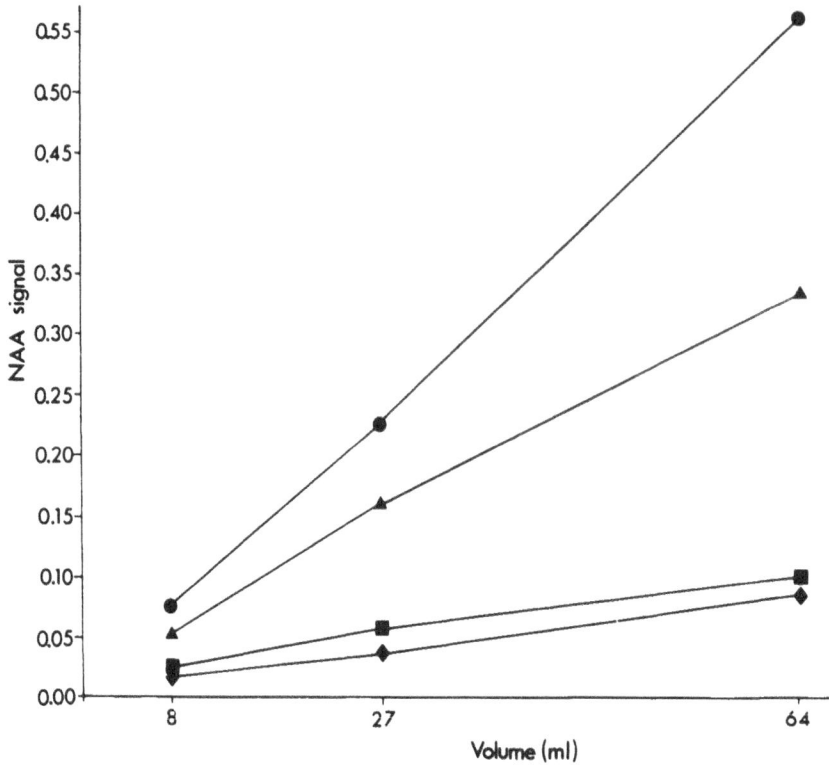

Figure 1. NAA signal obtained in a phantom containing a 10 mmol/l NAA solution is plotted against the selected volume size. The signals are obtained at four different echo times (46 ms, 92 ms, 136 ms and 272 ms).

circumstances). In the following, in vitro as well as in vivo studies are described with respect to implementation of this approach in practice (Christiansen et al., 1992).

CURRENT RESEARCH

The experiments have been carried out on a Siemens SP 63/84 whole body MR scanner operating at 1.5 T. For volume selective ^{1}H spectroscopy, STEAM pulse sequences with different echo times were used. We focused on methodological issues related to quantification as well as to the quality of the volume selection.

In Vitro Studies

In a number of studies on test objects, we found a reasonable signal linearity with the size of the selected volume and with the metabolite concentration. The question of contamination of signal originating from the outer volume was tested in a two-compartment test object (EEC Concerted Action, 1989) containing cyclohexane and methyl acetate in the inner and outer compartments, respectively. The results indicate that signal contamination from the outer volume is negligible. Finally the B_1 field homogeneity has been tested in a water phantom. The variation coefficient of the water signal obtained at 15 different locations was about 5%. Maximum deviations from the value obtained in the centre was 10%.

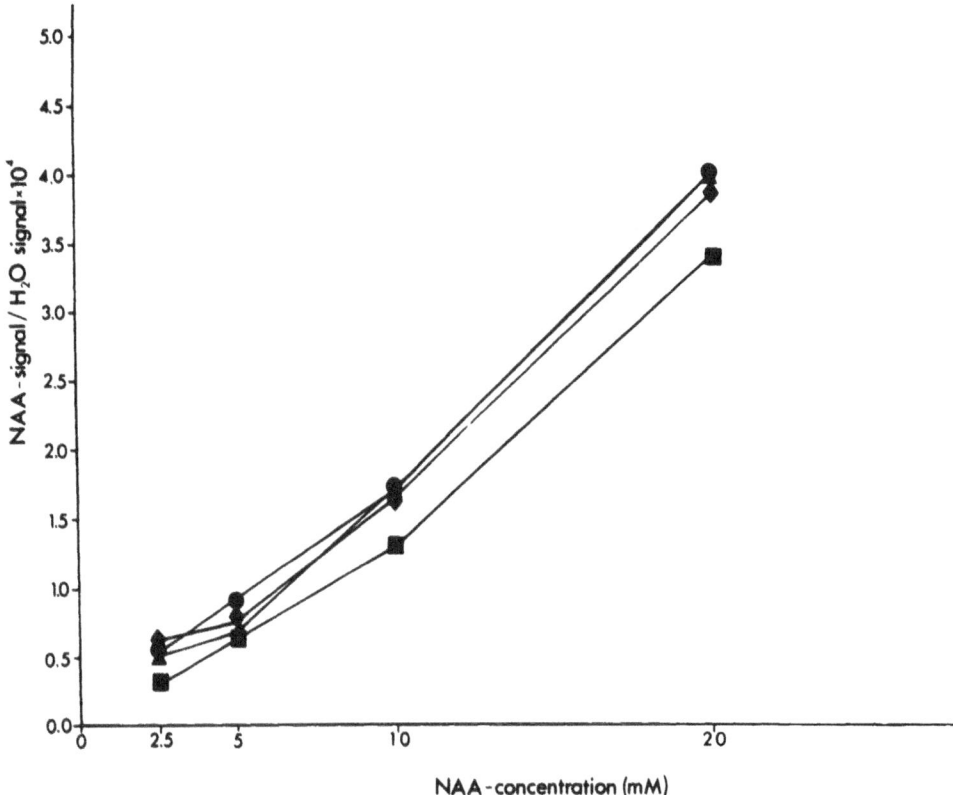

Figure 2. NAA signal obtained in phantoms where the NAA concentrations in the solutions are varied (2.5 mmol/l, 5 mmol/l, 10 mmol/l, and 20 mmol/l).

In Vivo Studies

The method was applied on five healthy volunteers. The selected volumes were located in the occipital region. We found a high linear correlation between the signal intensities of NAA, Cho, Cr + PCr, and selected volume sizes (8–27 ml). The same was true for the water signal.

Finally, based on selective measurements of T1 and T2 relaxation times and assuming a fractional water content of 75%, we calculated the concentrations in mmol/l ± 1 SD of NAA, Cho and Cr + PCr to be 11 ± 1.3, 1.7 ± 0.5 and 8 ± 1.4, respectively.

DISCUSSION

The results presented above indicate that the use of the unsaturated water signal as internal standard may give a reasonable first order approximation of metabolite concentration in the brain.

The method should be compared with those using external standards. The major draw back of our method is that the fractional water content has to be known. We assumed this to be 75% as an average for the mixture of grey and white matter within the selected volume.

In the present experimental conditions, we believe that in most physiological and pathophysiological conditions the variation in the average water content is less than 10%.

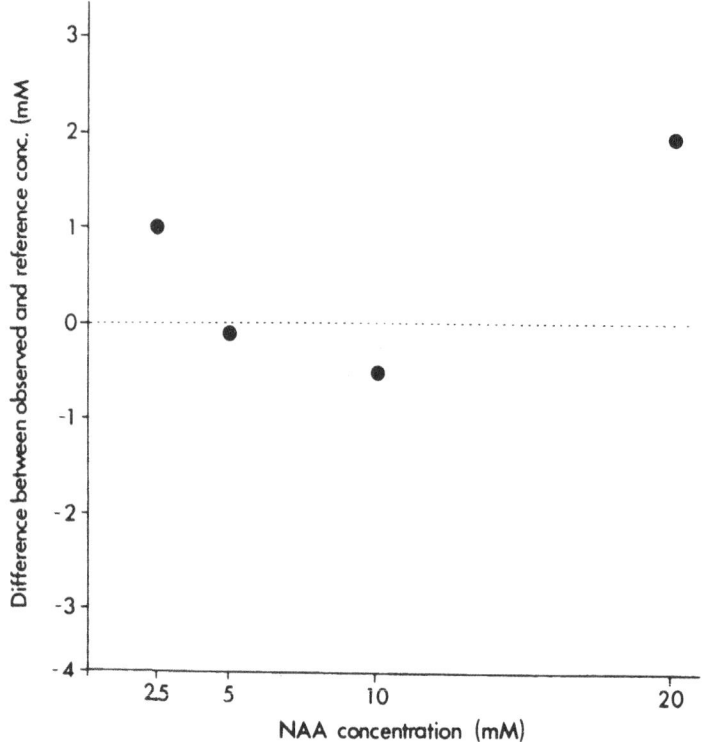

Figure 3. The differences between the calculated NAA concentrations and the reference values are plotted against the NAA concentrations in the solutions.

Using external standards the B_1 inhomogeneities have to be taken into account. Our results indicate a B_1 variation as high as 10%, suggesting that such errors are of the same magnitude as the uncertainties in the estimation of the tissue water content.

The internal standard approach may be hampered by MR-invisible water in the tissue. The possible magnitude of this source of error is not known and further research is warranted. On the other hand, the external standard method may be hampered by errors, in case imperfections in volume selection vary with location.

The two methods share the problems related to biological factors including tissue heterogeneity (partial volume effects), relaxation behaviour etc. The same is true regarding problems associated with post-processing of the spectra.

FUTURE DEVELOPMENTS

Further studies are needed in order to assess variations in tissue water content as well as to explore the question of MR-invisible water. The techniques should be improved to make it possible to reduce the size of the selected volume. Chemical shift spectroscopic imaging appears as an attractive solution, but a thorough quality assessment is needed in order to test the reliability of this approach for absolute quantification of metabolites in the brain.

We believe that such quantification techniques will offer valuable clinical information in patients with temporal lobe epilepsy.

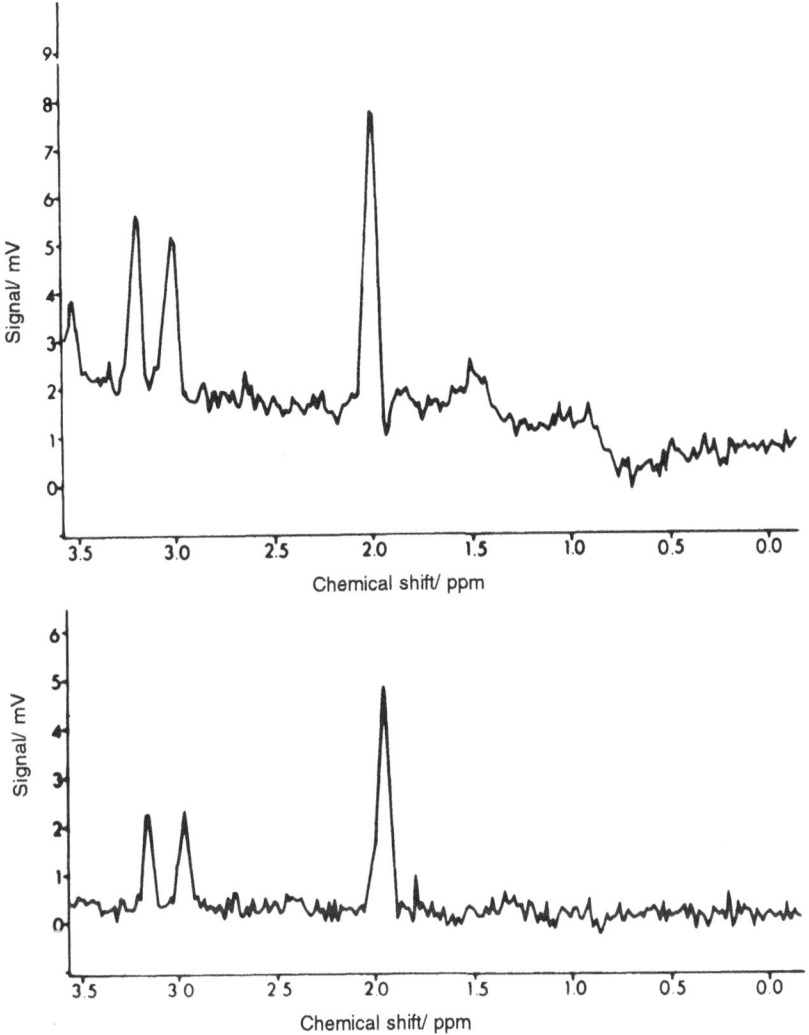

Figure 4. Examples of in vivo proton spectra obtained in a 8 ml volume in the occipital part of the human brain. The spectra are obtained at echo times of 136 ms (above) and 272 ms (below).

REFERENCES

Christiansen, P., Henriksen, O., Stubgaard, M., et al., 1992, In vivo quantification of brain metabolites by ^{1}H-MRS using water as an internal standard, Magn Reson Imaging 10: 001–012.

EEC Concerted Action Comac/BME. II 1.3.4., 1989, Eurospin 21: 22–25.

Frahm, J., Bruhn, H., and Gyngell, L., 1989, Localised proton NMR spectroscopy in different regions of the human brain in vivo, Magn Reson Med. 11: 47–63.

Luyten, P.R., Mariën, J.H., and Hollander, J.A., 1991, Acquisition and quantitation in proton spectroscopy, NMR Biomed. 4: 64–69.

Tofts, P.S., and Wray, S.A., 1988, A critical assessment of methods of measuring metabolite concentrations by NMR spectroscopy, NMR Biomed. 1: 1–10.

IMAGE-GUIDED PROTON MR SPECTROSCOPY IN EPILEPSY

P.J. Cozzone, J. Vion-Dury, S. Confort-Gouny, F. Nicoli, and B. Chabrol

Centre de Résonance Magnétique Biologique et Médicale
Faculté de Médecine de Marseille
27 Boulevard J. Moulin
13005 Marseille
France

INTRODUCTION

Localised proton magnetic resonance (MR) spectroscopy of the human brain is a new non-invasive technique which allows the detection of cerebral intermediary and oxidative metabolites (Hanstock et al., 1988). MR spectra can be obtained by using either single-volume acquisition sequences (such as STEAM, ISIS, VSE sequences) or multiple volume acquisition sequences such as the spectroscopic imaging (SI) technique which provides a display of metabolite maps (for a review, see Confort-Gouny et al., 1992a).

The cerebral metabolic impact of the epileptic seizures and status epilepticus is very severe, because epileptic seizures make the greatest metabolic demand on the brain and severely challenge its ability to maintain homoeostatic mechanisms (Wasterlain, 1989). The most recent publications emphasise that proton MR spectroscopy can detect the metabolic damage related to epileptic seizures in human brain ex vivo (cerebral biopsies) (Petroff et al., 1989) and in vivo (Matthews et al., 1990). Localised proton MR spectroscopy has demonstrated that epilepsy induces, in the epileptic focus, a loss of N-acetylaspartate in relation with the decrease in neuronal activity (neuronal loss?) and in some cases an increase of lactate in relation with the relative hypoxia which occurs during the seizures.

CURRENT RESEARCH

Our research is performed on a clinical Siemens SP 63 system equipped with a 1.5 T whole-body magnet. The sequence currently available on this system, for localised proton MR spectroscopy of the brain is the STEAM sequence, based on short (20 ms) stimulated echoes (Frahm et al., 1991) . Short echoes allow the detection of cerebral free amino acids. Figure 1 displays a typical spectrum obtained on a control subject.

Magnetic Resonance Scanning and Epilepsy, Edited by S.D. Shorvon et al.,
Plenum Press, New York, 1994

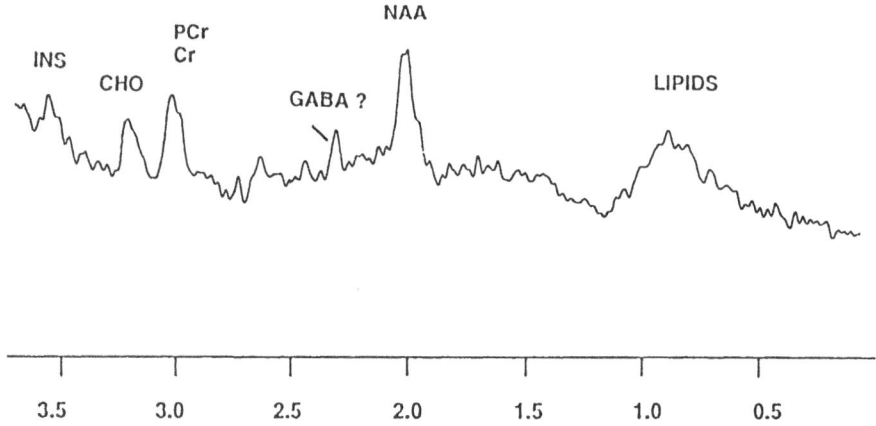

Figure 1. Localised proton MR spectroscopy of the human brain recorded on a control subject using a STEAM sequence (echo time:20 ms, voi size:8 ml). The assignment to taurine of the signal at 3.35 p.p.m. might be revised to scyllo-inositol according to Michaelis et al. (1992).

Metabolic data can be expressed as the ratio of the concentration (area of the MR signal) of a given metabolite to the sum of all the concentrations of the metabolites of interest detected on the spectroscopy. These metabolic ratios have been calculated on the 125 spectra recorded in 89 subjects (patients and controls) and processed by principal component analysis (PCA). The position of each patient displayed on a PCA map is in relationship to the respective weight of each metabolic parameter in the spectrum (Confort-Gouny et al., 1992b). Results obtained

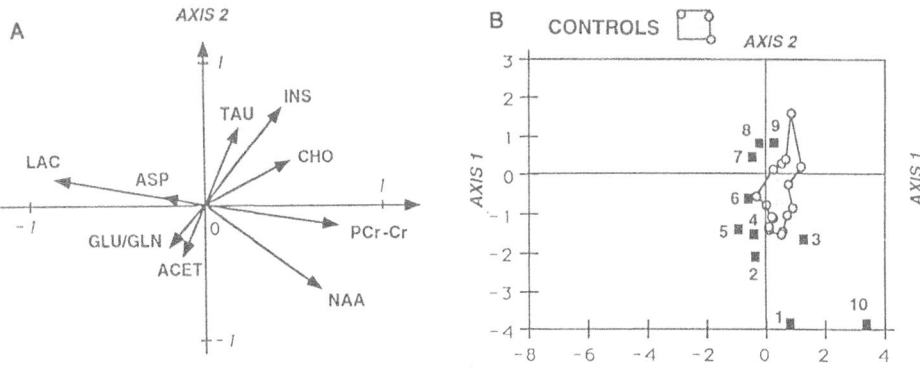

Figure 2. (A) Principal component analysis of 125 localised proton MR spectra recorded on 89 patients and normal volunteers. The contribution of each metabolic parameter (area of a given metabolite signal-Smet) to the two first axes is shown. (B) Individual positions of spectra on the PCA plot for patients presenting miscellaneous neurological diseases: 1 = epilepsy (permanent convulsive seizures); 2 = epilepsy (suspected focus), 3 and 5 = cerebral tuberculosis (respectively out and in the abscess); 4 = lesion of corpus callosum (abscess ?); 6 = mitochondrial encephalomyopathy, 7 = Parkinson's disease, 8 = haemispheric compression by hematoma, 9 = MELAS syndrome, and 10 = paraneoplastic encephalopathy (bronchic adenocarcinoma).

in epileptic patients are scattered on the PCA map and do not indicate clear trends in the alterations of metabolite levels.

In Figure 2B, position number 1 on the map, characterising the spectrum obtained from the temporo-occipital area of an epileptic patient with an anterior temporal lobe continuous seizure and treated by sodium valproate, can be explained by the presence of a new signal in the amino acid region. This new signal was tentatively assigned to gamma-aminobutyric acid GABA (Figure 3). Position number 2, characterising a spectrum recorded from the suspected parieto-occipital focus of a patient with secondarily generalised seizures, is compatible with a relative decrease in inositol, choline and NAA , in agreement with Sutherland and Peeling (1992).

It is noteworthy that, in particular conditions, localised proton MR spectroscopy can detect the presence of GABA, an inhibitory neurotransmitter controlling the spreading of epileptic discharges. Figure 3 displays a spectrum of a patient treated by sodium valproate, an anti-epileptic drug which induces an increase in intracerebral GABA concentration. Similar results have been already obtained in animals using another GABA-mimetic drug, vigabatrin (Preece et al., 1991).

DISCUSSION

For the first, time a non-invasive technique allows one to obtain a direct observation of the metabolism in the brain of epileptic patients without injection of radionuclides. In epilepsy, as in other neurological diseases, MR spectroscopy gives precise information about brain tissue suffering, as a metabolic complement to the electrical modifications observed during both the seizure and the post-critical period. The low sensitivity of localised MR spectroscopy limits the detection to the intermediary and oxidative metabolites present in the brain in millimolar or submillimolar concentration. Direct monitoring of neurotransmission impairment is still excluded at the present time. In addition, localised MR spectroscopy may provide a direct follow-up of the pharmacological effects of anti-epileptic drugs.

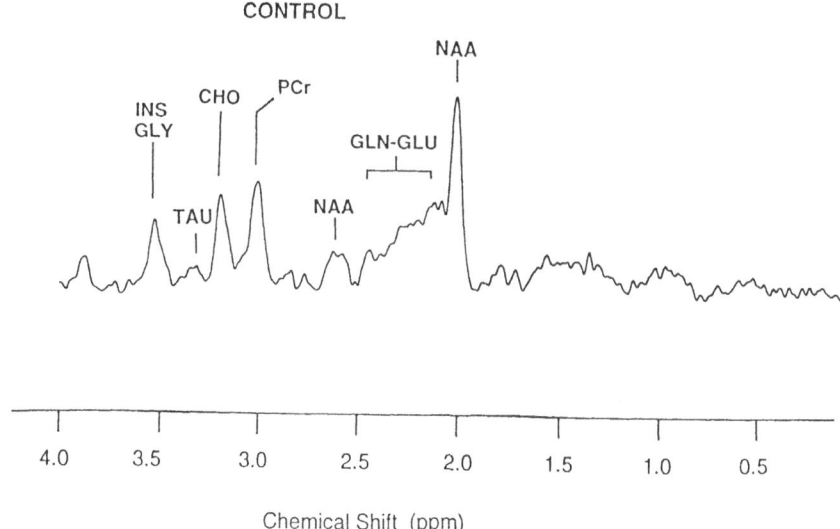

Figure 3. Localised proton MR spectrum recorded on the occipital cortex from the first patient (spectrum was recorded outside the epileptic focus) under treatment with high doses of sodium valproate. The signal at 2.25 p.p.m. might be assigned to GABA.

PROBABLE DEVELOPMENTS OVER THE NEXT FIVE YEARS

Localised MR spectroscopy will probably show usefulness in three aspects of clinical epileptology:

(1) Localisation of the epileptic focus, in the intractable epilepsies, can be achieved using spectroscopic imaging methods. Recently, Hugg et al. (1992) have demonstrated that, on the NAA map, one can pinpoint the area where neurons are lost with a better sensitivity (nine cases out of nine) than with any other computerized imaging techniques. This kind of analysis could be performed following a standard MR imaging procedure on epileptic patients, during the same examination, to provide a better evaluation of the metabolic configuration of the focus and of the surrounding parenchyma.

(2) As mentioned above, MR spectroscopy of epileptic brain is a new way to evaluate the impact of anti-epileptic drugs, either by determining the effects of the drug on GABA levels (when GABA is detected) or, more routinely, by assessing the impact of an antiepileptic treatment upon brain suffering.

(3) Epilepsy in infancy is often related to a metabolic encephalopathy. In recent publications (Grood et al., 1991; Confort-Gouny et al., 1993), MR spectroscopy of the brain has proved suitable in the definition of abnormal metabolic brain patterns associated with these metabolic encephalopathies. Consequently, MR spectroscopy could become an examination systematically integrated into the MRI procedure, in search of the etiological origin of this form of epilepsy. This strategy is implemented on a routine basis at our centre in Marseille.

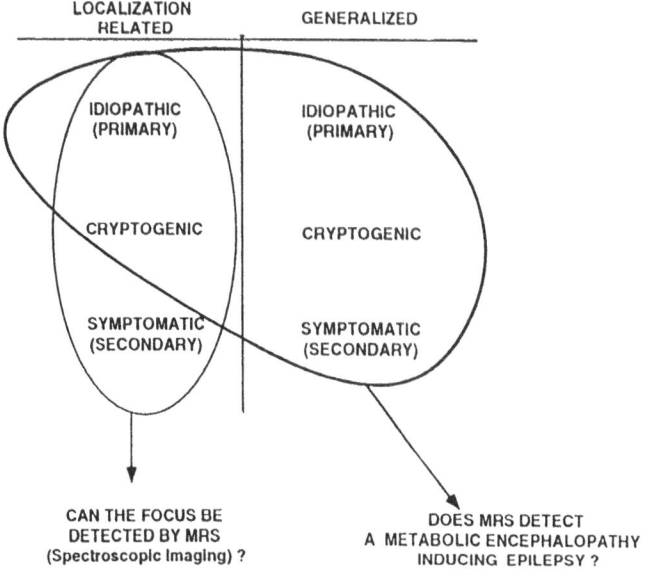

Figure 4. Possible future use of MR spectroscopy in the diagnosis of epilepsy.

In conclusion, proton MR spectroscopy of the brain will develop in the coming years as an indispensable tool in the study of some forms of epilepsy (Figure 4). This development will accelerate as (i) new technical and methodological breakthroughs continue to appear and are made available on MR spectrometers and (ii) an increasing number of clinical sites dedicate MR systems to the study of epilepsy.

ACKNOWLEDGEMENTS

This work is supported by the Administration de l'Assistance Publique à Marseille, the CNRS (URA 1186), the Direction de la Recherche et des Etudes Doctorales, the Association pour la Recherche sur le Cancer (ARC), the Association VML (Vaincre les Maladies Lysosomales), the Fondation pour la Recherche Médicale and the Ligue Nationale contre le Cancer.

REFERENCES

Confort-Gouny, S., Vion-Dury, J., and Cozzone, P.J., 1992a, Methodes de localisation du signal de RMN in vivo. Vers une approche métabolique des pathologies. J Radiol. (Paris) 73: 13–21.

Confort-Gouny, S., Vion-Dury, J., Nicoli, F. and Cozzone, P.J., 1992b, Metabolic characterization of neurological diseases by proton localised NMR spectroscopy of the human brain, CR Acad Sci (Paris) 315: 287–293.

Confort-Gouny, S., Chabrol, B., Vion-Dury, J., Mancini, J., and Cozzone, P.J., 1993, MRI and localised proton MRS in an early infantile form of neuronal ceroid lipofuscinosis, Pediatr Neurol 9: 57–60.

Frahm, J., Bruhn, H., Hänicke, W., Merboldt, K.D., Mursch, K., and Markakis, E. , 1991, Localised proton NMR spectroscopy of brain tumours using short echo time STEAM sequences. J Comp Assist Tomogr. 156: 915–922.

Grodd, W., Krageloh-Mann, I., Klose, U., and Sauter, R., 1991, Metabolic and destructive brain disorders in children: Findings with localised proton localised MR spectroscopy. Radiology, 481: 173–181.

Hanstock, C.C., Rothman, D.L., Prichard, J.W., Jue, T., and Shulman, R.G., 1988, Spatially localised 1H-NMR spectra of metabolites in the human brain, Proc Natl Acad Sci USA. 85: 1821–1825.

Hugg, J.W., Laxer, K.D., Matson, G.B., Maudsley, A.A., and Weiner, M.W., 1992, 1-H MR spectroscopic imaging detects neurons loss more sensitively than MRI in focal epilepsy. 11th Meeting of the Society of Magnetic Resonance in Medicine, Berlin, August 8–14, no. 1913.

Matthews, P.M., Andermann, F., and Arnold, D., 1990, A proton magnetic resonance spectroscopy study of focal epilepsy in humans. Neurology 40: 985–989.

Michaelis, T., Helms, G., Merboldt, K.D., Hänicke, W., Bruhn, H., and Frahm, J., 1992, First observation of the Scyllo-Inositol in proton NMR spectra of human brain, in vivo and in vitro. 11th Meeting of the Society of Magnetic Resonance in Medicine, Berlin, August 8–14, no. 541.

Petroff, O.A.C., Spencer, D.D., Alger, J.R., and Prichard, J.W., 1989, High-field proton magnetic resonance spectroscopy of human cerebrum obtained during surgery of epilepsy. Neurology 39: 1197–1202.

Preece, N.E., Williams, S.R., Jackson, G., Duncan, J.S., Houseman, J., and Gadian, D.G., 1991, 1-H NMR studies of vigabatrin induced increase in cerebral GABA, 10th Meeting of the Society of Magnetic Resonance in Medicine, San Francisco, August 10–16, no. 1000.

Sutherland, G.R. and Peeling, J., 1992, 1H Magnetic Resonance Spectroscopy of extracts of epilepsy neocortex and hippocampus. 11th Meeting of the Society of Magnetic Resonance in Medicine, Berlin, August 8–14, no. 1914.

Wasterlain, C., 1989, Epileptic seizures,in: "Basic Neurochemistry 4th", edn, G. Siegel, B. Agranoff, R.W. Alberts, and P. Molinoff, eds, Raven Press, New York.

TECHNIQUES FOR LOCALISATION AND SIGNAL IMPROVEMENT IN IN VIVO PROTON AND PHOSPHORUS MR SPECTROSCOPY

R. Sauter, M. Schneider, K. Wicklow, and H. Kolem

Siemens AG
Bereich Medizinische Technik
D-91050 Erlangen
Germany

INTRODUCTION

Magnetic resonance spectroscopy (MRS) is a unique tool providing non-invasive insight into human metabolism. At presence, the major limitations preventing a widespread clinical application of MRS are (i) the intrinsic low sensitivity of MR techniques, and (ii) the poor degree of integration and automation of techniques for localised MRS on commercially available MR scanners. On the other hand, the question for appropriate localisation techniques, exhaustively discussed in the early days of "whole body" MRS, can be considered solved: today, chemical shift resolved spectroscopic imaging (CSI, Brown et al., 1982; Maudsley et al., 1983) techniques have been established for ^{31}P MRS, whereas single-voxel techniques based on the stimulated echo (STEAM; Frahm et al., 1989) or the spin echo (SE; Bottomley, 1982) as well as hybrid techniques, combining CSI and single-voxel techniques are routinely used for ^{1}H MRS at many clinical MR scanners.

In in vivo ^{1}H MRS, sensitivity as well as specificity or the number of detectable metabolites can be increased significantly by acquiring the spectra with short echo times(TE) (Frahm et al., 1990). Short TE ^{1}H MRS generally reduces signal losses due to T2 relaxation, and especially for metabolites with complex multiplet patterns originating from intramolecular spin-spin coupling, dephasing due to J modulation is avoided. It is therefore desired to combine CSI techniques with short TE acquisition mode in order to improve the performance in spatial mapping of metabolites. Currently, we are evaluating regional differences in cerebral metabolite concentrations using a hybrid CSI technique which is based on a TE = 20 ms STEAM sequence. The data are compared to a SE-based TE = 135 ms hybrid CSI sequence. In agreement with previous findings using single-voxel techniques (Sauter et al., 1990), the TE = 20 ms hybrid CSI technique allows evaluation of resonances from glutamate, scyllo-inositols, myo-inositols and glucose, in addition to the resonances from N-acetylaspartate, creatines and

Magnetic Resonance Scanning and Epilepsy, Edited by S.D. Shorvon et al.,
Plenum Press, New York, 1994

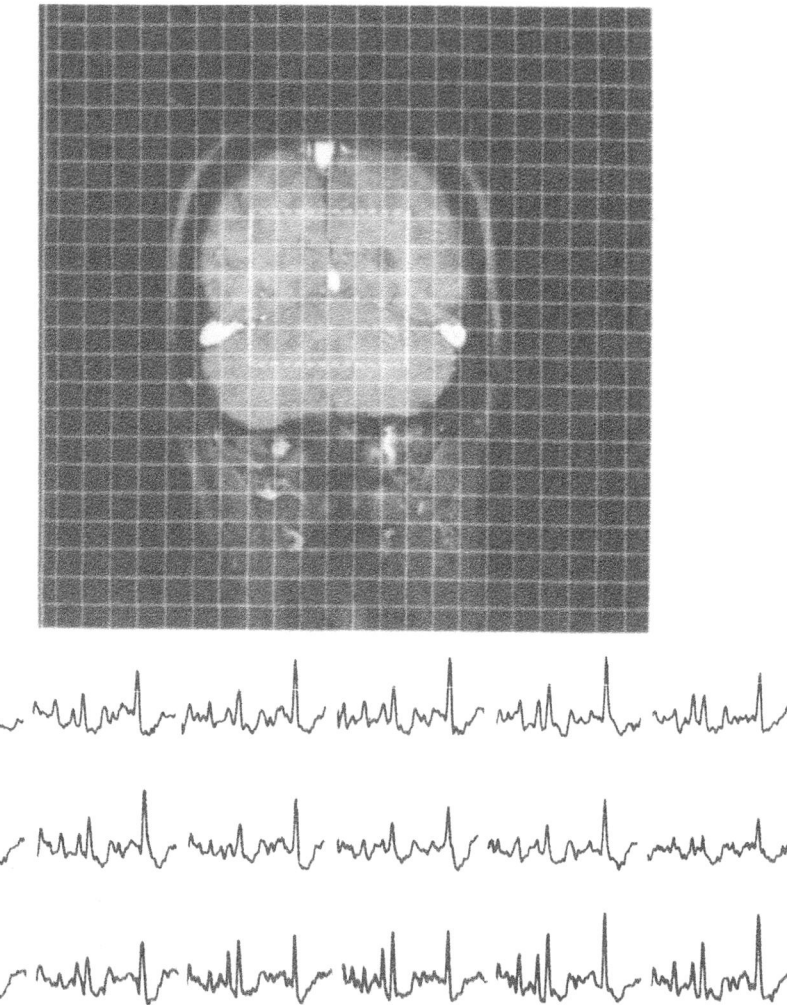

Figure 1. [1]H CSI examination of the brain of a healthy volunteer. The preselected volume of interest represents a coronal cut including occipital lobe and cerebellum. (a) MR image showing the preselected volume of interest (dotted box, 6 cm × 6 cm × 2 cm) and the in-plane spatial resolution for the CSI examination (grid, field of view = 32 cm × 32 cm, matrix size = 32 × 32, resulting voxel size = 2 ml). (b) Spectral map, showing all simultaneously acquired ^{1}H CSI spectra from within the preselected volume of interest. TE = 20 ms, TR = 1500 ms, number of acquisitions = 1, total acquisition time = 25.6 min.

cholines which are also detectable at longer echo times. Within a total acquisition time that is well tolerated by patients (26 min), a spatial resolution of 2 ml can be achieved (Figure 1).

By the application of (^{1}H–^{31}P) double-resonance techniques, the performance of in vivo ^{31}P MRS can be improved considerably (Bachert-Baumann et al., 1990; Kolem et al., 1992): Saturation of the ^{1}H spin system, by relaxation-induced transitions (nuclear Overhauser effect, NOE), effects higher population differences between ^{31}P energy levels, which translates to increased sensitivity, while line-narrowing due to ^{1}H decoupling in addition improves the amount of metabolic information obtained by ^{31}P MRS. We have combined ^{31}P CSI techniques with broad-band ^{1}H excitation pulses (applied prior to ^{31}P excitation) for NOE enhancement and a WALTZ-4 sequence (applied during ^{31}P data acquisition) for ^{1}H decoupling. We observed NOE-enhancement factors of up to 50%; due to ^{1}H decoupling, the resonances of phosphomonoester (PME) and phosphodiester (PDE) split into phosphorylcholine (PC) and phosphorylethanolamine (PE), and glycerophosphorylcholine (GPC) and glycerophospho-rylethanolamine (GPE), respectively. A spatial resolution of 16 ml can be achieved with 24 min total acquisition time. These (^{1}H–^{31}P) double resonance techniques have also been applied successfully to obtain ^{31}P spectra from liver and heart.

Currently, in requiring additional experimental software and hardware, the above-mentioned techniques for improved ^{1}H and ^{31}P MRS are complicating the procedures of MRS examination rather than facilitating the practical clinical application of MRS. On the other hand, the improved spatial and spectral resolution provided by these techniques, together with a better integration of these techniques in commercial MR scanners, are expected to increase the chances of MRS considerably to evolve into a clinical tool for diagnosis and therapy within the near future.

REFERENCES

Bachert-Baumann, P., Ermark, F., Zabel, H-.J., Sauter, R., Semmler, W., and Lorenz, W.J., 1990, In vivo Nuclear Overhauser effect in 31P-1H double- resonance experiments in a 1.5 T whole-body MR system, Magn Reson Med 15: 165.

Bottomley, P.A., US Patent 434688, 1982.

Brown, T.R., Kincaid, B.M., and Ugurbil, K., 1982, NMR chemical shift imaging in three dimensions, Proc Natl Acad Sci USA. 79: 3523.

Frahm, J., Bruhn, H., Gyngell, M.L., Merboldt K.D., Hänicke, W., and Sauter, R., 1989, Localised high-resolution proton NMR spectroscopy using stimulated echoes: initial applications to human brain in vivo, Magn Reson Med 9: 79.

Frahm, J., Michaelis, T., Merboldt, K.D., Bruhn, H., Gyngell, M.L., and Hänicke, W., 1990, Improvements in localised proton NMR spectroscopy of the human brain. Water suppression, short echo times and 1 ml resolution, J. Magn Reson. 90: 464.

Kolem, H., Schneider, M., Miyazaki, T., Wicklow, K. and Sauter, R., 1992, Meßzeitverkürzung bei in vivo Phosphor Chemical Shift Imaging durch Ausnutzung des Kern-Overhauser Effekts, 4. Internationales Kernspintomographie Symposium, Garmisch-Partenkirchen 1991, Referate, Schnetztor Verlag, Konstanz, 440.

Maudsley, A.A., Hilal, A.K., Perman, W.H., and Simon, H.E, 1983, Spatially resolved high resolution spectros-copy by "four-dimensional" NMR, J Magn Reson 51: 147.

Sauter, R., Schneider, M., Wicklow, K., and Kolem, H., 1990, Proton Spectroscopy of the human brain in vivo: improved specificity using single- voxel techniques with short echo times, "SMRM Book of Abstracts," p. 1083, Society of Magnetic Resonance in Medicine, Berkeley, CA.

43

PROTON OBSERVATION OF ^{13}C-LABELLED METABOLITES

P.G. Morris, R.S. Badar-Goffer, M.J.W. Prior, and H.S. Bachelard

Magnetic Resonance Centre
Department of Physics
University of Nottingham
University Park
Nottingham, NG7 2RD
United Kingdom

INTRODUCTION

The wide chemical shift range (> 200 p.p.m.) of the ^{13}C nucleus often allows metabolites to be identified directly and unambiguously from their ^{13}C MR spectra. The low natural abundance (1.1%) of this stable carbon isotope means that only metabolites such as triglyccrides or glycogen, which are highly concentrated in certain tissues, can be directly observed at natural abundance in vivo (Alger et al., 1981), and most applications of ^{13}C MR spectroscopy involve the administration of highly enriched substrates. The great advantage of this approach is that the metabolic time course of substrate use can be followed and used to determine fluxes through pathways, as well as to elucidate the pathways themselves. In recent years, these techniques, which were originally applied to studies of cell suspensions (e.g. yeast) (den Hollander et al., 1979), or hepatocytes (Cohen et al., 1979), have been extended to the study of brain metabolism in isolated tissue (Morris et al., 1986; Badar-Goffer et al., 1990), in experimental animals (Behar et al., 1986) and in humans (Gruetter et al., 1992a,b).

The substrate for in vivo brain studies is normally glucose. [13]C label from this source "flows" through glycolysis to pyruvate and thence to lactate, or else enters the tricarboxylic acid (TCA) cycle, accumulating in the C-4 carbon of glutamate, and redistributing to the C-2 and C-3 positions in subsequent turns of the TCA cycle, as well as to other key cerebral metabolites (Figure 1). The rate of appearance of label in C-3 of lactate and C-4 of glutamate gives a measure of the cerebral glycolytic and TCA cycle fluxes, respectively. Shulman's group at Yale have recently estimated the latter as 1.4 μmol/g per min in the rat (Fitzpatrick et al., 1990).

Although direct ^{13}C MR studies are possible, this approach suffers from several drawbacks, including excessive heating from the broad-band proton decoupling needed to collapse the ^{13}C multiplet structure. Composite pulse decoupling sequences, such as WALTZ 16, can

Magnetic Resonance Scanning and Epilepsy, Edited by S.D. Shorvon et al.,
Plenum Press, New York, 1994

alleviate this potential problem. However, the most serious objection, a lack of sensitivity, is less easily remedied. Large quantities of labelled material (up to 60 g) are required for human studies (Gruetter et al., 1992a), making these investigations extremely expensive—up to US $3000 per patient study. In addition, the spatial resolution is poor, often corresponding to regions of interest in excess of 100 cm^3.

The most promising alternative approach is to make use of the inherently higher MR sensitivity of protons to detect the ^{13}C atoms to which they are chemically bonded. The sensitivity is proportional to the third power of the magnetogyric ratio (an inherent property of the nucleus), giving a potential gain in sensitivity of 4^3 or 64. Unfortunately, the noise also depends on the MR operating frequency, a fact often ignored when estimating the potential benefits of inverse detection, and, assuming that the sample itself is the dominant source of noise, the improvement in signal-to-noise we can reasonably expect is of about a factor of 16.

CURRENT RESEARCH

Much technical effort is being expended in developing indirect detection techniques. The basis of all these methods is the scalar (J) coupling between protons and ^{13}C nuclei, which has a magnitude of typically 126 Hz. In the ^1H spectrum of Figure 2, the main resonance arising from the methyl protons of lactate is flanked by two satellites offset by ± 63 Hz. These represent the methyl protons attached to a ^{13}C-labelled C-3, whereas the central resonance is from the methyl protons attached to unlabelled (^{12}C) C-3 atoms. The relative areas immediately give the fractional enrichment of the lactate pool. This type of unedited ^1H experiment has been used to demonstrate that the elevated brain lactate, which persists in patients for several weeks following a stroke, is actively turning over (Rothman et al., 1990).

Such simple ^1H experiments do not allow the quantitation of glutamate, whose ^1H resonances occur in a more crowded region of the spectrum. To pick them out, proton observe carbon edit (POCE) experiments, originally used to observe cell suspensions, have been steadily refined. The basic sequence is illustrated in Figure 3. A non-selective ^{13}C inversion (180°) pulse is applied in alternate scans which are accumulated separately. Subtraction of the spectra yields a ^1H difference spectrum in which only those protons that are bonded to ^{13}C atoms appear (Bendall et al., 1981; Freeman et al., 1981). Although in theory this experiment should eliminate the troublesome water peak, the selectivity is far from perfect and additional steps must be taken to suppress it. These include selective presaturation of the water peak and replacement of the non-selective ^1H 90° and 180° pulses with semiselective "jump and return" pulses with excitation maxima in the region of interest (2.2 p.p.m.) and a null at the water peak (Fitzpatrick et al., 1990). Further improvements to the editing technique as well as to the spatial selection and particularly to the shimming (Gruetter and Boesch, 1992) have resulted in improved resolution that permits the glutamate C-3 and C-4 resonances to be resolved in human brain spectra (Chen et al., 1992).

These editing techniques must be combined with some form of spatial localisation–often either a simple surface coil (in which case it is preferable to use B_1 insensitive excitation pulses for both ^1H and ^{13}C channels), or else a field gradient-based method, such as ISIS (Ordidge et al., 1986). The latter methods have the advantage that they avoid excitation of the lipids in the scalp.

Another promising approach to indirect detection is the gradient-enhanced heteronuclear multiple quantum coherence technique, in which gradient pulses are used not only for selective volume excitation but also for coherence selection (Knuttel et al., 1990, van Zijl et al., 1992). This method provides extremely efficient elimination of the water peak permitting resonances that lie close to it, such as C-1 of glucose and C-2 of glutamate, to be observed.

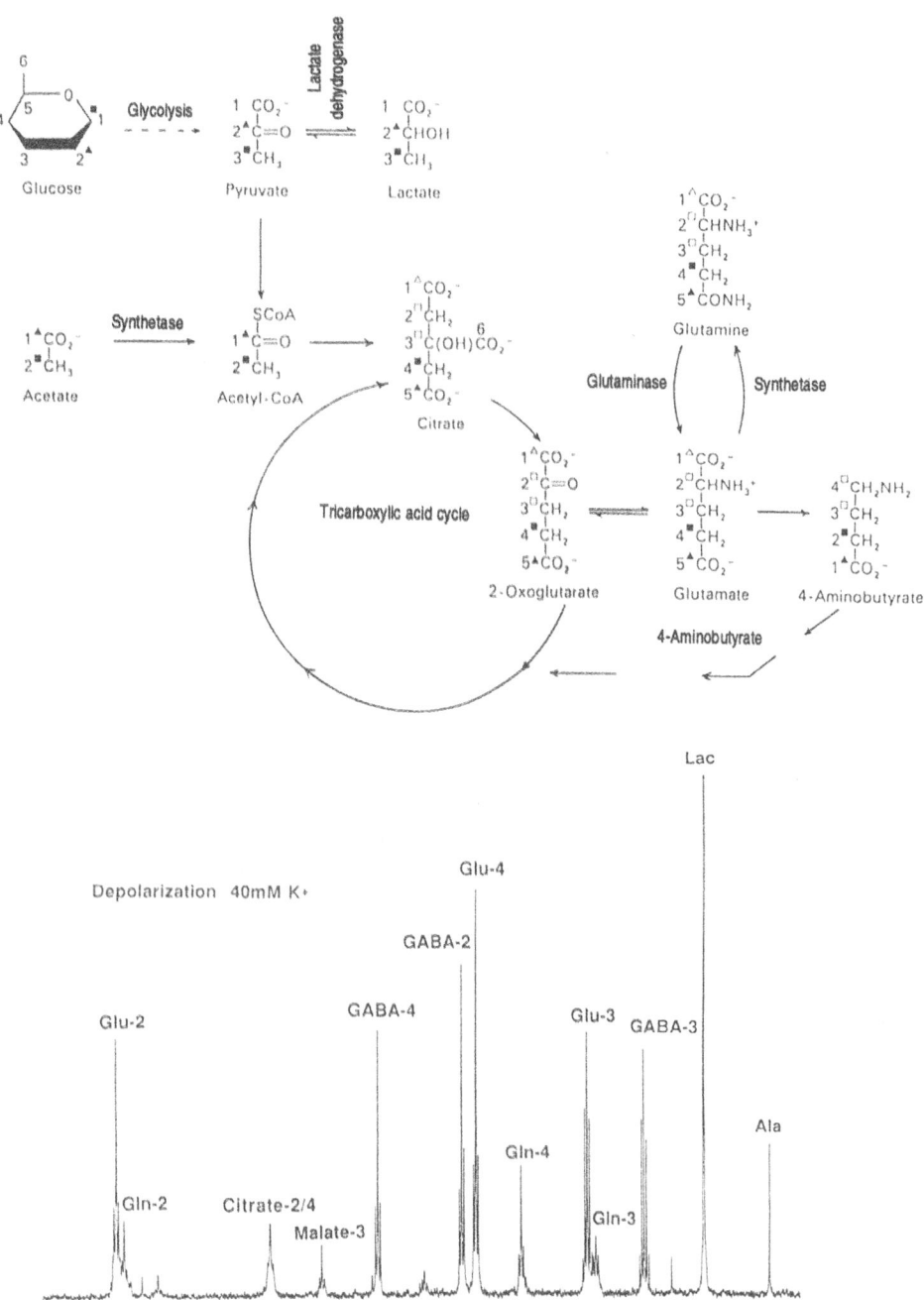

Figure 1. Top: labelling patterns from various precursors. Solid symbols, direct; open symbols, subsequent labelling. Bottom: ^{13}C MR spectrum of extract made from guinea-pig brain slices incubated with [1 -^{13}C] glucose under depolarising conditions (40 mmol-K$^+$/l, Bader-Goffer et al., 1990, 1992).

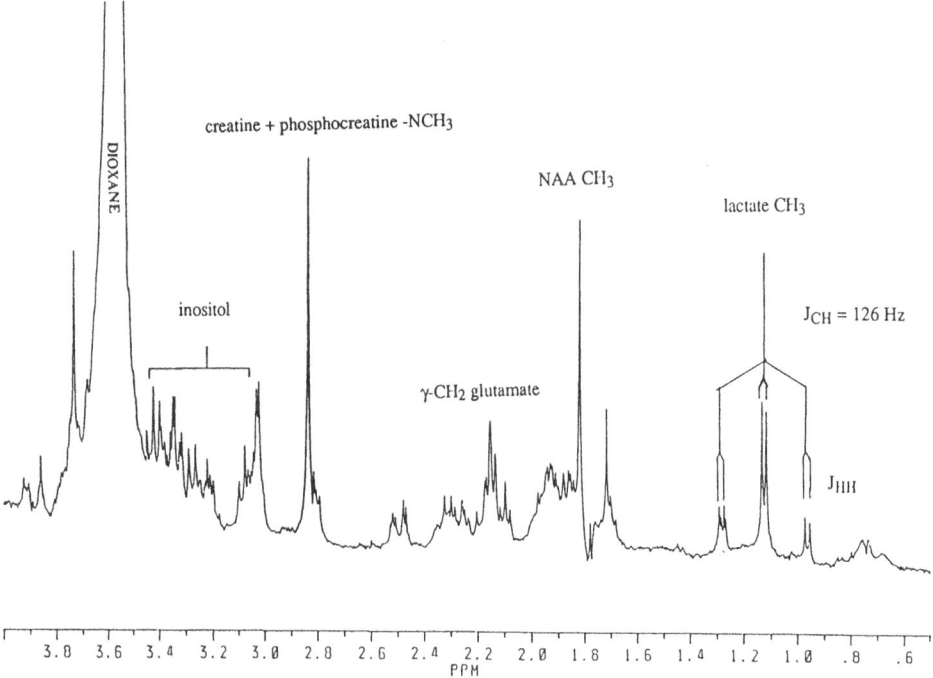

Figure 2. ^{1}H MRS spectrum of guinea-pig brain slice extract labelled from [1-^{13}C]glucose and [2-^{13}C] acetate under depolarising conditions.

DISCUSSION

Localised ^{13}C measurements of cerebral metabolism can now be made with sufficient spectral resolution to distinguish the C-2, C-3 and C-4 of glutamate and glutamine resonances (Gruetter et al., 1992b) and to measure cerebral glucose levels (Gruetter et al., 1992a). Localised ^{1}H spectroscopy can also be used to observe cerebral glucose and its metabolites directly at higher spatial resolution (see for example Bruhn et al., 1991). The indirect detection methods combine the advantages of both approaches, namely, the observation of labelled substrates at high spatial resolution. Measurements of regional cerebral metabolic rate clearly represent one exciting research avenue in the study of epilepsy, particularly if they can be made within active epileptic foci. The possibility of observing, by indirect ^{13}C MRS, the metabolic interaction between neuronal and glial cell populations (Badar-Goffer et al., 1992), and of exploring the role of elevated excitotoxic amino acid levels in mediating possible neuronal damage also represent exciting future possibilities.

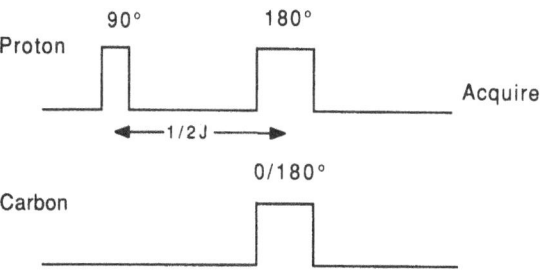

Figure 3. The basic POCE experiment.

PROBABLE DEVELOPMENTS OVER THE NEXT FIVE YEARS

We can expect to see a continuing refinement of indirect detection methods for the observation of ^{13}C-labelled metabolites. We can also expect that, as the anticipated sensitivity advantages of this method are realised, it will be possible to reduce the selected volume from 100 cm^3, certainly to $< 10 \text{ cm}^3$ and perhaps eventually to $< 1 \text{ cm}^3$. At this level of spatial resolution, chemical shift imaging methods, as opposed to localised spectroscopy, start to look attractive. Inevitably, there will be considerable effort in correlating indirect ^{13}C measurements with other types of neurospectroscopy, including ^{31}P measurements of bioenergetic status, and, especially, with the high-speed cerebral activation studies that are currently taking the imaging world by storm. All these developments will be aided by the use of the higher field clinical magnets (3 and 4 T) which are now becoming available. As the demand for these studies grows, so the cost of ^{13}C-labelled substrates is likely to fall (already [1-^{13}C]glucose can be purchased at one-tenth the cost of a decade ago), significantly reducing the cost per patient study. It does not seem likely that these methods will quickly establish themselves as routine investigatory tools. Nevertheless, the next five years promise to be extremely exciting ones, as they mature and start to be applied to key clinical issues, and especially to epilepsy.

REFERENCES

Alger, J.R., Sillerud, L.O., Behar, K.L., Gillies, R.J., Shulman, R.G., Gordon, R.E., Shaw, D., and Hanley, P.E., 1981, In vivo carbon-13 nuclear magnetic resonance studies of mammals, Science 214: 660–662.

Badar-Goffer, R.S., Bachelard, H.S., and Morris, P.G., 1990, Cerebral metabolism of acetate and glucose studied by 13C MRS spectroscopy, Biochem J. 266: 133–139.

Badar-Goffer, R.S., Ben-Yoseph, O., Bachelard, H.S., and Morris, P.G., 1992, Neuronal-glial metabolism under depolarizing conditions: a ^{13}C MRS study, Biochem J. 282: 225–230.

Behar, K.L., Petroff, O.A.C., Prichard, J.W., Alger, J.R., and Shulman, R.G., 1986, Detection of metabolites in rabbit brain by ^{13}C MRS spectroscopy following administration of [1-^{13}C]glucose, Magn Reson Med. 3: 911–920.

Bendall, M.R., Pegg, D.T., Doddrell, D.M., and Field, J., 1981, NMR of protons coupled to ^{13}C nuclei only, J Am Chem Soc. 103: 934–936.

Bruhn, H., Michaelis, T., Merboldt, K.D., Hanicke, W., Gyngell, M.L., and Frahm, J., 1991, Monitoring cerebral glucose in diabetics by proton MRS, Lancet 337: 745–746.

Chen, W., Rothman, D.L., and Shulman, R.G., 1992, Sensitivity and resolution improvements of POCE technique, "SMRM Book of Abstracts" p. 3833 Society of Magnetic Resonance in Medicine, Berkeley, CA.

Cohen, S.M., Ogawa, S., and Shulman, R.G., 1979, ^{13}C MRS studies of gluconeogenesis in rat liver cells: Utilization of labelled glycerol by cells from euthyroid and hyperthyroid rats, Proc Natl Acad Sci USA. 76: 1603–1607.

den Hollander, J.A., Brown, T.R., Ugurbil, K., and Shulman, R.G., 1981, ^{13}C nuclear magnetic resonance studies of anaerobic glycolysis in suspensions of yeast cells, Proc Natl Acad Sci USA. 76; 6096–6100.

Fitzpatrick, S.M., Hetherington, H.P., Behar, K.L., and Shulman, R.G., 1990, The flux from glucose to glutamate in the rat brain in vivo as determined by 1H- observed, ^{13}C-edited NMR spectroscopy, J Cereb Blood Flow Metab. 10: 170–179.

Freeman, R., Mareci, T.H., and Morris, G.A., 1981, Weak satellite signals in high resolution NMR spectra: separating the wheat from the chaff, J Magn Reson. 42: 341–345.

Gruetter, R., Novotny, E.J., Boulware, S.D., Rothman, D.L., Mason, G.F., Shulman, G.I., Shulman, R.G., and Tamborlane, W.V., 1992a, Direct measurement of brain glucose in humans by ^{13}C NMR spectroscopy, Proc Natl Acad Sci USA. 89: 1109–1112.

Gruetter, R., Novoty, E.J., Boulware, S.D., Rothman, D.L., Tamborlane, W.V. and Shulman, R.G. 1992b, Localised ^{13}C NMR of amino acids in the human brain in vivo, "SMRM Book of Abstracts", p. 1921 Society of Magnetic Resonance in Medicine, Berkely, CA.

Gruetter, R., and Boesch, C., 1992, Fast, noniterative shimming of spatially localised signals. In vivo analysis of the magnetic field along axes, J Magn Reson. 96: 323–334.

Knuttel, A., Kimmich, R., and Spohn, K.-H., 1990, Indirect ^{13}C tomography and volume-selective spectroscopy via proton MRS I. Spectroscopic techniques, J Magn Reson. 86: 526–541.

Morris, P.G., Bachelard, H.S., Cox, D.W.G., and Cooper, J.C., 1986, ^{13}C nuclear magnetic resonance studies of glucose metabolism in guinea-pig brain slices, Biochem Soc Trans. 14: 1270–1271.

Ordidge, R.J., Connelly, A., and Lohman, J.A.B., 1986, Image-selected in vivo spectroscopy (ISIS). A new technique for spatially selective NMR spectroscopy, J Magn Reson. 66: 283–294.

Rothman, D.L., Howseman, A.M., Graham, G.D., Lantos, G., Petroff, O.A.C., Brass, L.M., Fayad, P.B., Shulman, G.I., Shulman, R.G., and Prichard, J.W., 1990, Observation of lactate turnover in infarcted human brain with 1-^{13}C glucose infusion and ^{1}H NMR spectroscopy, "SMRM Book of Abstracts", p. 107 Society of Magnetic Resonance in Medicine, Berkeley, CA.

van Zijl, P.C.M., Chesnick, A.S., Moonen, C.T.W., Ruiz-Cabello, J. and van Gelderen, P, 1992, In vivo detection of [1-^{13}C]glucose and its metabolic products with proton sensitivity, "SMRM Book of Abstracts", p. 544 Society of Magnetic Resonance in Medicine, Berkeley, CA.

USE OF COMBINED ^{13}C -, ^{19}F - AND ^{31}P-MR SPECTROSCOPY IN RESEARCH ON BRAIN METABOLISM

H.S. Bachelard, R.S. Badar-Goffer, O. Ben-Yoseph, and P.G. Morris

Magnetic Resonance Centre
Department of Physics
University of Nottingham
University Park
Nottingham, NG7 2RD
United Kingdom

INTRODUCTION

The effects of metabolic insults which may be of importance in the consequences of convulsions can now be studied on mammalian brain preparations using multi-nuclear magnetic resonance spectroscopy. In the metabolising whole tissue, the energy state, pH and Mg^{2+} concentration are monitored using ^{31}P-MR spectroscopy, and free intracellular calcium [Ca^{2+}] can be measured from its binding to the ^{19}F-MR spectroscopy indicator, 5FBAPTA (Bachelard et al., 1988). At present metabolism of glucose to metabolic intermediates of glycolysis, the tricarboxylic acid cycle and to amino acids is followed by ^{13}C-MR spectroscopy of tissue extracts, rather than in whole tissue preparations, due to the relatively low sensitivity of ^{13}C-MR spectroscopy. Comparison of labelling patterns from [1-^{13}C]glucose and [2-^{13}C]acetate showed that ^{13}C-enrichment of glutamine and of citrate reflects mainly glial, rather than neuronal, metabolism (Badar-Goffer et al., 1990). It is therefore possible to monitor in the same preparations the energy state, changes in free intracellular cations (H^+, Ca^{2+} and Mg^{2+}), to follow fluxes through metabolic pathways and to discriminate to some extent between neuronal and glial metabolism.

CURRENT RESEARCH

Depolarisation using 40 mmol/l-K^+ caused a rapid reversible rise in intracellular [Ca^{2+}] with a fall in phosphocreatine (PCr) (Figure 1). ^{13}C-MR spectroscopy revealed the expected large increase in oxidative metabolism (the rate of ^{13}C-enrichment of most intermediates was accelerated) and the pattern of labelling indicated that this increase was occurring essentially from glucose in glia (Badar-Goffer et al., 1992).

Magnetic Resonance Scanning and Epilepsy, Edited by S.D. Shorvon et al.,
Plenum Press, New York, 1994

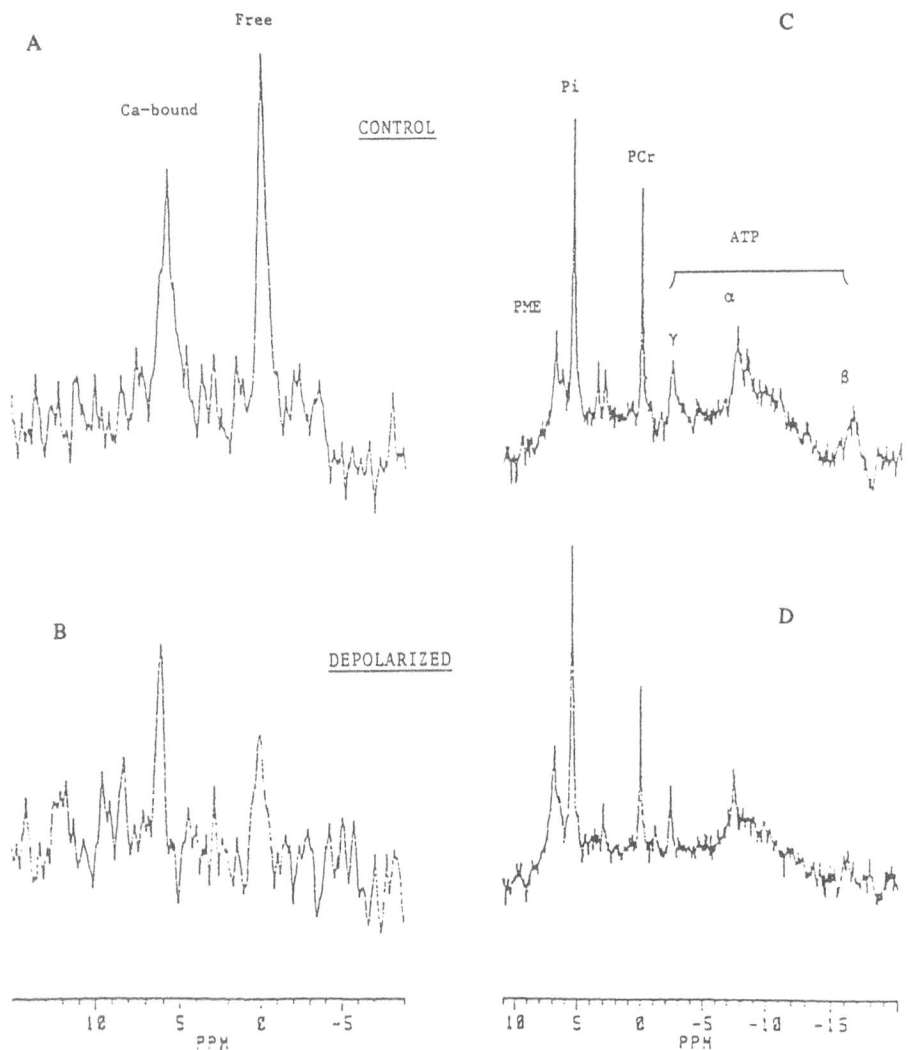

Figure 1. The effects of depolarisation (40 mmol/l-K$^+$) on free intracellular calcium [Ca^{2+}]i and the energy state in superperfused brain slices. The normal intracellular [Ca^{2+}] shown by the ^{19}F-BAPTA spectrum (A) is greatly increased by depolarisation (B) and the PCr is decreased by depolarisation (D) to 70% of its control value (C).

Hypoxia is known to cause decreased PCr without change in ATP, whereas severe hypoglycaemia causes decreases in both, i.e. PCr and ATP fall concomitantly. ^{13}C-MR spectra showed the build-up of glycolytic metabolites (lactate and alanine) and decreased enrichment of tricarboxylic acid intermediates and amino acids in severe hypoxia. An unexpected observation in the ^{13}C-MR spectra was the appearance of a new resonance which proved to be glycerol 3-phosphate (Figure 2), and was then also found to be present in ^{31}P-MR spectra (Figure 3). Its presence was confirmed by enzymatic analysis of tissue extracts, and the increase in glycerol 3-phosphate was calculated to be some 30-fold. Glycerol 3-phosphate is produced in a cytoplasmic reaction when NADH is high, so these

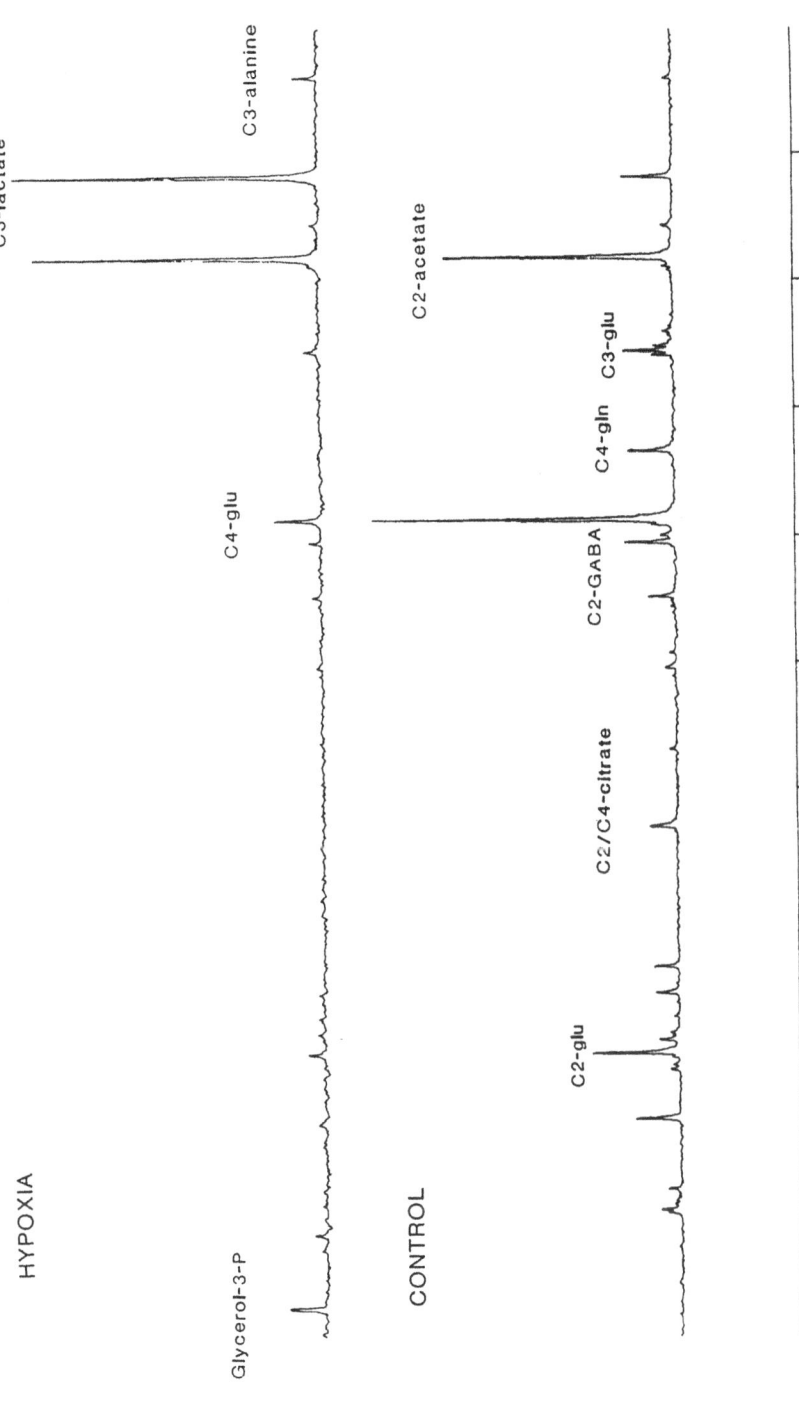

Figure 2. ^{13}C-MR spectra of extracts prepared from tissues incubated for 45 min with 5 mmol/l [1-^{13}C]glucose and [2-^{13}C]acetate. In severe hypoxia all resonances are decreased with the exception of lactate and alanine which are increased. The new resonance attributed to glycerol 3-phosphate can be seen only in the hypoxic spectrum at approx. 65 p.p.m. (Ben-Yoseph et al., 1993).

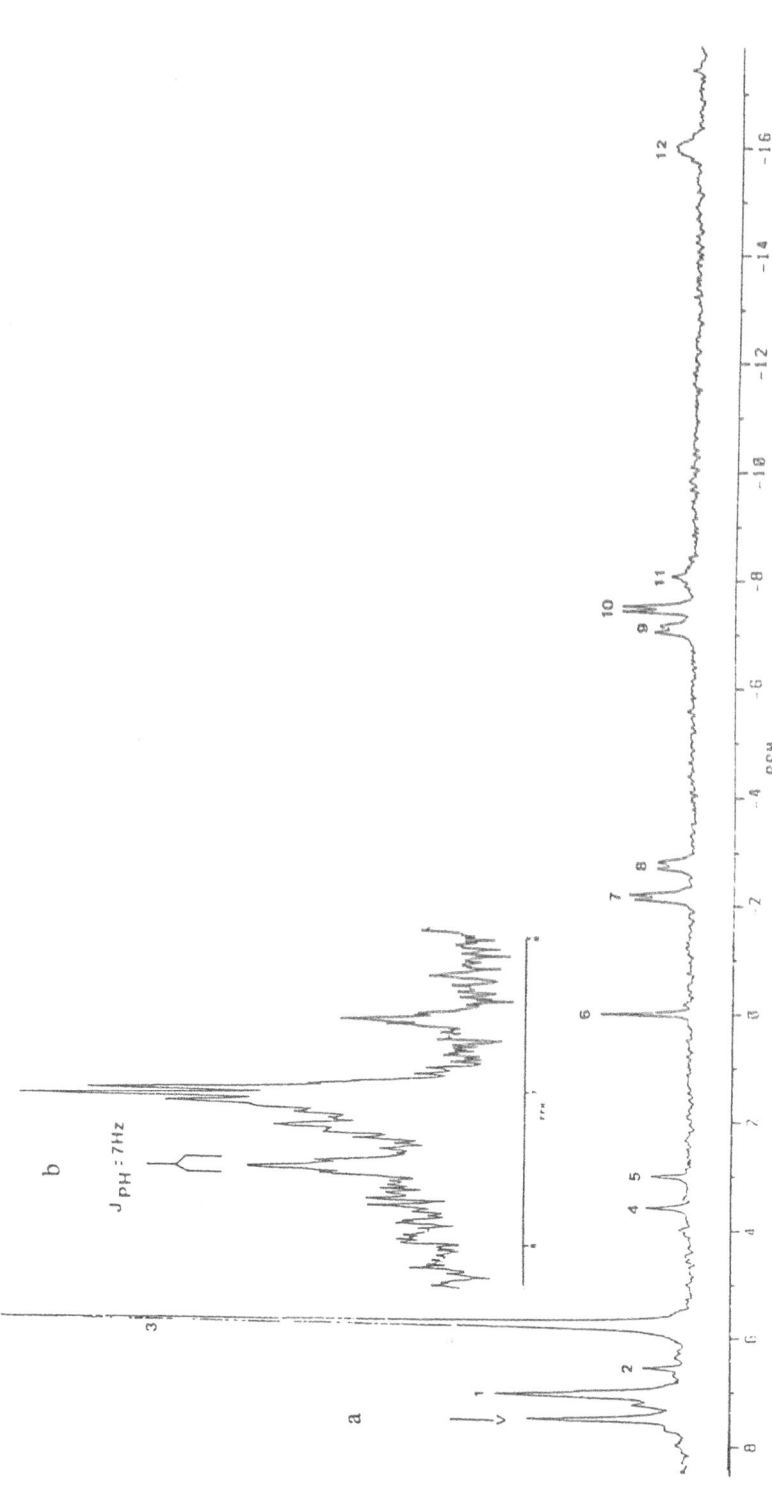

Figure 3. ^{31}P-MR spectrum of the hypoxic extract of Figure 2. 1,2: phosphomonoesters; 3: Pi; 4,5: phosphodiesters; 6: PCr; 7: γ-ATP; 8: β-ADP ; 9: α-ADP; 10: α-ATP; 11: [NAD/NADP]; 12: β-ATP. The arrowed resonance at 7.48 p.p.m. (a) is glycerol 3-phosphate, not observed in normoxia. The inset (b) shows an expanded view of the 6–8 p.p.m. region collected without broad-band decoupling, where the resonance appears as a triplet with a heteronuclear JPH constant of 7 Hz, thus confirming the resonance as glycerol 3-phosphate (Ben-Yoseph et al., 1992).

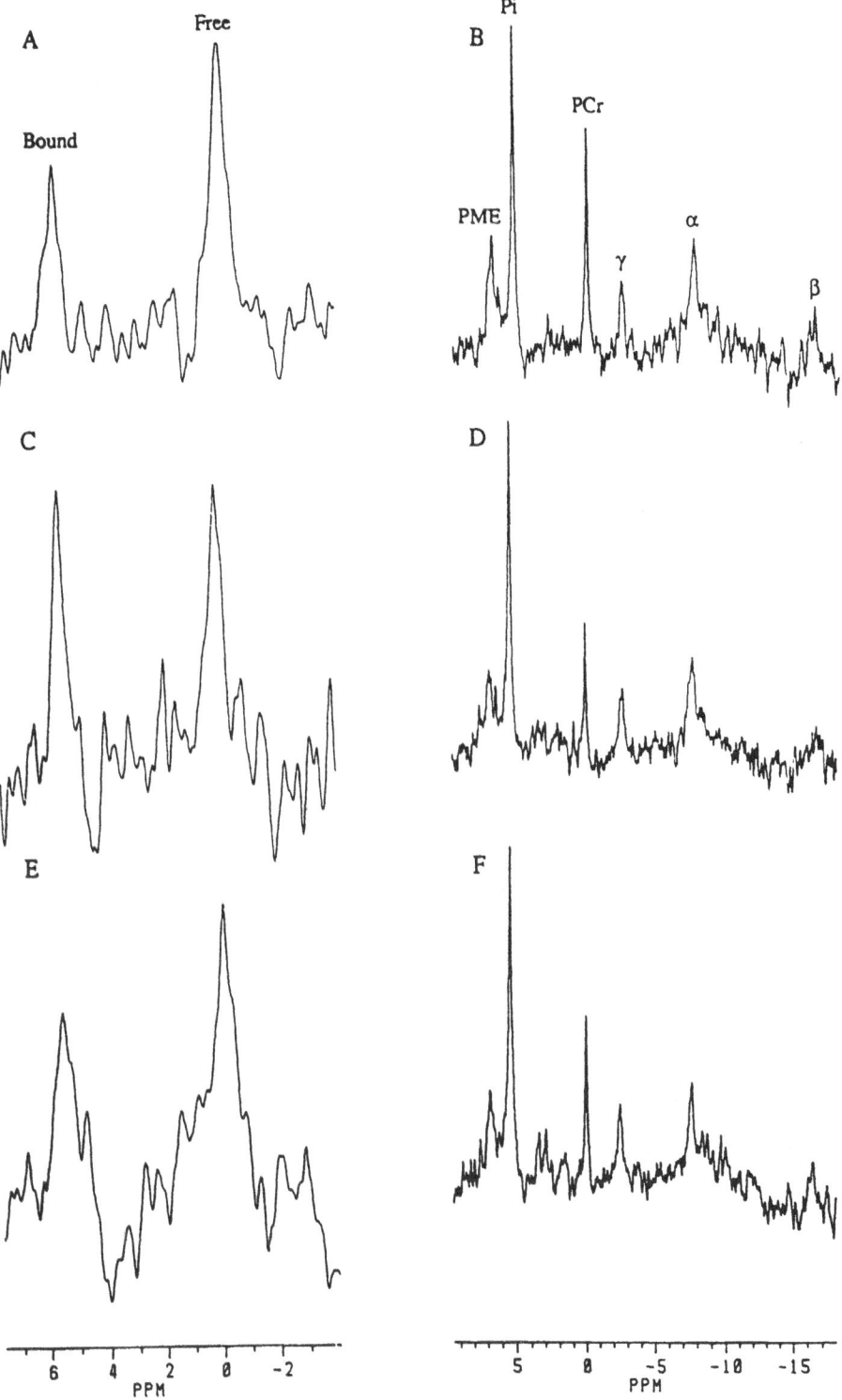

Figure 4. Effects of NMDA on intracellular [Ca^{2+}] and the energy state. ^{19}F- (A) and ^{31}P- (B) MR spectra under control conditions, in the presence of 10 μmol/l NMDA in the absence of Mg^{2+} (C and D), and in the presence of 10 μmol/l-NMDA in the presence of Mg^{2+} (E and F). Intracellular [Ca^{2+}] is increased by NMDA in the absence (C) but not in the presence (E) of Mg^{2+}, whereas PCr is decreased under both conditions (D and F) (Ben-Yoseph et al., 1990).

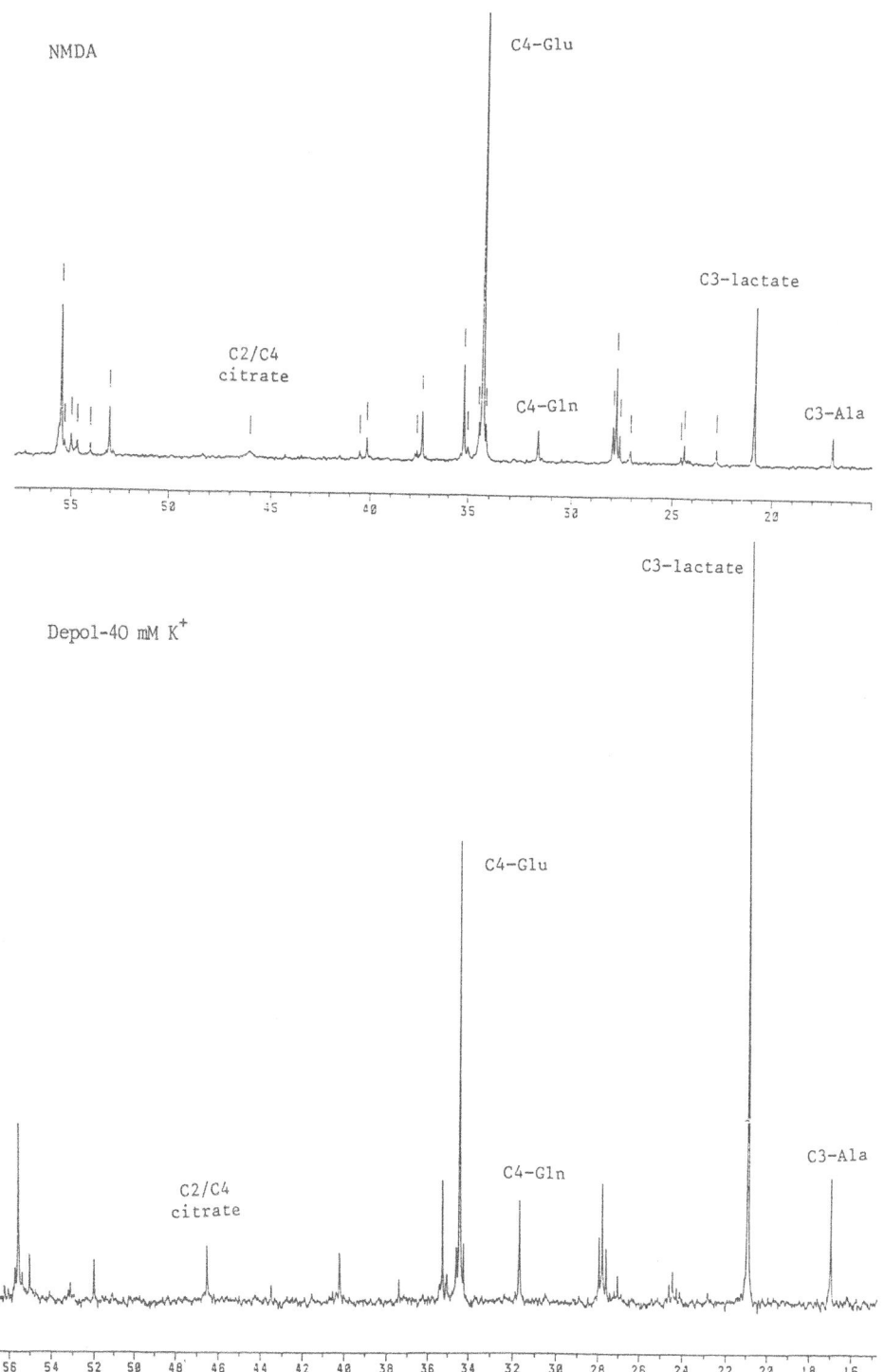

Figure 5. Comparison of the effects of depolarisation (40 mmol-K$^+$/l) and NMDA on intermediary metabolism using [1-^{13}C]glucose and ^{13}C-MR spectroscopy. The stimulation of glycolysis by NMDA is less marked and the pattern is different from that observed using depolarisation—see text (unpublished results).

results suggest a novel method of monitoring the cytoplasmic redox state non-invasively (Ben-Yoseph et al., 1992).

No change in intracellular [Ca^{2+}] could be detected in hypoxia and the results using low glucose were equivocal. However, when low glucose was present under hypoxic conditions there were further decreases in PCr and ATP and a four-fold increase in intracellular [Ca^{2+}] (unpublished results).

The excitotoxic hypothesis of neuronal damage caused by elevated acidic amino acids (glutamate and aspartate) in perturbed conditions such as epilepsy and ischaemic stroke invokes involvement of the N-methyl-D-aspartate (NMDA) subtype of glutamate receptor. Our studies showed that the increase in intracellular [Ca^{2+}] caused by low (10 μmol/l) concentrations of NMDA in the absence of Mg^{2+} was irreversible and slower than a decrease in PCr, with no change in ATP. NMDA caused no change in intracellular [Ca^{2+}] in the presence of Mg^{2+} (as would be expected because this calcium channel is normally blocked by Mg^{2+}), but a similar decrease in PCr was observed (Figure 4, Table 1). We suggested therefore that NMDA may perturb neuronal metabolism by a mechanism independent of the Mg^{2+}-gated calcium channel (Ben-Yoseph et al., 1990).

The increased intracellular [Ca^{2+}] and decreased PCr (but not ATP) caused by NMDA in the absence of Mg^{2+} were similar to the changes seen on depolarisation in the presence of Mg^{2+} (Figure 1), although the changes caused by depolarisation were reversible whereas those caused by NMDA were not. We therefore compared the effects of NMDA with those of depolarization on ^{13}C-labelling patterns. The results (Figure 5) showed that the effects of NMDA on ^{13}C-labelling patterns are different from those caused by depolarisation and that the results are independent of Mg^{2+}. The main differences observed were in percentage ^{13}C-enrichment of lactate, alanine, citrate and glutamine. Pool sizes of the amino acids were slightly lower on depolarisation, but greatly decreased with NMDA. The pool size of lactate was also much lower with NMDA. We tentatively interpreted these results to indicate that NMDA is producing an excitation of glycolysis in some but not all neurons independently of the presence of Mg^{2+}, whereas depolarisation causes a large stimulation of glycolysis and the triaboxylic acid cycle essentially in glia. These studies provide further evidence to support the possibility that the neurotoxic effects of NMDA may be mediated by mechanisms not directly related to opening of calcium channels, and are not due to depolarisation of the tissues. The enrichment patterns

Table 1. The Effects of NMDA on the Energy State, Intracellular Ca^{2+} and Mg^{2+} in the Presence and Absence of [Mg^{2+}]$_e$

NDMA (μM)	[Mg^{2+}] (mM)	n	[Mg^{2+}]$_i$ (mM)	[Ca^{2+}]$_i$ (nM)	PCr (% of control)
0	1.2	10	0.30 ± 0.06	362 ± 59	100
10	0	4	0.33 ± 0.03	571 ± 1.4* (slow)	58 ± 8* (fast)
400	0	2	N.D.[a]	567	58
10	1.2	1	0.30	356	57
400	1.2	1	0.34	344	59
10	1.2	4	0.37	N.D.[b]	78 ± 9*
400	1.2	4	N.D.[a]	N.D.[b]	75 ± 6*

Values (mean ± S.D.) were calculated from spectra accumulated between 1 and 2 h after addition of NMDA to superfusing media. There were no changes in ATP or ADP. Control values from enzymic analyses were (μmol/100 mg protein): PCr, 3.23; ATP, 1.37; ADP, 0.16.

N.D.[a]: not determinable due to low β-ATP resonance;
N.D.[b]: not determinable due to absence of preloaded 5FBAPTA in the tissue.

and pool sizes suggest a possible interpretation, i.e. that a population of neurons is damaged but that the remaining cells are metabolising normally (unpublished results).

PROBABLE DEVELOPMENTS OVER THE NEXT FIVE YEARS

The relatively low sensitivity of ^{13}C-NMR spectroscopy can be improved some 30-fold by indirect ^{1}H-MR observation of ^{13}C-labelled metabolites (see Chapter 43), to the extent that some of the studies reported here are becoming feasible in metabolising whole tissues and in the human brain in vivo. Some success has already been achieved in humans (Rothman et al., 1989). The combination of multi-nuclear MR spectroscopy will prove of great value in exploring the metabolic basis for, and consequences of, disorders such as stroke and epilepsy.

ACKNOWLEDGEMENTS

These studies were supported by the MRC.

REFERENCES

Bachelard, H.S., Badar-Goffer, R.S., Brooks, K.J., Dolin, S.J., and Morris, P.G., 1988, Measurement of free intracellular calcium in the brain by 19F-NMR spectroscopy, J Neurochem. 51: 1311–1313.

Badar-Goffer, R.S., Bachelard, H.S., and Morris, P.G., 1990, Cerebral metabolism of acetate and glucose studied by ^{13}C-n.m.r. spectroscopy. A technique for investigating metabolic compartmentation in the brain, Biochem J. 266: 133–139.

Badar-Goffer, R.S., Ben-Yoseph, O., Bachelard, H.S., and Morris, P.G., 1992, Neuronal-glial metabolism under depolarizing conditions. A ^{13}C-n.m.r. study, Biochem J. 282: 225–230.

Ben-Yoseph, O., Bachelard, H.S., Badar-Goffer, R.S., Dolin, S.J., and Morris, P.G., 1990, Effects of N-methyl-D-aspartate on [Ca2+]i and the energy state in the brain by 19F- and 31P- nuclear magnetic resonance spectroscopy, J Neurochem. 55: 1446–1449.

Ben-Yoseph, O., Bachelard, H.S., Badar-Goffer, R.S., and Morris P.G., 1993, Glycerol 3-phosphate and lactate as indicators of the cerebral cytoplasmic redox state in severe and mild hypoxia respectively: a ^{13}C- and ^{31}P-MR study, Biochem J. 291: 915–919.

Rothman, D.L., Howsman, A., Novotny, E.J., Hanstock, C.C., Lantos, G., Petroff, O.A.C., Prichard, J.W. and Shulman, R.G., 1989, Feasibility of proton-observe carbon-decouple editing of glutamate in the human brain, "Proceedings of the 8th Annual Meeting of the Society of Magnetic Resonance in Medicine," p. 372.

MALIGNANT TUMOURAL LESIONS INVESTIGATED BY MRS

W. Semmler,[1,2] P. Bachert,[1] and G. van Kaick[1]

[1] German Cancer Research Center
Heidelberg
[2] Institute for Diagnostic Research
Berlin
Germany

INTRODUCTION

Magnetic resonance spectroscopy (MRS) is a non-invasive technique applicable for in vivo detection of metabolites in tissue and for the observation of drug pharmacokinetics. MRS has become increasingly important in the study of in vivo chemistry of healthy brain and brain tumours. Chemical shift imaging (CSI) provides information on tumour metabolic heterogeneity and the involvement of surrounding tissue. With the use of ^{31}P MRS the turnover of high-energy phosphates and intermediates of phospholipid metabolism and the intercelluar pH can be observed. In ^{1}H-decoupled ^{31}P spectra, resonances of phosphocholine and phosphoethanolamine are resolved in the phosphomonoester (PME) and of glycerophosphoryl-choline and glycerophosphorylethanolamine in the phosphodiester (PDE) resonance band. ^{1}H MRS allows to detect N-acetylaspartate (NAA), inositols, choline (Cho), creatine/phosphocreatine, glutamate/glutamine, lactate and a number of other small metabolites. First results on drug monitoring with ^{7}Li and ^{19}F MRS in brain have been reported, but these techniques have not yet been used to study brain tumours.

CURRENT RESEARCH

Four goals were defined for in vivo MRS studies on human tumours: (1) tumour characterization, (2) monitoring of tumour growth, (3) tumour therapy monitoring, and (4) drug monitoring.

Magnetic Resonance Scanning and Epilepsy, Edited by S.D. Shorvon et al.,
Plenum Press, New York, 1994

TUMOUR CHARACTERISATION

^{31}P and ^{1}H MRS are used to characterise different brain tumours. Bruhn et al., (1989) stated that by means of in vivo ^{1}H MRS benign and malignant tumours and furthermore different tumour histologies, e.g. astrocytomas, meningiomas, gliomas etc. can be differentiated. Lazeyras et al. (1992) claim that tumour grading might be possible by means of ^{1}H MRS, whereas other authors concluded that this is not the case (Heindel et al., 1988; Ott et al., 1990; Hagberg et al., 1992). Recent results are still not conclusive. Naruse et al. (1992) observed new ^{1}H MR resonances in spectra of patients with glioblastoma.

MONITORING OF TUMOUR GROWTH

In vivo MRS data on tumour growth observed in humans are scarce. Animal experiments show a change of PME, PDE and inorganic phosphate (P_i) ^{31}P MR signal intensities concomitant with tumour growth. In necrotic tissue ATP levels are depleted and PME and P_i levels are enhanced (Ng et al., 1982; Naruse et al., 1985).

THERAPY MONITORING

Brain tumour monitoring has been performed by means of ^{31}P and ^{1}H MRS. Arnold et al. (1988) observed changes in ^{31}P MR spectra of patients after chemotherapy with BCNU indicating that the tumour metabolism changes during the therapy. MRS studies on malignant brain tumours undergoing fractionated stereotactical irradiation allow intraindividual comparison of the biochemistry of non-involved hemisphere and irradiated tumour. Surprisingly strong changes of NAA and choline intensities were observed after 2 Gy (Semmler et al., 1990). Embolisation of meningiomas is a common pre-surgical technique and can be monitored by means of ^{31}P MRS. In ^{31}P MR spectra increases in P_i intensity but also localised increases in PME, and PDE levels were observed (Knopp et al., 1992). ^{1}H MRS has been used to observe the lactate concentration in meningiomas before and after embolisation, and showed an increase of lactate levels post-embolization. One day after embolisation the lactate signal vanished (Jüngling et al., 1992).

DRUG MONITORING

MRS drug monitoring has not been performed in human brain tumours so far; however, ^{7}Li and ^{19}F MRS have been used to study the accumulation of psychoactive drugs in patients with schizophrenia and depression (Komoroski et al., 1989, 1990).

DISCUSSION

Currently, MRS cannot be used for tumour characterisation, and the different histologies cannot be assigned to specific MR spectral patterns. Because there is no tumour-specific metabolism, one might expect only qualitative changes in the MR spectra. However, with improvements in techniques, this may change. In this context, Naruse et al., (1992) have reported a specific resonance in human brain tumour spectra.

In animal studies, different stages of tumour development can be identified and this work can be extrapolated to clinical practice. For example, high PME and PDE intensities might indicate a late stage of tumour development and elevated PME and P_i and depleted nucleotide triphosphate levels can be attributed to necrotic tumour regions. Tumour therapy monitoring is feasible by MRS techniques, in which early effects, in particular, can be observed.

PROBABLE DEVELOPMENT OVER THE NEXT FIVE YEARS

MRS has proven to be a powerful tool for in vivo observation of the metabolism in tumours and in other diseases of the brain. Improved localisation and data evaluation methods will result in the widespread application of MRS techniques in studies on human neurochemistry, and its chemical relevance can then be judged. An important step forward will be the understanding of the complete information content of localised in vivo MR spectra originating from the complex superposition of multiple resonances.

REFERENCES

Arnold, D.L., Shoubridge, E.A., Villemure, J.G., and Feindel, W., 1988, Phosphorus magnetic resonance spectroscopy of cerebral gliomas following treatment with intravenous BCNU, "SMRM Book of Abstracts," P.333, Society of Magnetic Resonance in Medicine, San Francisco, California.

Bruhn, H., Frahm, J., Gyngell, M., Merbold, K.D., Hänicke, W., Sauter, R., and Hamburger, C., 1989, Noninvasive differentiation of tumours using localised H-1 MR spectroscopy in vivo: initial experience in patients with cerebral tumours, Radiology 172: 541–548.

Hagberg, G., Radü E., and Seelig, J., 1992, Brain tumours measured with STEAM ^{1}H-MRS using an echotime of 50 ms, "SMRM Book of Abstracts," p.3601, Society of Magnetic Resonance in Medicine, Berlin, Germany.

Heindel, W., Bunke, J., Glathe, S., Steinbrich, W., and Mollevanger, L., 1988, Combined [1]H-MR imaging and localised ^{31}P-spectroscopy of intracranial tumours in 43 patients, J Comput Assist Tomogr. 12: 907–916.

Jüngling, F., Wahkloo, K., and Hennig, J., 1992, Localised proton spectroscopy of meningeoma after embolization, "SMRM Book of Abstracts," p.8605, Society of Magnetic Resonance in Medicine, Berlin, Germany.

Knopp, M.V., Bachert, P., Ende, G., Blankenhorn, M., Kolem, H., Semmler, W., Heß, T., Forsting, M., Santor, K., and Lorenz, W.J., 1992, Nuclear Overhauser enhanced ^{31}P chemical shift imaging for monitoring embolisation therapy of meningiomas, "SMRM Book of Abstracts," P.8605, Society of Magnetic Resonance in Medicine, Berlin, Germany.

Komoroski, R.A., Newton, J.E.O., Karson, C.N., Cardwell, D., Jagannathan, N.R., and Sprigg, J.R., 1989, Detection of psychoactive drugs in vivo in human brain using ^{19}F NMR spectroscopy, "SMRM book of Abstracts," p.444, Society of Magnetic Resonance in Medicine, Amsterdam, The Netherlands.

Komoroski, R.A., Newton, J.E.O., Walker, E., Cardwell, D., Jagannathan, N.R., Ramaprasad, S., and Sprigg, J., 1990, In vivo NMR spectroscopy of Lithium-7 in humans, Magn Reson Med. 15, 347–356.

Lazeyras, F., Charles, H.C., Boyko, O., Fredericks, R., Schold, C., and Coleman, R.E., 1992, New perspectives in tumour grading by combined short echo/long echo ^{1}H spectroscopic imaging, "SMRM Book of Abstracts," p.3604, Society of Magnetic Resonance in Medicine, Berlin, Germany.

Naruse, S., Horikawa, Y., Tanaka, C., Higuchi, T., Ueda, S., Hirakawa, K., Nishikawa, H., and Watari, H., 1985, Observations of energy metabolism in neuroectodermal tumours using in vivo ^{31}P-NMR, Magn Reson Imag. 3: 117–123.

Naruse, S., Furuya, S., Ide, M., Umeda, M., Tanaka, C., Horikawa, Y., Ueda, S., Kinoshita, Y., and Yokata, A., 1992, Specific metabolites in brain tumours detected by ^{1}H chemical shift imaging, "SMRM Book of Abstracts," p.1952, Society of Magnetic Resonance in Medicine, Berlin, Germany.

Ng, T.C., Evanochko, W.T., Hiramoto, R.N., Ghanta, V.K., Lilly, M.B., Lawson, A.J., Corbett, T.H., Durant, J.R., and Glickson, J.D., 1982, ^{31}P NMR-Spectroscopy of in vivo tumours, J Mag Reson. 49: 271–286.

Ott, D., Ernst, T., and Hennig, J., 1990, Clinical value of [1]H Spectroscopy of brain tumours, "SMRM Book of Abstracts," p.105, Society of Magnetic Resonance in Medicine, NY.

Semmler, W., Bachert-Baumann, P., Gademann, G., Bellemann, M., Gückel, F., Lorenz, W.J., and van Kaick, G., 1990, In-vivo-Tumourtherapieverlaufskontrolle mit Hilfe der [1]H-MR-Spektroskopie unter Teilhirnbestrahlung, Zentrabl Radiol. 141: 421.

Section 7

New Techniques and Prospects

ANALYSIS OF CORTICAL PATTERNS

M.J. Cook, S.L. Free, D.R. Fish, S.D.Shorvon, K. Straughan, and
J.M. Stevens

Institute of Neurology
Imperial College
St. Mary's Hospital
London
United Kingdom

INTRODUCTION

Analysis of cortical structure is complicated by the complex geometry of the gyral patterns. Image analysis methods are one approach to the problem, and the anatomical detail provided in MR images is ideally suited to these methods. Disruption of normal gyral patterns, alteration of cortical ribbon volumes and simplification of the normal pattern of white matter digitations are features of many pathologies responsible for epilepsy. Many image analysis techniques used in the physical sciences are applicable to these problems. One developing technique is the physical implementation of mathematical morphology (Serra, 1982), which attempts to define images in terms of their shape content. An image is probed with a sequence of filter shapes of different but related sizes, and the response can be represented graphically and numerically. These shape descriptors can define size and shape of features as well as their spatial relationships. Fractal analysis of the gyral patterns is another method, which we have applied to a small group of patients in an attempt to define subtle simplification of gyral patterns.

CURRENT RESEARCH

Fractal geometry describes properties of shape which allow the quantification of the complexity of a structure over a range of scales (Mandelbrot, 1983). Perfect fractal structures have identical structure, and hence complexity, over all scales. Many naturally occurring structures exhibit fractal scaling properties, but over a limited range of scales (Kaye, 1989). Normal cerebral gyral patterns in MR images may be characterised by a simple dimension over a suitable range of scales. We applied this method to a group of 16 patients with frontal lobe epilepsy (FLE) and normal structural imaging. These patients have a high incidence of lesions which cause disruption of gyration, and the aim was to provide

Magnetic Resonance Scanning and Epilepsy, Edited by S.D. Shorvon et al.,
Plenum Press, New York, 1994

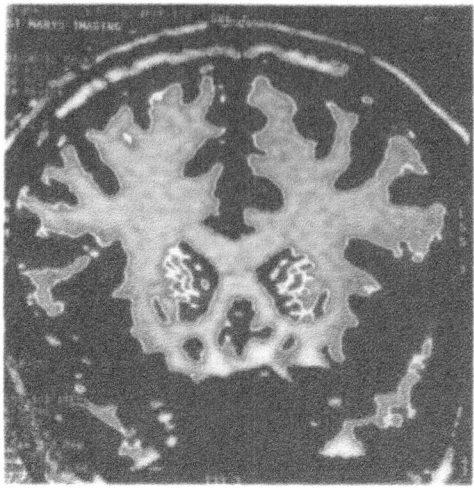

Figure 1. Coronal SPGR image with thresholding applied to define the grey–white interface. The fractal dimension is calculated from this area.

quantification of subtle degrees of abnormality. Using a box-counting method, the complexity of the grey–white interface was characterised. The log of the box count is plotted against the log of the box size (Figure 2), and the gradient of this line expressed as the fractal dimension. A normal range of fractal dimension (mean = 1.45 ± 0.06 SD) was defined using normal volunteers, in both the axial and coronal planes. Ten of these 16 patients with FLE had a fractal dimension of < 1.27 (mean − 3 SD), and in four cases there was bilateral asymmetrical reduction. The plane in which the maximal reduction occurs may vary according to the distribution of the lesion.

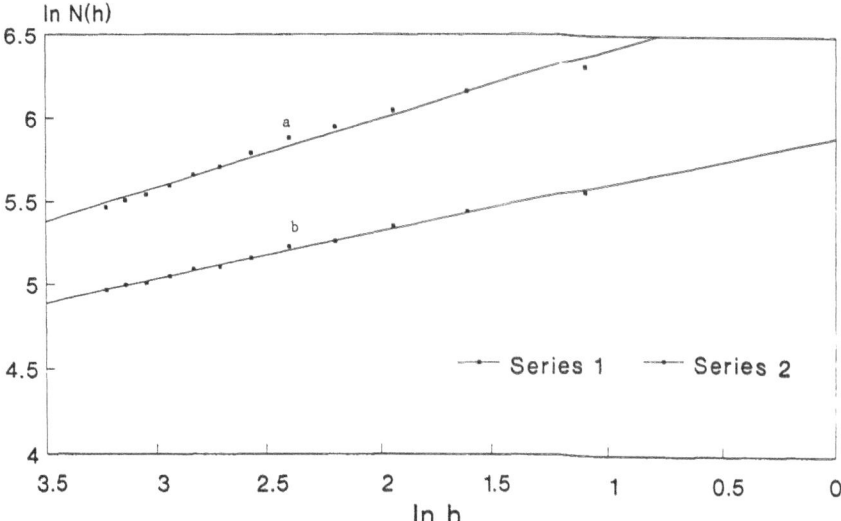

Figure 2. Plots of box-counts for normal and patient with epilepsy. X-axis is the log 1/box-size, and Y-axis is the log box count. The gradient of this line is the fractal dimension and represents the complexity of the contour. Calculated from coronal image, applied to grey–white interface of one hemisphere. (Coronal T1 weighted image, 1.5 mm thick). Normal study marked **a**. Abnormal study (marked **b** on graph), patient with epilepsy and no demonstrable focal abnormalities on visual inspection of images. Less steep gradient shows reduced complexity of this interface in this patient, corresponding to a low fractal dimension.

DISCUSSION

Description of shape is a valuable evolving technique in MR image processing, and addresses some of the problems encountered in imaging in epilepsy. Application to the cortical gyral patterns will permit description of complexity, in addition to standard anatomical features. One method, fractal analysis, has shown useful results, and other methods may allow categorisation of a wide group of pathologies. Automation of this type of analysis is possible, and applied in the physical sciences (Flook, 1978). In addition to the lateralisation of lesions, these methods may allow definition of extent and unsuspected bilaterality. This type of classification would be suitable for collaborative multicentre studies.

PROBABLE DEVELOPMENT OVER THE NEXT FIVE YEARS

Widespread availability of powerful computing facilities and sophisticated image processing software, combined with the high spatial resolution and excellent tissue contrast of high-field MR imaging, will lead to rapid development in this area. Compilation of libraries of normal anatomy, and more flexible descriptors of shape should permit accurate definition of a wide range of abnormalities currently outside visual detection.

REFERENCES

Flook, A.G. , 1978, The use of dilation logic on the Quantimet to achieve fractal dimension characterisation of textured and structured profiles, Powder Tech. 21: 295–298.

Kaye, B.H. , 1989, "A Random Walk Through Fractal Dimensions," VCH, New York.

Mandelbrot, B.B., 1983, "The Fractal Geometry of Nature", Freeman, New York.

Serra, J., 1982, "Image Analysis and Mathematical Morphology," Academic Press, London.

DIGITAL IMAGE PROCESSING FOR EPILEPSY

S.L. Free,[1] K. Straughan,[1] M.J. Cook,[2] S.D. Shorvon,[2] D.R. Fish,[2] and J.M. Stevens[3]

[1] Imperial College
[2] Institute of Neurology
  Queen Square
[3] St. Mary's Hospital
  London
  United Kingdom

INTRODUCTION

In a recent series of patients with intractable epilepsy studied at Queen Square the advent of high-quality MR volume imaging enabled the pick-up rate for many abnormalities to be raised significantly (Free et al., 1992). Of 128 patients studied, 110 were CT negative and 29 had a previously negative MR scan. In 92 of the CT-negative cases an abnormality was identified on volume MR, including hippocampal volume loss, foreign tissue lesions, macrogyrias and band heterotopias. However, this still leaves 18 cases in which no abnormality was shown. In some cases of cortical dysplasia clinical opinion was equivocal, and in others the extent of the abnormality was unclear. The use of high-quality volume imaging gives us the opportunity of extending our understanding of these abnormalities with the techniques of digital image processing.

Digital image processing involves using computer software to manipulate, enhance, interrogate and classify information represented in a digital format, such as magnetic resonance images of the brain. There are numerous analysis techniques available which have been applied in many medical and non-medical situations. It is important to have clinical input in deciding which features to investigate and the identification of which techniques may be most useful. This could take the form of the quantification of features presently described qualitatively by radiologists. Also, the application of mathematical models of shape and structure to isolate, for example, cortex characteristics in a form which gives diagnostic information not available to the human observer. One such application is the analysis of the grey–white matter interface as a fractal structure, described in Chapter 46.

One technique of increasing interest in image analysis is the use of mathematical morphology, using predefined shapes for image filtering. These shape filters are chosen with reference to the size and structure of the feature of interest. The results of applying a particular

Magnetic Resonance Scanning and Epilepsy, Edited by S.D. Shorvon et al.,
Plenum Press, New York, 1994

filter process called "opening" are illustrated in Figure 1. In this sequence a circular filter of increasing diameter is applied to the object, in this example the extracted white matter from a coronal brain image. The opening filter results in the removal of detail from the object which is too small to contain the applied shape filter. As the size of the circle filter is increased the amount of detail lost from the object also increases. There is a direct relationship between the size and shape of the filter at each step to the size and shape of features lost in the object. Thus a sequence of the filter steps shown here characterises the size and shape of the components of the object, in this example, the digitations of the white matter.

The difficulty in applying these techniques often is not in the application of the measuring process but in the decision about which object one wants to measure and the reproducibility of identifying this particular region in a multitude of cases. The segmentation of MR images is a continuing and growing area of research (Cline et al., 1992) and presently most techniques combine automated extraction with some level of intelligent operator intervention.

It is not only the shape of features in MR images which can be characterised. If the normal physical nature of a tissue is disturbed, this will often be manifest as an alteration in the expected spatial variations in tissue intensity, or the image texture, within the MR image. As the disturbance becomes more subtle these variations also become more subtle, and their spatial relationship more significant. Image texture is a concept that is relatively straightforward to appreciate visually but difficult to define theoretically. However, this does not prevent the mathematical description of texture and the use of quantifiable texture analysis techniques. Statistical methods identify the relationships between neighbouring pixels over the specific region of interest, often considering the probability that certain intensities are found in specific spatial locations with respect to each other. These techniques usually result in numerical feature descriptors which can be used for tissue characterisation (Magnin et al., 1986).

Despite the successes of digital image processing in many areas there are difficulties which should not be overlooked. Image quality is vital; it is often possible to extract features from poor quality images and attempt to characterise them but it can be of no clinical help.

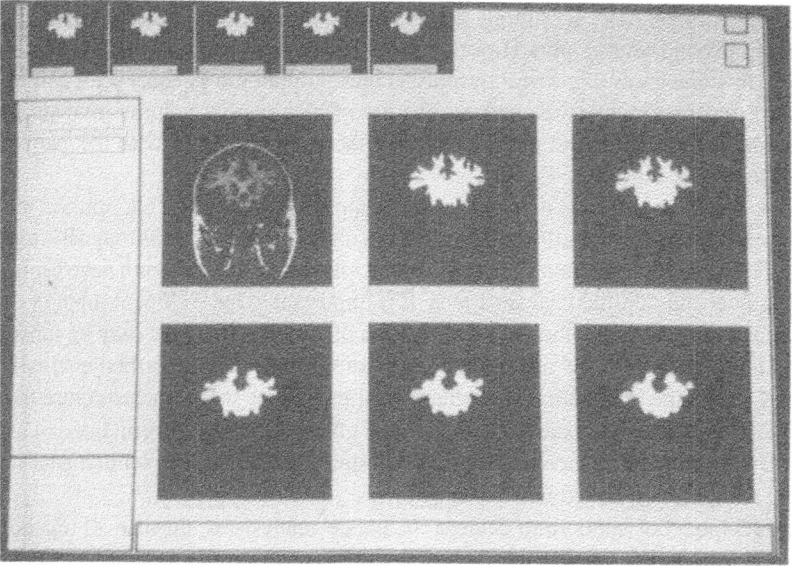

Figure 1. Morphological opening filters of different sizes characterise the white matter extracted from the MR image of a normal brain.

Consideration must be given to image intensity characteristics, especially with different acquisition sequences and slice thickness effects. With imaging features which provoke discussion between radiologists it is important that other means are available for comparison of any image analysis measures. The use of a large control group is necessary if meaningful distinctions are to be made about the nature of abnormalities. MRI is the only imaging option which allows the collection of normal data in a proactive manner.

Clinical input to these approaches to image analysis is very important. However clinical staff, inexperienced with computers, often find "in house" software difficult to use. The flexibility and responsiveness of software in research and development militates against user-friendliness. Commercial hardware and software packages, although often more limited in their range of applications are usually specifically tailored to the clinical user. They are also more often focused on particular functions which they implement well. One example, of a growing market, is the Allegro system produced by ISG Technologies Inc., Canada. This integrated hardware and software system primarily focuses on the display of volume data in two and three dimensions. The user is able to identify particular features on a slice by slice basis and reconstruct these into a three-dimensional object. This system has been used at Queen Square to visualise three-dimensional reconstructions of the cerebral cortex and the white matter. These processes have revealed more clearly the nature, location and extent of suspected gyral disruptions, especially in planes oblique to the image acquisition plane. Other features which have been investigated in this way include the hippocampi, dysembryoplastic lesions and foreign tissue lesions.

It is hoped that the use of commercial image visualisation packages can involve the clinical user more closely with the development of image analysis applications which, in turn, can assist in the investigation of imaging abnormalities in epilepsy.

REFERENCES

Cline, H.E., Lorensen, W.E., Kikinis, R,. and Jolesz, F., 1992, Three-dimensional segmentation of MR images of the head using probability and connectivity, J Comput Assist Tomogr. 14: 1037–1045.

Cook, M.J., Free, S., Fish, D.R., Shorvon, S.D., Straughan, K., and Stevens, J.M., 1992, Analysis of cortical patterns, NATO Workshop on MRI in Epilepsy, October.

Free, S., Cook, M.J., Fish, D.R., Shorvon, S.D., Straughan, K., and Stevens, J.M., 1992, Volumetric imaging in temporal and extratemporal epilepsies, 11th Annual Meeting SMRM, Berlin, August.

Magnin, I.E., Cluzeau, F., Odet, C.L., and Bremond, A., 1986, Mammographic texture analysis: An evaluation of risk for developing breast cancer, Optical Engineering 25: 780–784.

AN MRI-BASED PROBABILISTIC ATLAS OF NEUROANATOMY

A.C. Evans, M. Kamber, D.L. Collins, and D. MacDonald

Montreal Neurological Hospital and Institute
McGill University
3801 University Street
Montreal, Quebec
Canada H3A 2B4

INTRODUCTION

Three-dimensional MRI imaging techniques offer new possibilities for qualitative and quantitative studies of gross neuroanatomy, functional neuroanatomy and for neurosurgical planning. The digital nature of the data allows for the reconstruction of realistic three-dimensional models of an individual brain which can be sliced at arbitrary orientations for optimal visual inspection of often complex neuroanatomy and pathology. This is particularly relevant in the assessment of potential neuroanatomical correlates of temporal lobe epilepsy. Re-formatting of contiguous thinly sliced (1–2 mm thick) volumetric MRI data along planes parallel and perpendicular to the temporal plane allow finer visual discrimination and greater standardisation in qualitative procedures than previously possible. Perhaps more exciting are the applications of quantitative analysis where, for instance, accurate measurements of hippocampus and/or amygdala volumes provide important indicators of unilateral mesial temporal sclerosis which compare favourably with EEG and more invasive methods of lateralising the epileptogenic focus (Jack et al., 1990; Cascino et al., 1991; Watson et al., 1992; Cendes et al., 1993 a,b). For instance, by combining volumetric measurements of both hippocampus and amygdala, Cendes et al., (Chapter 9) quote correct lateralisation of focus in 93 of 100 temporal lobe epilepsy cases. The study of epilepsy arising from cortical abnormalities has been limited in the past by the difficulties of visualising the cortical surface from a set of conventional two-dimensional MRI slices. New acquisition techniques with gradient echo as opposed to spin echo techniques allow for an improved signal-to-noise ratio in thin slices in times compatible with clinical examinations. Whole brain coverage with thin slice data is now possible, such that partial volume effects are minimised with consequent improvements in fine detail. Numerous authors have reported dramatic improvements in the assessment of cortical dysplasia and grey matter heterotopias, particularly for more subtle abnormalities (Palmini et al., 1991a,b,c ; Barkovich and Kjos, 1992a,b,c). The impact of this improved raw data when

Magnetic Resonance Scanning and Epilepsy, Edited by S.D. Shorvon et al.,
Plenum Press, New York, 1994

combined with new techniques for generating three-dimensional surface renderings in reasonably interactive circumstances is yet to be fully realised but initial experience is promising. At present, most studies have relied upon visual inspection to identify abnormalities in gyration on three-dimensional surface-rendered MRI. Such methods are quite acceptable for gross pathologies but, in a manner similar to mesial temporal volumetrics, the identification of more subtle distortions may require quantitative analysis of left/right differences and comparison of individual gyral surface area or gyral/sulcal locations with previously established population norms. Cook et al., (Chapter 47) have approached the problem by application of fractal analysis to two-dimensional MRI images from normal and frontal lobe epilepsy (FLE) patients. The grey-white matter interface was extracted by image processing procedures as a continuous contour and the fractal dimension, an index of contour complexity, derived. Results indicate that 10 of 16 FLE patients had a fractal index more than 3 standard deviations (3SD) below normal. In its present form, the method provides a non-specific indicator of cortical abnormality, yielding an overall index of complexity rather than identifying specific abnormalities, and is implemented in two dimensions rather than three dimensions. Nevertheless, it illustrates the potential of quantitative analysis for detecting aberrant cortical morphology. For a more directed analysis of cortical folding, a model of normal neuroanatomical variability, expressed in three-dimensional coordinates, is necessary. Keyserlingk and co-workers have developed methods for digitising sulcal patterns from post-mortem brains and constructed a map, with cuboid elements of 4 mm or 8 mm edge length, of major sulcal anatomy from 30 such brains (Keyserlingk et al., 1983, 1985, 1988; Niemann et al., 1988). The advent of high resolution MRI scanning offers finer spatial and contrast resolution in normal brain in vivo. At the Montreal Neurological Institute, MRI and PET imaging techniques are combined with three-dimensional graphics and computational analysis in the study of functional neuroanatomy of cognitive and sensorimotor processing. As part of this "brain mapping" programme, we have collected a database of over 300 MRI volumes from young normal subjects and are presently engaged in a series of projects whose long-term goal is the construction of a probabilistic description of normal neuroanatomy derived from high-resolution (1 mm thick slices) MRI data. In this chapter we briefly describe the current brain mapping environment at our institute and the current development of the MRI atlas project in both volumetric and surface domains.

CURRENT RESEARCH

In current brain mapping research, three-dimensional MRI and PET data are mapped into a standardised brain-based coordinate space such that all brains have the same orientation and extent in three orthogonal directions. The PET data consist of sparsely distributed intensity peaks which reflect small changes in cerebral blood flow elicited by a specific cognitive or sensorimotor stimulus. As these images have no inherent anatomical information, each plane of the re-sliced volume is directly compared with an anatomical atlas and/or a co-registered MRI image. The most commonly employed coordinate space is that developed by Talairach and colleagues (Talairach et al., 1967; Talairach and Tournoux, 1988). This stereotactic transformation is based on the identification of the anterior-posterior commissural (AC-PC) line, extended to the cortical edge in the anteroposterior (AP) direction, and a set of perpendiculars to this line from the AC and PC points to the cortical edge. Strict application of the method (e.g. Lemoine et al., 1991) requires the proportional scaling to be partitioned into three piecewise linear components in the AP direction (pre-AC, AC-PC, post-PC), two in the CC direction (above/below AC-PC) and to be independent for each hemisphere. This is intended to overcome problems introduced by non-linear morphometric variability among individuals. Most centres have either retained a single scale along each dimension or have applied full non-linear warping techniques to address the non-linearity issue directly. At our institute, the Talairach space is used both for anatomical analysis with MRI data and for functional activation studies with PET, using a pre-registered MRI image for defining the required transformation (Evans et al., 1991a, 1992a). Since the AC and PC points are close (approximately 25 mm apart), and difficult to identify reliably even on MRI, significant errors can be introduced which are magnified at the cortex level. We therefore select a series of five well-separated mid-line landmarks which yield a least-square fit approximation to the AC-PC line (Evans et al., 1992a). Validation studies in 37 MRI volumes from young normal subjects indicate an angular discrepancy of $-0.24 \pm 2.9°$ and a vertical translational error of 1.2 ± 1.0 mm. Recently, we have implemented an automated method for mapping data into stereotactic space, using a general multi-scale feature-matching technique discussed in more detail below (Collins et al., 1992a,b).

The continued growth of brain mapping research has drawn attention to the inadequacies of the present methodologies. In particular, the current standard atlas of Talairach and Tournoux (1988) was derived from the post-mortem sectioning of the brain of a single 60-year-old female. Slice separation is variable, typically 3–4 mm, and atlas data from orthogonal planes are inconsistent. Given (i) the known variability in human cortical anatomy, (ii) the prevailing differences between local implementations of the stereotactic transformation at individual centres and the original piecewise-linear Talairach framework, and (iii) that most brain-mapping studies are performed on young normal subjects, the precise anatomical localisation of focal activation derived from PET using the Talairach atlas alone is problematic and can lead to over-interpretation of the results (Drevits et al., 1988). These uncertainties and the availability at our institute of a large database of MRI volumes obtained from young, normal subjects has lead to a programme to construct a three-dimensional probabilistic atlas of young, normal, gross neuroanatomy, defined within stereotactic space. Figure 1 shows a composite MRI dataset from 305 young normals (239 males; 66 females; mean age 23.4 ± 4.1) after transformation of each MRI volume into Talairach space and intensity normalisation. All subjects were right-handed and each MRI volume was acquired as 64 contiguous 2 mm-thick images (Evans et al., 1992b). The transformed atlas is composed of 80 slices separated by 1.5 mm in Talairach coordinates. Transverse image dimensions are 256×256, corresponding to a pixel size of 0.77 mm $\times$ 0.86 mm, in X and Y respectively. The average intensity MRI dataset obtained from the database illustrates the effect of anatomical variability in different brain areas and serves as a low-resolution, large sample atlas of gross neuroanatomy in Talairach space. The dataset has been distributed to over 30 centres for use alongside the Talairach atlas.

Although useful as a qualitative indicator of local anatomical variability, the composite MRI-intensity atlas is insufficient as a quantitative tool. For this purpose, the MRI intensity for each voxel in each MRI volume must be replaced by an anatomical label, e.g. caudate, pre-central gyrus or calcarine sulcus, and a probability assigned for each voxel having a particular label. This requires a precise segmentation of each MRI volume into component structures, features and tissue types. Manual labelling, in addition to being prohibitively time-consuming, would introduce intra- and inter-observer variations in labelling strategy which would confound the overall goal. Completely automatic and accurate image segmentation at the regional level is as yet an unsolved problem. At our institute, three overlapping projects are addressing the problem of anatomical variability, aimed at the automatic labelling of three-dimensional MRI datasets by tissue type, by specific neuroanatomical volume and by gyral/sulcal surface anatomy.

Tissue Classification

We have implemented a three-dimensional tissue-classification algorithm which segments double-echo MRI volumes into voxels labelled as grey matter, white matter and CSF. The classification algorithm employs the ID3 decision-tree classifier (Quinlan, 1986) operating on $3 \times 3 \times 3$ voxel neighbourhoods and T1-weighted and T2-weighted intensity features for

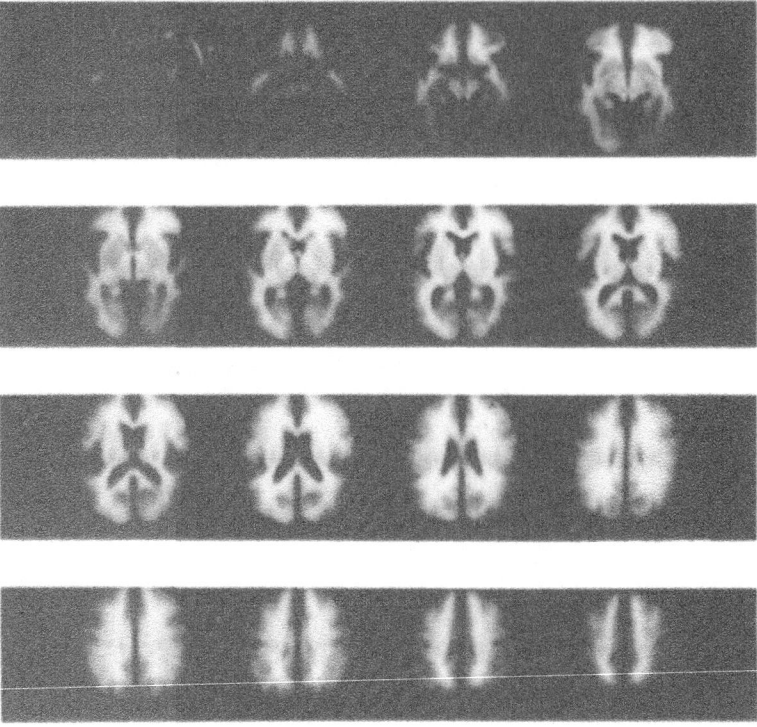

Figure 1. Mean MRI dataset drawn from 305 young normal volunteers. The dataset can be used as an anatomical atlas for locating functional activation data in Talairach space. It also provides a visual impression of local anatomical variability and an indication of how well a particular functional measurement can be localised. (Montreal Neurological Institute, N = 305)

each voxel. This algorithm represents tissue classification rules in the form of a binary decision-tree where each tree node represents a test on a feature and each leaf represents a tissue class. A top-down divide-and-conquer strategy is used to grow the tree by recursively partitioning user-provided tissue training samples into progressively smaller subsets which eventually correspond to tissue classes (Kamber et al., 1992).

The above segmentation procedure was applied to 12 three-dimensional spin-echo double-echo MRI datasets previously transformed into stereotactic space (Kamber et al., 1992). The proportion of all datasets for which a voxel was assigned to a given tissue class represents a probability function for membership in that class when taken across the population. Figure 2 illustrates orthogonal planes through this stereotactic grey-matter probability mask. The data can be used, for example, as a constraint on subsequent classifications by rejecting a particular voxel classification which has a probability lower than some pre-set threshold, e.g. peri-orbital fat could not be classified as cerebral white matter.

Regional Segmentation

Tissue classification only identifies gross components of the brain and does not specifically label individual brain structures automatically. For such segmentation (a priori), information is needed to augment the intensity/gradient/texture features of the MRI data, in the form of explicit geometric models or rules constraining the spatial relation of labelled structures. At

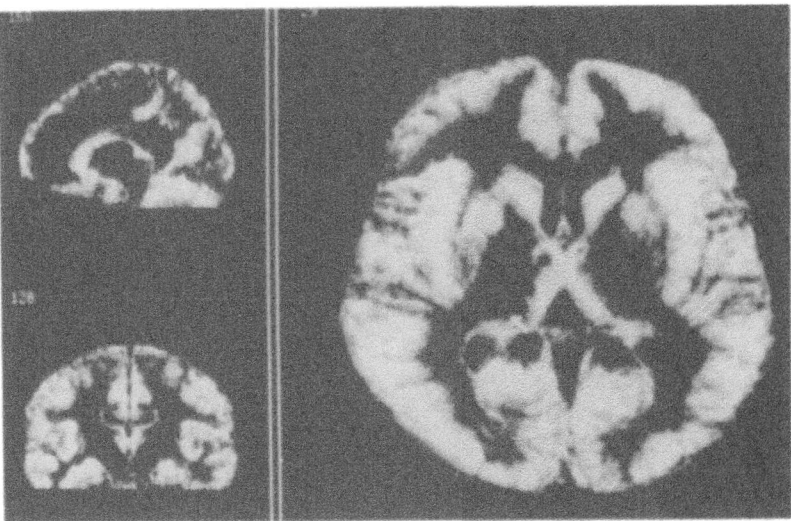

Figure 2. Grey matter probability map from 12 normal subjects. three-dimensional tissue classification identified grey matter voxels in each subject. Transformation to a standardised coordinate space allowed a composite probability for each voxel. Similar maps have been derived for other tissue classes (Kamber et al., 1992).

our institute, a three-dimensional volume-of-interest (VOI) atlas has been constructed by manual outlining of individual brain regions on 64 2 mm-thick adjacent MRI slices. Sixty structures in each hemisphere are identified including deep grey matter structures, major gyri, ventricles and white matter zones. The data exist as a tessellated geometrical model which can be re-sliced along any two-dimensional plane or warped in three dimensions to fit an image volume. We have employed this three-dimensional model in two ways for regional segmentation of individual MRI datasets.

Landmark-Driven Matching of VOI Atlas to Image

In this approach, the VOI atlas is deformed to match the individual image volume by manual identification of corresponding three-dimensional landmarks in the VOI atlas space and target MRI space, using the "thin-plate" spline algorithm (Bookstein, 1989) for non-linear deformation of atlas coordinates. The warping procedure identifies the non-linear transformation which will bring homologous points in each space into exact superimposition, decomposing that transformation into a series of principal warps of decreasing scale. To investigate this procedure, the algorithm was applied in three dimensions to fit the VOI atlas to each of 16 three-dimensional MRI datasets (Evans et al., 1991b). Using an interactive three-dimensional display system (Evans et al., 1989, 1991a), 26 clearly identifiable landmarks were tagged in the master MRI volume (from which the VOI atlas was originally constructed) and in each of the 16 target MRI volumes. For each target MRI/master MRI pair the 26 landmark-pairs were used to define the required deformation for the master MRI which was then applied to its co-extensive VOI atlas. Figure 3 shows an illustrative slice through one of the matched VOI/MRI volumes at the level of the peri-ventricular grey matter regions. In general, the warped atlas fitted the central brain regions well, owing to the number of landmarks identifiable in the peri-ventricular regions (caudate, thalamus, anterior/posterior commissures, corpus callosum, lateral ventricles). The lack of specific cerebellar landmarks resulted in unsatisfactory fits of that region. Such problems must be

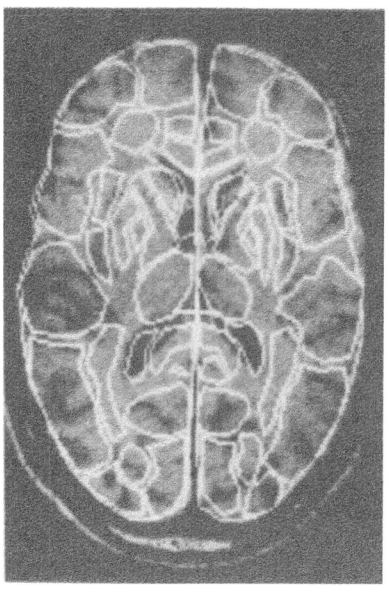

Figure 3. An example of the fit between VOI atlas and target MRI dataset in a plane passing through the basal ganglia.

dealt with by imposing additional cerebellar constraints. An important consideration is the extent to which such non-linear techniques are necessary for automatic identification of brain regions. A direct comparison of the simple linear scaling method and this approach was performed as follows. For each dataset employing the 26 landmarks as before, the matched VOI atlas was inverse-warped back to the master MRI space by the full non-linear warp or by application of only the linear terms in the expansion. By restricting the number of terms in the warping algorithm to only linear transformations, including anisotropic scaling, the mapping operation was reduced to a linear model in which the solution was effectively a least-square residual between master and target ensembles. Mapping the VOI atlas on to a single MRI volume by both linear and non-linear solutions would have allowed a direct comparison of the two solutions for that volume. However, as each brain had different dimensions, the pooling of results across all subjects would not have been straightforward. Instead, by first fitting the VOI atlas to an MRI volume with the non-linear solution and then applying the inverse solution to the fitted VOI atlas, but allowing only linear terms, the two methods could be compared. The difference between the starting coordinates of the VOI atlas in master space and its coordinates after the forward and inverse warps reflected the influence of the extra non-linear terms in a way that allowed comparison across the 16 different subjects. The centre of gravity for each of the structures in the VOI atlas used to assess the local inadequacy of the linear model and the results, shown Table 1, indicate that a substantial component of normal anatomical variation cannot be accommodated within a linear model. The overall three-dimensional centre of gravity shift between linear and non-linear models of 6–7 mm is considerable for applications which seek to localise specific structures with respect to other anatomical fiduciary markers based on principles of linear stereotaxy, e.g. biopsy or depth electrode placement. The same principle was also applied directly to each target MRI volume rather than to the corresponding customised VOI atlas. An average MRI volume was formed from all 16 datasets following either linear or non-linear deformation and the two compared as shown in Figure 4. The sharper appearance of the non-linear average MRI is a qualitative demonstration of

Table 1. Root Mean Square Distance (mm) of Regional Three-Dimensional Centre-of-Gravity from Target Position following Linear Warping of VOI Atlas to Target Space Indicating Residual Anatomical Variability not Handled by the Linear Model (See Text). 60 Regions in Total (14 Shown); 16 Subjects.

Distance (R)	(SD)	Region
6.34	(3.15)	Superior frontal gyrus
7.69	(2.27)	Middle frontal gyrus
5.86	(2.40)	Inferior frontal gyrus
5.83	(2.14)	Precentral gyrus
5.05	(2.35)	Postcentral gyrus
4.50	(1.91)	Superior temporal gyrus
4.47	(1.65)	Middle temporal gyrus
5.19	(2.07)	Inferior temporal gyrus
5.38	(2.19)	Amygdala
5.22	(2.26)	Hippocampus
9.18	(3.52)	Head of caudate nucleus
7.14	(2.99)	Putamen
7.80	(3.15)	Globus pallidus
7.63	(2.94)	Thalamus
6.52	(3.16)	Total (note: 60 structures)

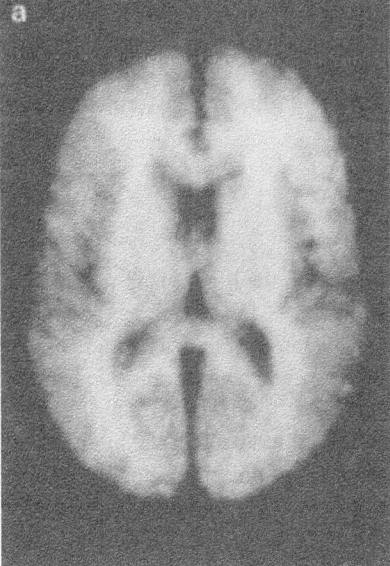 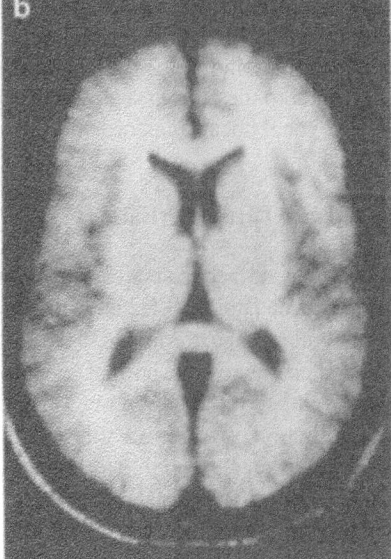

Figure 4. Comparison of the average MRI brain obtained from 16 subjects using a linear (a) and non-linear (b) model of anatomical variability.

the non-linear variability in brain anatomy, complementing the atlas-based analysis of Table 1.

Automatic Matching of Image to VOI Atlas

A problem of some concern with interactive landmark-based approaches is the subjectivity of landmark choice, i.e. the dependence of the resultant deformation on the number and distribution of landmarks selected and the behaviour of the algorithm in regions distant from any landmark. An alternative approach which avoids the need for potentially time-consuming landmark tagging, but sacrifices explicitly-defined point correspondence, is that of feature matching. Image features are local properties of the image intensity which can be extracted automatically by neighbourhood operators, e.g. edges, zones of relatively homogeneous intensity or particular shapes.

We are presently developing a new procedure for automatic identification of individual brain regions which combines this automatic approach with the concept of stereotactic space and the VOI atlas. The matching procedure first calculates a three-dimensional gradient volume from each original MRI volume and then evaluates the cross-correlation function between the two gradient volumes (Collins et al., 1992a,b). The maximum cross-correlation value, indicating the required transformation, is found by non-linear optimisation using the SIMPLEX algorithm. The algorithm operates in a multi-scale loop, beginning with a heavily-smoothed version of each image and successively sharpening the images at each iteration. The use of blurred images for obtaining approximate transformation parameters reduces the likelihood of encountering local minima during the search and is approximately four times faster than single-stage high-resolution optimisation. For automatic regional segmentation, the VOI atlas and the MRI volume upon which the VOI atlas was originally defined are resident in stereotactic space. Mapping an individual MRI volume into this space by feature-matching against the resident MRI also fits it to the VOI atlas. An inverse transformation fits the VOI atlas to the new MRI in its original space (Collins et al., 1992a, b). The multi-scale nature of the feature-matching algorithm facilitates the recursive application of the linear cross-correlation optimisation to individual neigbourhoods defined on a three-dimensional grid with a dimension equal to the current scale. Hence, an overall non-linear transformation is obtained by successive local linear transformations.

Cortical Surface Parameterisation

The cortical surface is an area of particular interest in the brain mapping domain—both its intrinsic neuroanatomical features and the relationship of functional neuroanatomy to the superficial gyral/sulcal patterns and to the underlying cytoarchitecture. The study of variability in cortical anatomy across the normal population merits special consideration and new methods are being developed for this purpose. Many methods already exist for visualising the cerebral cortex by extraction of surfaces with isovalues, with or without subsequent polygonalisation. These techniques are susceptible to artefacts introduced by noise or signal inhomogeneities and do not enforce topological continuity, i.e. there can be holes in the surface. Moreover, the unstructured representation of the cortex as between 10^5 and 10^7 cuberilles or polygons is not best suited for point-to-point comparison of equivalent surfaces across a population.

This goal has motivated attempts to use analytical representations to replace the isosurface. Such parametric representations are continuous, relatively compact and can often be expressed at different scales, i.e. resolutions, in a hierarchical fashion. The problem of quantifying, as opposed to visualising, the cortical surface and measuring its variability across subjects is difficult to express in mathematical terms because the boundaries of gyri and the extent of sulci are ill-defined. Moreover, many secondary gyri have a highly variable appearance or may be absent altogether. Even major sulci may have variable branching patterns. Van Essen and Maunsell (1980) advanced the notion of mapping the cortex, with examples in macaque and cat brains. Since then, various approaches have been made to apply such techniques to MRI data from the human brain. Jouandet et al., (1989) outline the cortex manually on successive cortical slices whereas Carman (1990) and Sereno and Dale (1992) have employed similar surface tension models to define the cortical anatomy.

At our institute, we have developed a procedure which combines the advantages of polygonal, parametric and hierarchical representations with a fast converging elastic deformation model (MacDonald et al., 1993). The vertices of a starting parametric surface, defined by a polygonal mesh, are moved towards a boundary surface, defined by a feature description, i.e., intensity or gradient magnitude, along a direction normal to the current parametric surface and for a distance controlled by a weighting factor for each boundary point. The weighting is linear such that zero weighting leaves the point unmoved and unit weighting moves directly to the boundary surface. The algorithm proceeds iteratively, adjusting all mesh points at each iteration, until equilibrium is obtained with all mesh edges of almost equal length. The simplicity of the model allows a simple control of the surface resolution, by sub-sampling of the boundary points, and hence the degree of sulcal detail apparent in the fitted surface.

The boundary points are usually isosurface voxels obtained by intensity or gradient thresholding, but can also include additional manually defined boundary points reflecting specific surface targets with increased weighting. The mesh form of the parametric surface guarantees a continuous single surface topology and also allows a direct one-to-one mapping of the cortical surface to any simple parametric representation. Figure 5 illustrates mapping from a three-dimensional cortical manifold to a spherical projection, both viewed from above. Corresponding sulci and gyri are evident and can be identified by traditional cartographic lines of latitude and longitude. Application of this transformation to a large number of MRI datasets and morphometric analysis across a normal population require definition of specific orienting landmarks in native or parametric space. At present, we use the existing Talairach transformation but this may be superseded by landmarks in the parametric space.

Similar procedures can be applied to each hemisphere separately to avoid the gross distortions involved in fitting the inter-hemispheric fissure. As the deformation from cortical

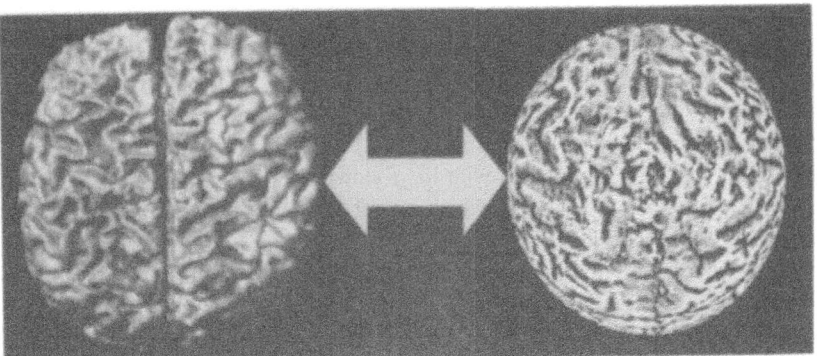

Figure 5. An example of cortical parameterisation or "surface-flattening". The surface is first extracted from three-dimensional MRI data by intensity or gradient thresholding. The parameter surface, in this case a sphere, is expanded iteratively to overlay the extracted surface using a minimum distance criterion (see text). The one-to-one correspondence allows an inverse mapping of cortex to parameter surface. Dark areas on the parameter surface correspond to high negative curvature (sulcal floors) whereas light areas indicate high positive curvature (gyral ridges). (Montréal Neurological Institute)

surface to a simple parametric surface will also be severe in the vicinity of other major fissures, we are presently exploring the possibility of using the average cortical surface, drawn from a 305-brain MRI composite, as a starting surface instead of a sphere. The problem of surface modelling is then reduced to modelling local folding with respect to the average surface rather than to a simple object, i.e. a more realistic topology at the expense of a direct cartographic analogy.

DISCUSSION

Quantitative neuroimaging applications are appearing with increasing frequency, mostly using two-dimensional images. A continuing problem has been the difficulty in obtaining equivalent two-dimensional images within or across patients for comparative analysis. Recent technical developments make three-dimensional approaches both feasible and preferable, as all the anatomical information is available and the necessary presumption of topological equivalence across datasets is satisfied. However, suitable normative data are needed before diagnostic inferences can be drawn from three-dimensional imaging studies of pathological brain. This paper has discussed progress towards a probabilistic atlas of neuroanatomy.

The averaged MRI image, shown in Figure 1, contains striking features not normally apparent on individual MRI images. In the central regions, the noise reduction consequent to image averaging outweighs the resolution loss caused by anatomical variability. Hence, for example, the dorsomedial nucleus of the thalamus is visible and the contrast between cingulum bundles and adjacent grey matter is enhanced. At the cortex, anatomical variability leads to a loss of contrast for secondary sulci but major sulci are well defined. Interestingly, the ascending arm of the cingulate sulcus appears highly conserved. Comparison of left and right hemispheres, performed by reflecting one hemisphere around the mid-line of stereotactic space and subtracting the images, reveals some interesting features consistent with previous work (Geschwind and Levitsky, 1968; Rubens et al., 1976; Witelson, 1977; Galaburda et al. , 1978; Chang Chui and Damasio, 1980; Weinberger et al., 1982). There is clear evidence of left occipital petalia and right frontal petalia (Le May and Kido, 1978). Heschl's gyrus is seen to be differently represented with a second sulcus evident on the left.

The MRI atlas of Figure 1 has the advantage that no subjective decisions have been taken about the borders of structures of interest. Any visually apparent differences, preserved across 305 brains, are likely to be real anatomical differences rather than artefacts of the choice of boundary in each hemisphere. However, no quantitative information is provided. The application of a landmark-driven atlas provides regional segmentation and information about brain morphometrics. However, it is also susceptible to artefacts arising from the subjective choice of landmarks and errors in identifying truly homologous coordinates for those landmarks. The automatic feature-matching approach will allow a completely objective mapping of the VOI atlas to each MRI and statistics on local volumetrics with the following caveat. The present VOI atlas is composed of a finite set of contour nodes which cannot be arbitrarily deformed. Fine structural details will not be detected and an atlas-based method will not give as accurate a measurement of regional volume as a trained investigator using a manual technique to outline the structure on successive MRI slices. It remains to be seen whether the objectivity and increased reproducibility of an automated approach outweigh this decreased ability to delineate fine structure when comparing regional volumes between hemispheres or between normals and patient groups.

The extraction and labelling of cortical anatomy in an automatic or semi-automatic fashion is still at an early stage. The results shown in Figure 5 were obtained without subjective decisions. We have applied the same procedure to the 305 brains of the database in sequence and are presently building an average parametric surface. Ultimately, this work will lead to a probabilistic description of the flattened cortical surface. Comparison of an individual's flattened surface with the probabilistic surface may facilitate the automatic identification of subtle dysplasias and other cortical anomalies.

The data presented here represent a limited analysis of the raw data available in the 305-brain database. The manual labour involved in hand-segmentation of each dataset is prohibitive and thorough analysis awaits completion of the automatic three-dimensional matching/segmentation work. The goal of a probabilistic three-dimensional description of normal neuroanatomy will take many years to achieve. It is most probable that the major components, i.e. the initial model, the matching/segmentation procedure and the database being segmented, will all be repeatedly updated during that time. However, technical improvements in computers and brain imagers combined with the knowledge gained at each iteration should produce an accelerating cycle. Numerous national and international initiatives to create such widely applicable databases are already under way, and one can expect increasing cooperation and exchange of data to build up a compendium of datasets for different age ranges and pathological conditions. Intermediate results, such as the averaged young normal brain presented here, have immediate application.

REFERENCES

Barkovich, A.J., and Kjos, B.O., 1992a, Gray matter heterotopias: MR characteristics and correlation with developmental and neurological manifestations, Radiology 182: 493–499.

Barkovich, A.J., and Kjos, B.O., 1992b, Non-lissencephalic cortical dysplasia: Correlation of imaging findings with clinical deficits, AJNR 13: 95–103.

Barkovich, A.J., and Kjos, B.O., 1992c, Schizencephaly: Correlation of clinical findings with MR characteristics, Radiology 182: 493–499.

Bookstein, F., 1989, Principal warps: Thin-plate splines and the decomposition of deformations, IEEE Transactions on Pattern Analysis and Machine Intelligence, 11: 567–585.

Carman, G.J., 1990, Mapping of the cerebral cortex, PhD Thesis: Caltech.

Cascino, G.D., Jack, C.R. Jr, Parisi, J.E., Sharbrough, F.W., Hirschorn, K.A., Meyer, F.B., Marsh, W.R., and O'Brien, P.C., 1991, Magnetic resonance imaging-based volume studies in temporal lobe epilepsy: pathological correlations, Ann Neurol. 30: 31–36.

Cendes, F., Andermann, F., Gloor, P., Evans, A.C., Jones-Gotman, M., Watson, C., Melancon, D., Olivier, A., Peters, T., Lopes-Cendes, I., and Leroux, G., 1993a, Volumetric measurements of amygdala and hippocampal formation in temporal lobe epilepsy, Neurology in press.

Cendes, F., Andermann, F., Dubeau, F., Gloor, P., Evans, A.C., Jones-Gotman, M., Olivier, A., Andermann, E., Robitaille, Y., and Melancon, D., 1993b, Early childhood prolonged febrile convulsions, atrophy and sclerosis of mesial structures in temporal lobe epilepsy: An MRI volumetric study, Neurology 43: 1083–1087.

Chang, Chui, H., and Damasio, A.R., 1980, Human cerebral asymmetries evaluated by computed tomography, J Neurochem Neurosurg Psychiat. 43: 873–878.

Collins, D.L., Dai, W., Peters, T.M., and Evans, A.C., 1992a, Model-based segmentation of individual brain structures from MRI data visualisation in Biomedical Computing, Proceedings of the International Society of Optical Engineering (SPIE), 1808: 10–23.

Collins, D.L., Peters, T.M., and Evans, A.C., 1992b, Non-linear multi-scale image registration and segmentation of individual brain structures from MRI , Proceedings of IEEE Symposium on Advanced Medical Image Processing in Medicine: 105–110.

Drevits, W.C., Videen, T.O., MacLeod, A.K., Haller, J.W., and Raichle, M.E., 1988, PET images of blood flow changes during anxiety: Correction, Science 256: 1696.

Evans, A.C., Marrett, S., Collins, D.L., and Peters, T.M., 1989, Anatomical-functional correlative analysis of the human brain using three-dimensional imaging systems, Medical, Imaging III: 264–274.

Evans, A.C., Marrett, S., Torrescorzo, J., Ku, S., and Collins, L., 1991a, MRI-PET correlative analysis using a volume of interest (VOI) atlas, J Cereb Blood Flow Metabol. 11: A69-A78.

Evans, A.C., Dai, W., Collins, L., Neelin, P., and Marrett, S., 1991b, Warping of a computerised three-dimensional atlas to match brain image volumes for quantitative neuroanatomical and functional analysis, Proceedings of the International Society of Optical Engineering (SPIE): Medical Imaging V 1445: 236–247.

Evans, A.C., Marrett, S., Neelin, P., Collins, L., Worsley, K., Dai, W., Milot, S., Meyer, E., and Bub, D., 1992a, Anatomical mapping of functional activation in stereotactic coordinate space, NeuroImage 1: 43–63.

Evans, A.C., Collins, D.L., Milner, B., 1992b, An MRI-based stereotactic brain atlas from 300 young normal subjects, "Proceedings of the 22nd Annual Symposium, Society for Neuroscience," Arnheim 179.4: 408.

Galaburda, A.M., LeMay, M., Kemper, T.L., and Geschwind, N., 1978, Right-left asymmetries in the brain. Structural differences between the hemispheres may underlie cerebral dominance, Science 199: 852–856.

Geschwind, N., and Levitsky, W., 1968, Human brain: left-right asymmetries in temporal speech regions, Science 161: 181–187.

Jack, C.R. Jr, Sharbrough, F.W., Twomey, C.K., Cascino, G.D., Hirschorn, K.A., Marsh, W.R., Zinsmeister, A.R., and Scheithauer, B., 1990, Temporal lobe seizures: lateralisation with MR volume measurements of the hippocampal formation, Radiology 175: 423–429.

Jack, C.R. Jr, Sharbrough, F.W., Cascino, G.D., Hirschorn, K.A., O'Brien, P.C., and Marsh, W.R. 1992, Magnetic resonance image-based hippocampal volumetry: correlation with outcome after temporal lobectomy, Ann Neurol, 31: 138–146.

Jouandet, M.L., Tramo, M.J., Herron, D.M., Hermann, A., Lostus, W.C., Bazell, J., and Gazzaniga, M.S., 1989, Computer-generated two-dimensional maps of the human cerebral cortex in vivo, J Cognit Neurosci. 1: 88–117.

Kamber, M., Collins, D.L., Francis, G.S., Shinghal, R., and Evans, A.C., 1992, Model-based three-dimensional segmentation of multiple sclerosis lesions in MRI data Visualisation in Biomedical Computing, Proceedings of the International Society of Optical Engineering (SPIE): 1808: 590–600.

Keyserlingk, D.Gv., De Bleser, R., and Poeck, K., 1983, Stereographic reconstruction of human brain CT series, Acta Anat. 123: 240–246.

Keyserlingk, D.Gv., Niemann, K., Wasel, J., Reinold, J., and Poeck, K., 1985, A new method in computer-assisted imaging in neuroanatomy, Acta Anat. 123: 240–246.

Keyserlingk, D.Gv., Niemann, K., and Wasel, J., 1988, A quantitative approach to spatial variation on human cerebral sulci, Acta Anat. 131: 127–131.

Le May, M. and Kido, D.K., 1978, Asymmetries of the cerebral hemispheres on computed tomograms, J Comput Assist Tomogr. 2: 471–476.

Lemoine, D., Barillot, C., Gibaud, B., and Pasqualini, E., 1991, An anatomical-based three-dimensional registration system of multimodalityand atlas data in neurosurgery, Lecture Notes in Computer Science 511: Information Processing in Medical Imaging, Colchester A.C.F. and Hawkes D.J.: eds, Springer-Verlag, Heidelberg, pp 154–164.

MacDonald, D., Avis, D., and Evans, A.C., 1993, Automatic parameterisation of human cortical surfaces, "Proceedings of the Annual Symposium on Information Processing in Medical Imaging (IPMI)", in press.

Niemann, K., Keyserlingk, D.Gv., and Wasel, J., 1988, Superposition of an averaged three-dimensional pattern of brainstructures on CT scans, Acta Neurochir. (Wien) 93: 61–67.

Palmini, A., Andermann, F. et al., 1991a, Diffuse cortical dysplasia, or the "double cortex" syndrome: the clinical and epileptic spectrum in 10 patients, Neurology 41: 1656–1662.

Palmini, A., Andermann, F. et al., 1991b, Focal neuronal migration disorders and intractable partial epilepsy: a study of 30 patients, Ann Neurol. 30: 741–749.

Palmini, A., Andermann, F. et al., 1991c, Focal neuronal migration disorders and intractable partial epilepsy: results of surgical treatment, Ann Neurol. 30: 750–757.

Quinlan, J.R., 1986, Induction of decision trees, Machine Learning 1: 81–106.

Rubens, A.B., Mahowald, U.W., and Hutton, J.T., 1976, Asymmetry of the lateral (sylvian) fissures in man, Neurology 26: 620–624.

Sereno, M.I., and Dale, A.M., 1992, A technique for reconstructing and flattening the cortical surface using MRI images, Society for Neuroscience Abstracts 18: 585.

Talairach, J. and Tournoux, P., 1988, Co-planar stereotactic atlas of the human brain: three-dimensionalimensional proportional system: an approach to cerebral imaging, Georg Thieme Verlag, Stuttgart, New York.

Talairach, J., Szikla, G., Tournoux, P., Prossalentis, A., Bordas-Ferrer, M., Covello, L., Jacob, M., Mempel, A., Buser, P., and Bancaud, J., 1967, "Atlas d'anatomie stereotaxique du telencephale," Masson, Paris.

Van Essen, D.C., and Maunsell, J.H.R., 1980, Two-dimensional maps of the cerebral cortex, J Comparative Neurol. 191: 255–281.

Watson, C., Andermann, F., Gloor, P., Jones-Gotman, M., Peters, T., Evans, A., Olivier, A., Melanson, D., and Leroux G., 1992, Anatomical basis of amygdaloid and hippocampal volume measurement by magnetic resonance imaging, Neurology 42: 1743–1750.

Weinberger, D.R., Luchins, P., Morihisa, J., and Wyatt, R.J., 1982, Asymmetrical volumes of the right and left frontal and occipital regions of the human brain, Neurology 11: 97–102.

Witelson, S.F., 1977, Anatomical asymmetry in the temporal lobes: its documentation, phylogenesis and relationship to functional asymmetry, Ann NY Acad Sci. 299: 328–354.

OTHER METHODS

Functional Imaging, Magnetisation Transfer, and Relaxation Times

Paul Tofts

Institute of Neurology
Queen Square
London, WC1N 3BG
United Kingdom

FUNCTIONAL IMAGING

Functional imaging has previously been the prerogative of PET, whereas MRI has been confined to anatomical and pathological descriptions. Recently, methods for imaging cerebral blood volume, and changes in blood oxygenation and blood flow, have been demonstrated using standard MRI equipment.

Cerebral blood volume (CBV) can be imaged by tracking a bolus injection of a susceptibility contrast agent. A bolus of gadolinium-DTPA, injected over 4 seconds, produces a transient reduction, lasting about 15 s, in $T2^*$. This can be observed as a reduction in signal in a gradient echo image on a conventional imager (Edelman et al., 1990) or in an echo-planar image (Belliveau et al., 1991). The time integral of the signal reduction is proportional to blood volume; this can be calculated for each pixel and displayed as a functional image of blood volume. Regions in cerebral infarcts, metastases and arteriovenous malformations showed different patterns from those of oedema around a lesion, and from those of normal brain (Edelman et al., 1990). Using photic stimulation at 8 Hz a change in CBV could be imaged in the visual cortex (Belliveau et al., 1991).

Changes in blood oxygenation (PO_2) can be imaged by observing the change in T2 caused by the presence of paramagnetic deoxyhaemoglobin in the blood, which is a natural contrast agent. An increase in oxygenation causes an increase in $T2^*$, and in the signal observed in a gradient echo or echo-planar image (Kwong et al., 1992). By activating parts of the brain (e.g. the visual or motor cortex) an increase in PO_2 and hence signal can be produced. Difference images map the appropriate parts of the cortex. With suitable choice of slice thickness and orientation, a signal increase of 15% in the motor cortex can be observed.

Changes in blood flow can be imaged using a T1-weighted sequence of sufficient speed (e.g. an echo-planar or gradient echo sequence with a pre-inversion pulse). T1 is reduced by

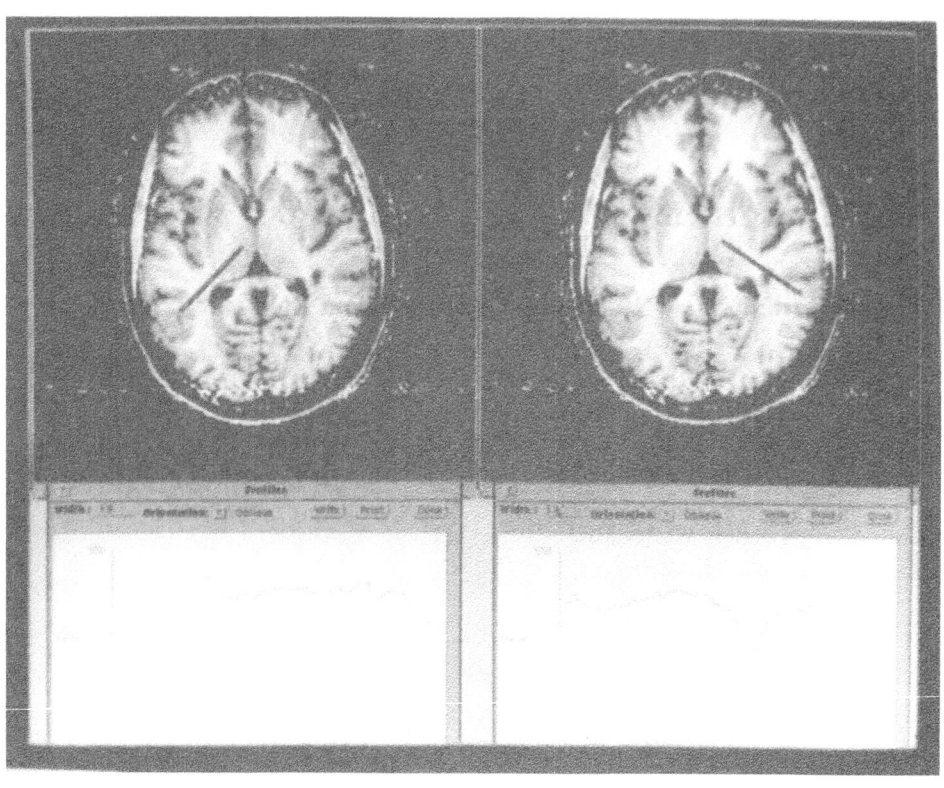

Figure 1. Magnetisation transfer contrast image in a patient with multiple sclerosis. This was calculated on a pixel-by-pixel basis from images without and with off-resonance presaturation. In normal white matter (left-hand image and profile) the MTC (i.e. signal reduction) is about 40% (vertical scale is MTC x 10); in the lesion (right-hand image) MTC is reduced to about 25%.

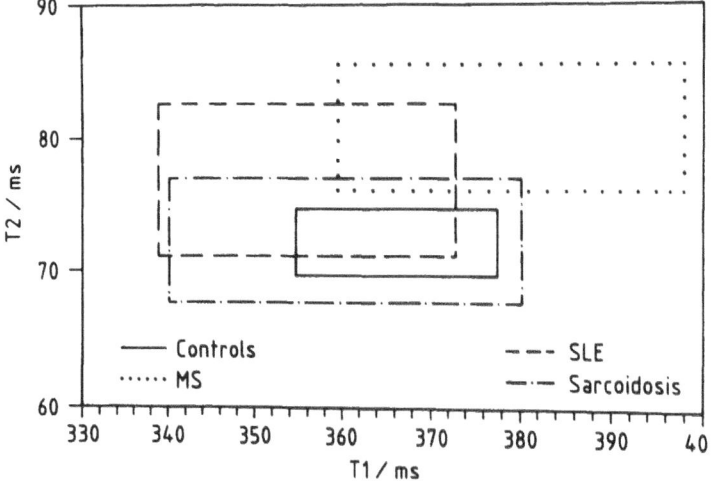

Figure 2. Subtle changes in relaxation times T1 and T2 are detected in the normal appearing white matter in patients with multiple sclerosis, when compared to controls and patients with sarcoidosis and systemic lupus erythematosus. Boxes are ± 1 standard deviation. (From Miller et al., 1989.)

the inflow of fresh, unsaturated, blood bringing magnetisation into the slice (Kwong et al., 1992).

Changes in blood volume, oxygenation and flow are usually correlated, and therefore activation of the cortex produces an effect in all three types of functional image. Blood oxygenation and flow have the advantage of not needing injection of a contrast medium, and therefore can be repeated easily, with scope for signal averaging to improve signal-to-noise ratio. They have the possible disadvantage that changes in function, arising from activation, are observed, rather than the absolute measurement given by the bolus injection method. Echo planar imaging is fast enough to measure the brain time constants for blood oxygenation change (4 s) and flow change (9 s) (Kwong et al., 1992). Highfield (4 T) images show increased contrast-to-noise ratio and spatial detail. Superimposition of a functional image on a conventional anatomical image indicates the location of the activated area.

Improvements in slice position and orientation will increase the contrast that can be obtained. Other parts of the brain will show activation. The techniques will be used to identify important parts of the cortex prior to surgery. Because the technique can be used on standard MR imagers, widespread use will be made of functional imaging by MRI.

MAGNETISATION TRANSFER

Magnetisation transfer (Wolff and Balaban, 1989) contrast enables bound water to be probed. Free water (about 80% of the total, with $T2 \simeq 50$ ms) is NMR visible and is the subject of conventional images. Bound water (about 15% of the total, $T2 \simeq 0.1$ ms) is attached to large proteins and cellular structures and is generally NMR invisible. Magnetisation can be transferred between the two pools of water, and the principal mechanism of T1 relaxation of the free water is through the bound water. If the bound water is saturated by applying RF power about 1–5 kHz from the resonant frequency of the free water, the magnetisation of the free water, and hence its signal, is reduced by a factor called the magnetisation transfer contrast (MTC). In white matter this is 40%; in CSF it is 0%; in oedematous lesions it is intermediate as a result of the reduced structure and amount of bound water. Thus MTC gives a direct indication of the amount of structured material.

Magnetisation transfer can be used to increase contrast in sequences designed to make lesions visible as bright objects, by suppressing the signal from normal tissue (this contains more bound water than the lesion). In multiple sclerosis, MTC is reduced in the lesions and in the normal appearing white matter (Dousset et al., 1992); this has been attributed to demyelination.

The specificity of MTC remains to be established; any loss of tissue structure will decrease MTC. Loss of structure will also increase T2, and the amplitude of the slow component in a bi-exponential analysis of multi-echo data.

The relative merits of MTC and T2 will be elucidated for characterising tissue breakdown. Power limitations in MTC measurements will be investigated to provide the maximum contrast within safety guidelines. Absolute measurements of the transfer constant k will be correlated with ultrastructural tissue changes in experimental lesions.

RELAXATION TIMES

Relaxation times (T1 and T2) are the NMR parameters most widely used to differentiate one tissue from another. They enable white–grey structural interfaces to be observed in T1- or T2-weighted images. The differences in relaxation times are visible to the eye in a qualitative way, because one tissue with one relaxation time gives a visibly different signal from an

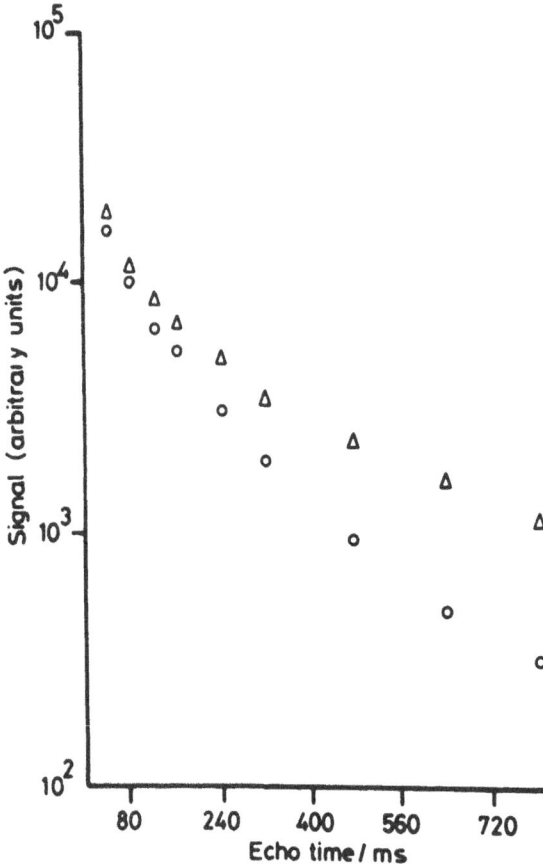

Figure 3. The decay of transverse magnetisation in an experimental oedematous lesion. Circles are 2 days after production of the lesion, triangles 4 days after production. Non-linearity at long echo times arises from extracellular fluid. (From Barnes et al., 1986.)

adjacent tissue with a different relaxation time.

Some changes in relaxation time may not be visible, either because the difference is too small, or because the affected tissue has diffuse (rather than focal) edges. In this case a quantitative measurement of signal intensity, or relaxation time, is needed to establish whether or not the tissue is abnormal. A review of relaxation times, covering mechanisms of relaxation, factors influencing their change, instrumental precision and accuracy, and clinical measurements, can be found in Tofts and Du Boulay (1990).

Relaxation times can be measured extremely accurately (1–4%), given the right sequence and sufficient imaging time. Relaxation times increase as water becomes more free to rotate (this time averages the local fields that cause relaxation). Thus any pathology that involves loss of cellular structure, or oedema, gives increased relaxation times. In fact relaxation times are the most sensitive indicator we have of changes in the tissue pathology, because they are so sensitive to the physical state of the water. In patients with multiple sclerosis and other white matter diseases, the lesions have raised relaxation times (which make them visible), and also the normal-appearing white matter between the lesions has subtly raised relaxation times which are invisible to the eye, but which respond to quantitative measurements (up to 15%, Miller et al., 1989; Tofts and Du Boulay, 1990). Multi-echo data, where the decay of transverse magnetisation is observed, enables intra- and extracellular water, with their distinct T2 values, to be separately identified (Barnes et al., 1986).

Values of accuracy and precision in the measurement of relaxation times which are less than the normal variation (5%) will be achievable in a reasonable time on standard imagers. Other white matter diseases in which there are diffuse changes will be shown to have altered relaxation times. The reproducibility of relaxation time measurements in grey matter may improve with careful reposition techniques, smaller voxels, and an increased familiarity with cortical anatomy.

REFERENCES

Barnes, D., McDonald, W.I., Tofts, P.S., Johnson, G., and Landon, D.N., 1986, Magnetic resonance imaging of experimental cerebral oedema, J Neurol Neurosurg Psychiat. 49: 1341.

Belliveau, J.W., Kennedy, D.N., McKinstry, R.C., Buchbinder, B.R., Weisskoff, R.M., Cohen, M.S., Vevea, J.M., Brady, T.J., and Rosen, B.R., 1991, Functional mapping of the human visual cortex by magnetic resonance imaging, Science 254: 717.

Connelly, A., Jackson, G.D., Frackowiak, R.S.J., Belliveau, J.W., Vargha-Khadafa, F., and Gadian, D., 1993, Functional mapping of activated human primary cortex with a clinical MR imaging system, Radiology, 188: 125.

Dousset, V., Grossman, R.I., Ramer, K.N., Schnall, M.D., Young, L.H., Gonzales- Scarano, F., Lavi, E., and Cohen, J.A., 1992, Experimental allergic encephalomyelitis and multiple sclerosis: lesion characterisation with magnetisation transfer imaging, Radiology 182: 483.

Edelman, R.R., Mattle, H.P., Atkinson, D.J., Hill, T., Finn, J.P., Mayman, C., Ronthal, M., Hoggewoud, H.M., and Kleefield, J., 1990, Cerebral blood flow: assessment with dynamic contrast-enhanced $T2^*$-weighted MR imaging at 1.5T, Radiology 176: 211.

Kwong, K.K., Belliveau, J.W., Chesler, D.A., Goldberg, I.E., Weisskoff, R.M., Poncelet, B.P., Kennedy, D.N., Hoppel, B.E., Cohen, M.S., Turner, R., Cheng, H-M., Brady, T.J., and Rosen, B.R., 1992, Dynamic magnetic resonance imaging of human brain activity during primary sensory stimulation, Proc Natl Acad Sci USA, 89: 5675.

Miller, D.H., Johnson, G., Tofts, P.S., Macmanus, D., and McDonald, W.I., 1989, Precise relaxation time measurements of normal-appearing white matter in inflammatory central nervous system disease, Magn Reson Med. 11: 331.

Tofts, P.S,. and du Boulay, E.P.G.H., 1990, Towards quantitative measurements of relaxation times and other parameters in the brain, Neuroradiology, 32: 407.

Wolff, S.D., and Balaban, R.S., 1989, Magnetisation transfer contrast (MTC) and tissue water proton relaxation in vivo, Magn Reson Med. 10:135.

50

MR IMAGING OF DIFFUSION

J.V. Hajnal[1] and G.M. Bydder[2]

[1]Nuclear Magnetic Resonance Unit
Picker International
East Lane
Wembley, Middlesex, HA7 7PP
[2]Royal Postgraduate Medical School
Hammersmith Hospital
London, W12 0HS
United Kingdom

INTRODUCTION

Diffusion-weighted MRI is an imaging technique in which image contrast depends principally on the degree to which tissue water molecules are free to move within cells and to pass through cell membranes. The molecules move along random paths, repeatedly colliding with one another as they drift about. This random motion is known as diffusion and it takes place to a greater or lesser extent in all fluids and tissues.

MRI detects the presence of water through the magnetic properties of the hydrogen nucleus. If during an MRI scan large magnetic field gradients are applied for short periods, interleaved with the standard image acquisition gradients, the MR signal can be made highly sensitive to the molecular motions produced by diffusion (Stejskal and Tanner, 1965a; Le Bihan et al., 1986, 1988; Thompsen et al., 1987; Le Bihan et al., 1988; Chein et al., 1990).

The random nature of this motion results in a loss of coherence of the NMR signal, diminishing its amplitude. Where the diffusion of water molecules is relatively unimpeded by tissue structures, diffusion-weighted images appear dark, whereas regions in which cells are effective in confining the molecules appear bright. This ability to differentiate between tissues according to their cellular structure is expected to provide an important adjunct to conventional forms of imaging.

FREE AND RESTRICTED DIFFUSION

All this random movement of molecules may seem difficult to visualise and harder still to describe in a quantitative way. In fact, a mathematical description exists in which a single quantity known as the diffusion coefficient (D) is used to characterise the molecular motion.

Magnetic Resonance Scanning and Epilepsy, Edited by S.D. Shorvon et al.,
Plenum Press, New York, 1994

The larger the value of D the greater the rate of diffusive motion and vice versa. Viscosity is an important factor that determines the magnitude of D; variations in viscosity may lead to contrast between tissues and in disease.

When barriers exist which impede the free movement of molecules the situation becomes more complicated (Stejskal and Tanner, 1965). On very short time-scales molecules diffuse as if they are in a homogeneous fluid, but over progressively longer times more of them diffuse far enough to encounter a barrier which hinders their further movement away. A practical approach to describing this behaviour is to replace D by an apparent diffusion coefficient D^*, the magnitude of which depends on the time interval T_d (the diffusion time) over which diffusion is monitored. Depending on the symmetry of the barriers to diffusion, D^* may or may not be directionally dependent. The manner in which D^* varies with T_d depends on the nature of the barriers including their geometry, permeability and spacing. In general D^* is smaller than the unrestricted value of D and decreases monotonically from a value close to D when T_d is near to zero to a small limiting value as T_d becomes large. (D is independent of T_d.)

The decrease in D^* with T_d is the basic contrast mechanism in restricted diffusion imaging. By choosing the pulse timing of diffusion sensitive imaging sequences appropriately, T_d can be selected to reveal highly restricted diffusion in one tissue or a particular direction within a tissue (D^* small) while still retaining relatively free diffusion ($D^* \simeq D$) in another tissue or another direction within a tissue. Thus T_d is a key parameter for determining the extent to which diffusion reveals cellular structure.

DIRECTIONAL DIFFUSION IN MYELINATED WHITE MATTER

The choice of direction of the applied gradients is another essential factor in this form of imaging. This is because only the diffusive motions in that direction give rise to contrast. One tissue type in which there is a clear directional dependence is myelinated white matter. Myelin provides an almost impenetrable barrier to the diffusion of water molecules. If suitable gradients are applied *perpendicular* to an axon (a direction in which there is very restricted diffusion) D^* appears small and there is little attenuation of the MR signal. This gives a light appearance on the image. If the gradients are applied *along* the direction of the axon where there is little restriction to diffusion D^* appears large and a dark appearance results on the image.

This directional dependence of diffusion enables specific white matter tracts to be highlighted. A typical examination involves selecting both a gradient direction and an appropriate imaging plane to reveal tracts running in the plane, perpendicular to the plane or at some oblique angle to it.

In view of the additional factors which affect image contrast, anisotropically restricted diffusion (ARD) images need to be labelled, not only by such parameters as TR and TE but also by the direction of the applied gradients and the diffusion time (T_d) (which determines the extent to which restrictions are probed). The overall sensitivity of the images to diffusion depends on the strength, duration and separation of the gradient pulses applied. A diffusion sensitivity parameter, b, which incorporates these factors is used to indicate the degree of diffusion contrast. The larger the value of b the greater the sensitivity of the image to diffusion. The diffusion time T_d is quoted in milliseconds and the diffusion sensitisation parameter b in s/mm^2. In the absence of diffusion sensitising gradients the imaging sequences employed in this study were only slightly sensitive to diffusion, having b values of less than 5 s/mm^2.

In the volunteer and clinical studies described in this article cardiac gating on alternate beats with a delay of 200–600 ms from the R wave was employed. All studies were performed at 0.15 T. Images were of 128×128 matrix size and 8 mm slice thickness.

CHOICE OF T_d AND b

In some ways the parameters T_d and b play roles analogous to the window level and width functions used to optimise the display of MR images. T_d sets the threshold scale at which $D*$ becomes small in comparison to D, resulting in relatively bright regions on the images. Assuming that, in the absence of restriction, cellular water has a diffusion coefficient similar to free water and using a practical range for T_d (from 1 to 100 ms) the range of scale lengths that can be probed by diffusion weighted sequences is about 2.5 µm to 25 µm or 10^{-3} mm. These distances are appropriate for studying effects due to cell structure and are comparable to myelinated axon diameters of about 1–15 µm or 10^{-3} mm.

Standard whole-body imaging machines may be unable to achieve shorter T_d values (with useful values of b) without modification to their gradient system. In consequence some tissues or directions within tissues may always exhibit highly restricted diffusion.

The parameter b sets the overall level of attenuation, and determines the dynamic range of the images. For example, with T_d of 50–100 ms, a b value of 1510 s/mm^2 is sufficient to suppress virtually all signals except those from highly restricting structures such as appropriately oriented axons.

Studies demonstrating the use of anisotropic diffusion to highlight white matter tracts in vivo were performed by Moseley et al. (1990a). In systematic studies of the cat brain using a small bore system the essential requirements for implementing this technique were determined. The gradient strength employed (up to 56 mT/m) was considerably greater than that available on most commercial whole body systems. Because of the higher gradient strength it was possible to use shorter echo times (80 ms) than in our human studies. Values of b up to 1413 s/mm^2 were used.

PATHOLOGICAL CONSIDERATIONS

Most reports of pathological lesions such as tumour, oedema, cysts and chronic infarction suggest that $D*$ is increased compared with brain although it has been shown in animal models that diffusion-weighted images may demonstrate a decrease in $D*$ in acute infarction (Moseley et al., 1990b). ARD images may show features that are not apparent with conventional sequences.

In multiple sclerosis, ARD images may demonstrate larger areas of apparent abnormality than standard imaging approaches. The lesions may be of high signal and oriented along the direction of the tracts (Doran et al., 1990; Hajnal et al., 1991).

Children in whom there appears to be little or no myelin, as assessed with the inversion-recovery sequence, may demonstrate anisotropic diffusion at large b values. This suggests that ARD may be more sensitive than highly T1-weighted imaging for demonstrating myelination (Rutherford et al., 1991).

In AIDS, focal lesions such as toxoplasmosis and peri-ventricular high-signal intensity changes on T2-weighted images are seen as areas of high signal which demonstrate variable loss of dependence on orientation. In other cases the ascending and descending tracts of the internal capsule fail to demonstrate directional contrast and are relatively hypointense suggesting less restricted water mobility.

DISCUSSION

ARD-sensitive sequences produce images quite unlike any previously obtained with MRI and an intensive period of work will be required to establish their ultimate clinical role. The specific demonstration of white matter tracts should improve the capability of MR to localise lesions.

The capacity to manipulate diffusion contrast should add another valuable option to the range of parameters already available for MR imaging. Anisotropic diffusion in normal white matter of the brain has been reported by a number of authors, but clinical studies using this technique are just beginning and the basis for image interpretation has yet to be established. Important basic information on the changes of D^* in disease has been obtained in animal and human studies. In acute stroke D^* is initially decreased in the first few hours following infarction and then returns to normal values (MacFall et al., 1990; Moonen et al., 1990). The possible mechanisms for this are a matter for conjecture at the present time. This finding has been applied to the detection of early infarction in clinical studies and changes in D^* have been seen before T2 weighted images display evidence of disease (Levy and Bryan, 1990). Increased D^* has been seen in experimental tumour (Hooper et al., 1990) as well as in clinical cases (Ebisu et al., 1990; Harada et al., 1990). Abscess oedema (presumably vasogenic) also shows an increase in D^* which may return towards normal in time (Chenevert et al., 1990). Chronic multiple sclerosis shows a variable increase in D^* (Larsson, et al., 1990a). An increase in D^* produces a reduction in signal intensity so that it is possible that the highlighting of some lesions is a result of greater reduction in D^* in surrounding white matter in a particular orientation than that occurring within the lesion. It will take time to accumulate clinical experience and to choose appropriate diffusion as well as T1 and T2 weighting for any given disease. It is also possible that small-scale susceptibility effects may be important (Zhong and Gore, 1990).

The gradient pulses that make the imaging sequences sensitive to diffusion also sensitise them to motion such as blood flow and bulk body motion. These may produce artefacts. In many cases careful attention to patient immobilisation is sufficient, but it is also worth considering methods of making the sequences more tolerant to these types of motion. Techniques such as gradient moment nulling are likely to be effective in achieving this (Pattany et al., 1987; Larsson et al., 1990b) but at a cost of decreasing b. With the gradient coils that are generally available at present, it is unlikely that greater than first or second order compensation will be worthwhile. Echo-planar approaches to diffusion may also be of considerable value because of their ability to collect all the data for a single image in a matter of milliseconds (Turner et al., 1989).

Another disadvantage, which is also ultimately dependent on available gradient power, is the tendency to require large echo times to achieve adequate values of b. Clinical examinations performed to date have generally used echo times of 80–200 ms and required averaging over two to four data collections to achieve an acceptable signal-to-noise ratio. These longer echo times limit the use of this technique to tissues with larger values of T2, making it difficult to observe restricted diffusion in tissues such as muscle which might be expected to reveal interesting anisotropic properties. An approach to this problem is the use of small gradient coil sets which also have the advantage that they reduce problems due to eddy currents. They have the disadvantage that in adults they may only be of use in examining the head and limbs.

The link between diffusion of water molecules, microscopic structure of the axon and gross anatomy of the brain provided by ARD imaging is yet another fascinating facet of MRI. ARD imaging may have a wide variety of applications in anatomical localisation, neuropathological correlation and the detection of subtle pathological changes, although much research remains to be done in understanding the mechanism and degree to which diffusion is restricted in different disease processes.

REFERENCES

Chenevert, T.L., et al., 1990, Quantitative perfusion and diffusion measurement of human brain lesions in vivo, "SMRM Book of Abstracts," p.314, Society of Magnetic Resonance in Medicine, Berkeley, CA.

Chien, D., et al., 1990, MRI diffusion of the human brain, J Comput Assist Tomogr. 14: 514–520.

Doran, M., et al., 1990, Use of directional diffusion weighted sequences to demonstrate normal and abnormal white matter tracts, J Comput Assist Tomogr. 14: 865–873.

Ebisu, T., et al., 1990, Clinical use of diffusion/perfusion imaging with three orthogonal gradients, "SMRM Book of Abstracts," p.390, Society of Magnetic Resonance in Medicine, Berkeley, CA.

Hajnal, J.V., et al., 1991, MRI of anisotropically restricted diffusion of water in the nervous system: technical, anatomic and pathologic considerations, J Comput Assist Tomogr. 15: 1–18.

Harada, K., et al., 1990, Diffusion of the brain using a sequence employing gradient sensitisation in three orthogonal directions, "SMRM Book of Abstracts," p.375, Society of Magnetic Resonance in Medicine, Berkeley, CA.

Hooper, J., et al., 1990, Application of diffusion imaging to monitor tumour growth and response to chemotherapy, "SMRM Book of Abstracts," p.371, Society of Magnetic Resonance in Medicine, Berkeley, CA.

Larsson, H.B.W., et al., 1990a, In vivo measurement of water self diffusion in patients with chronic multiple sclerosis, "SMRM Book of Abstracts," p.150, Society of Magnetic Resonance in Medicine, Berkeley, CA.

Larsson, H.B.W., et al., 1990b, In vivo measurement of diffusion in the CNS using a flow compensated spin echo sequence, "SMRM Book of Abstracts," p.389, Society of Magnetic Resonance in Medicine, Berkeley, CA.

Le Bihan, D., et al., 1986, MR imaging of intravoxel incoherent motions. Application to diffusion and perfusion in neurologic disorders, Radiology 161: 401–407.

Le Bihan, D., et al., 1988, Separation of diffusion and perfusion in intravoxel coherent motion MR imaging, Radiology 168: 497–505.

Levy, L. and Bryan, R.N., 1990, Acute stroke: Appearance on diffusion weighted MRI, in "Future Directions in MRI of Diffusion and Microcirculation," D. Le Bihan, Ed. "SMRM Book of Abstracts," p.240–246, Society of Magnetic Resonance in Medicine, Berkeley, CA.

MacFall, J.R., et al., 1990, Restricted diffusion measurement in sub-acute rat stroke, "SMRM Book of Abstracts," p.1119, Society of Magnetic Resonance in Medicine, Berkeley, CA.

Moonen, C.T.W., et al., 1990, Restricted and anisotropic displacement of water in healthy cat brain and in stroke by NMR diffusion imaging. "SMRM Book of Abstracts," p.1121, Society of Magnetic Resonance in Medicine, Berkeley, CA.

Moseley, M.E., et al., 1990a, Diffusion-weighted MR imaging of anisotropic water diffusion in cat central nervous system, Radiology 176: 439–445.

Moseley, M.E., et al., 1990b, Early detection of regional cerebral ischemia in cats: comparison of diffusion and T2 weighted MRI and spectroscopy, Magn Reson Med. 14: 330–346.

Pattany, P.M., et al., 1987, Motion artefact suppression technique (MAST) for magnetic resonance imaging, J Comput Assist Tomogr. 11: 369–377.

Rutherford, M.A., et al., 1991, MR imaging of anisotropically restricted diffusion in the brain of neonates and infants, J Comput Assist Tomogr. 15: 188–198.

Stejskal, E.O. and Tanner, J.E., 1965a, Spin diffusion measurements: spin echoes in the presence of a time dependent field gradient, J Chem Phys. 42: 288–292.

Stejskal, E.O. and Tanner, J.E., 1965b, Use of spin echo in pulsed magnetic field gradient to study anisotropic restricted diffusion and flow, J Chem Phys. 43: 3579–3603.

Thompsen, C., et al., 1987, In vivo measurement of water self diffusion in the human brain by magnetic resonance imaging, Acta Radiol Scand. 28: 353–361.

Turner, R.B., et al., 1989, Echo planar diffusion and perfusion imaging at 2T, "SMRM Book of Abstracts," p.139, Society of Magnetic Resonance in Medicine, Berkeley, CA.

Zhong, J., and Gore, J.C., 1990, Studies of restricted diffusion in heterogeneous media containing variations in susceptibility., in "Future Direction in MRI of Diffusion and Microcirculation," D. Le Bihan, Ed. "SMRM Book of Abstracts," p.166–179, Society of Magnetic Resonance in Medicine, Berkeley, CA.

51

FAST IMAGING AND SERIAL SCANNING

R. Bowtell, R.J. Coxon, J. Firth, P.A. Gowland, P. Gibbs, and P. Mansfield.

Magnetic Resonance Centre
University of Nottingham and
Department of Neurosurgery
Queen's Medical Centre
Nottingham, NG7 2RD
United Kingdom

INTRODUCTION

The application of conventional magnetic resonance imaging (MRI) techniques to humans is often hampered by the long data acquisition times of several minutes per image. These lead to the production of motion artefacts in images and to slow patient throughput. Echo planar imaging (EPI) (Mansfield, 1977) obviates these problems because it allows the generation of two or even three-dimensional images in times of the order of 20–150 ms. Such acquisition times mean that by using EPI it is possible to follow rapid dynamic processes in the body and also to optimise image appearance interactively .

The timing diagram of the EPI sequence is shown in Figure 1. After slice selection, the application of a trapezoidally modulated gradient generates a series of gradient echoes. These echoes are progressively phase encoded by a second orthogonal blipped gradient. Each individual echo is then equivalent to the signal gathered in one pass of a conventional Fourier imaging technique, but in EPI all the echoes are gathered after a single spin excitation and the imaging time is therefore drastically reduced. In Figure 1 the sequence is shown preceded by a chemically selective RF pulse followed by a phase scrambling gradient. These act to suppress the signal from fat or water, so that the resulting image shows the distribution of water or fat alone. The EPI sequence can also be preceded by other combinations of gradient and RF pulses in order to sensitise the spin system to other parameters, such as the relaxation times T1 and T2 and the self-diffusion coefficient, before its state is read out by the EPI "module". This modular approach means that EPI can yield the full range of contrast accessible to conventional imaging techniques.

The price paid for the high speed of EPI is that it imposes stricter demands on scanner hardware than other techniques. This results from the fact that all the echoes need to be gathered before the NMR signal has decayed away. This means that typically each echo must be sampled in 1 ms and it is therefore necessary to use a large oscillating gradient in order to achieve

Magnetic Resonance Scanning and Epilepsy, Edited by S.D. Shorvon et al.,
Plenum Press, New York, 1994

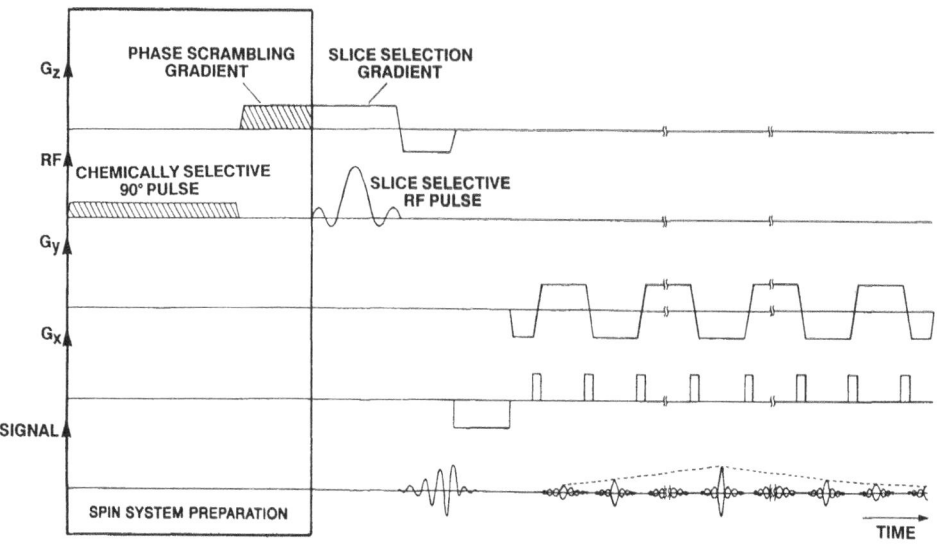

Figure 1. EPI sequence diagram.

adequate resolution. The switched gradient also has to be rapidly reversed, so that the time over which switching takes place is a small fraction of the echo time. In a typical head-imaging experiment of 128 ms duration, a 128×128 (matrix) image with 2.0 mm in plane resolution is generated by using a gradient of strength 12 mT/m, which is reversed in 350 µs. In order to produce such large switched gradients it is necessary to use high-power gradient coil drivers or resonant systems (Mansfield et al., 1991) as well as optimised gradient coil designs (Turner, 1986). Actively screened gradient coils (Mansfield and Chapman, 1986) are usually employed so as to prevent the production of eddy currents in the magnet heat shields.

EPI generally requires the use of large bandwidths in signal acquisition (approx 128 kHz for the experiment quoted above), because many points have to be sampled across the echo train. In EPI the frequency per point may be less than 10 Hz, and as a result image distortion can easily occur if the applied magnetic field is not highly homogeneous or if there are significant magnetic susceptibility differences within the region of interest.

CURRENT RESEARCH

Experience in normal volunteers and in patients with a variety of intracranial pathology has shown that the range of T1 and T2 dependent contrast which EPI offers allows excellent discrimination of different brain tissues. At 0.5 T images with resolutions of better than 2 mm have been produced, and this has permitted delineation of pathology, including small areas of demyelineation in multiple sclerosis (Worthington and Mansfield, 1990). At higher static magnetic field, images with a voxel size of $1.0 \times 1.5 \times 5$ mm have recently been demonstrated. These compare well with standard spin echo (SE) images (Stehling et al., 1991b.). Further improvements in spatial resolution can be achieved by sacrificing temporal resolution and adopting a two- or four-pass sequence (Cohen and Weisskoff, 1991).

In recent work inversion recovery EPI has been used to follow the uptake of gadolinium-DTPA in tumours (Gowland et al., 1992). Here the high temporal resolution provided by EPI meant that it was possible to examine both vascular uptake in the tumour and diffusion across the blood-brain barrier in a single experiment.

From the experimental results it was possible to make an assessment of tumour vascularity which correlated with that obtained by other techniques.

EPI has also allowed CSF dynamics to be monitored in real time (Stehling et al., 1991a). When imaging with the echo-planar sequence, rapid in-plane flow leads to dephasing of the NMR signal and the production of voids in images, whereas flow perpendicular to the imaging plane introduces fresh unsaturated spins into the selected slice and so produces bright regions in images. In head images CSF flow has been observed via both these effects. In particular, turbulent flow in a CSF jet has been seen in cases of hydrocephalus.

Recently it has been shown that MRI techniques can be made sensitive to changes in cerebral blood flow and blood oxygenation, via the local increase in T2 which occurs in heterogeneous regions where the blood deoxyhaemoglobin content is low (Ogawa et al., 1990). The high speed of echo planar imaging allows the haemodynamic alterations which accompany neuronal activation to be followed in real time (Bandettini et al., 1992), and in conjunction with its high sensitivity to T2 decay make it the method of choice for functional mapping.

DISCUSSION

It is anticipated that the application of EPI to the investigation of patients with epilepsy will be advantageous. The ability of the sequence to generate relatively high resolution three-dimensional datasets spanning the head in a time of the order of 5 s, will speed up the process of data gathering. The interactive optimisation of image contrast which EPI allows will make it easier to maximise lesion observation. It may also be possible to look for changes in neuronal activation after an epileptic episode, via echo planar imaging, using the natural T2 contrast due to changes in blood flow.

PROBABLE DEVELOPMENT OVER THE NEXT FIVE YEARS

The increasing availability of commercial scanners which are capable of implementing the echo planar imaging sequence, and the advent of high field (3–4 T) whole-body imaging systems, which offer the possibility of improved resolution and signal-to-noise ratio in echo planar images, as well as increased T2 contrast, both mean that EPI is likely to have major applications in the investigation of epilepsy in future years.

REFERENCES

Bandettini, P.A., Wong, E.C., Hinks, R.S., Tikofsky, R.S., and Hyde, J.S., 1992, Time course EPI of human brain function during task activation, Magn Reson Med. 25: 390–397.
Cohen, M. S., and Weisskoff, 1991, Ultra-fast imaging, Magn Reson Imag. 9: 1–37.
Gowland, P. A., Mansfield, P., Bullock, P., Stehling, M., Worthington, B., and Firth, J.,1992, Dynamic studies of Gadolinium uptake in brain tumours using inversion recovery echo-planar imaging, Magn Reson Med. 26: 241–258.
Mansfield, P., 1977, Multi-planar image formation using NMR spin echoes, J Phys C. 10: L55–58.
Mansfield, P. and Chapman, B., 1986, Active magnetic screening of gradient coils in NMR imaging, J Magn Reson. 66: 573–576.
Mansfield, P., Harvey, P. R., and Coxon, R. J., 1991, Multi-mode resonant gradient coils circuit for ultra high speed NMR imaging, Meas Sci Technol. 2: 1051–1058.
Ogawa, S., Lee, T.M., Nayak, A.S., and Glynn, P., 1990, Oxygenation sensitive contrast in magnetic resonance imaging of rodent brain at high magnetic fields, Magn Reson Med. 14: 68–78.
Stehling, M.K., Firth, J.L., Worthington, B.S., Guilfoyle, D.N., Ordidge, R.J., Coxon, R., Blamire, A.M., Gibbs, P., Bullock, P., and Mansfield, P., 1991a, Observation of cerebrospinal fluid flow with echo-planar magnetic resonance imaging, Br J Radiol. 64: 89–97.

Stehling, M. K., Turner, R., and Mansfield, P., 1991b, Echo-planar imaging: magnetic resonance imaging in a fraction of a second, Science 254: 43–50.

Turner, R., 1986, A target field approach to optimal coil design, J Phys D 19: L147–151.

Worthington, B.S., and Mansfield, P., 1990, The clinical applications of echo planar imaging in neuroradiology, Neuroradiology 32:367–370.

NMR STUDIES OF BRAIN ACTIVATION

J. W. Prichard

Department of Neurology
Yale University School of Medicine
New Haven, Connecticut 06510

INTRODUCTION

The first in vivo study of brain activation by nuclear magnetic resonance (NMR) methods was done early in the development of in vivo NMR techniques to help validate them (Prichard, et al., 1983). Observations on status epilepticus induced by bicuculline in rabbits showed that ^{31}P magnetic resonance spectroscopy (MRS) could reliably demonstrate in vivo the reduction of phosphocreatine and elevation of inorganic phosphate that were known to occur in that condition, as shown in Figure 1.

Later ^{31}P and ^1H MRS studies of status epilepticus extended MRS capabilities and revealed two aspects of experimental status epilepticus that had not been described earlier: lactate and intracellular pH in the brain could become dissociated when seizure discharge was relatively moderate, and lactate remained elevated long after vigorous seizure discharge ceased (Petroff et al., 1984, 1986), as shown in Figure 2.

Lactate/pH dissociation detected by other techniques was later described in experimental brain tumors and 24 hours after reversible global cerebral ischaemia (Paschen et al., 1987), and workers using in vivo NMR techniques have more recently observed it in neonatal anoxia (Hida et al., 1991). Another group that studied bicuculline-induced status epilepticus in cats did not observe the dissociation, probably because they did not examine the level of seizure intensity at which it occurs (Schnall et al., 1988). Still other groups have used MRS methods to study epileptic activation of immature brain (Younkin et al., 1986; Young et al., 1990).

In an effort to determine whether similar metabolic changes occur in domains of brain activation less drastic than status epilepticus, a study was done of brief activation of rabbit brain by electrical shocks delivered via electrodes on the cortex or optic nerves (Prichard et al., 1987). Cortical electrical shock raised brain lactate without causing clearly detectable lowering of pH, and lactate elevation persisted long after the electroencephalogram had returned to normal. Optic nerve shocks also raised cerebral lactate, suggesting that the effect did not depend on passing intense current directly through the region observed by MRS.

Magnetic Resonance Scanning and Epilepsy, Edited by S.D. Shorvon et al.,
Plenum Press, New York, 1994

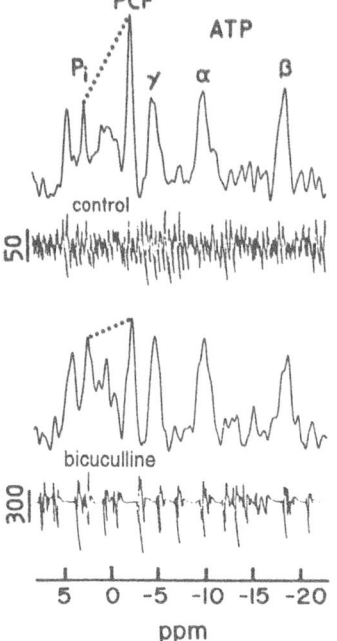

Figure 1. Phosphorus (^{31}P) NMR spectra of living rabbit brain before (above) and during (below) bicuculline-induced status epilepticus. The paralysed, pump-ventilated animal was studied with a surface coil in a 1.9 T Oxford Research Systems spectrometer. Labelled resonances are from inorganic phosphate (Pi), phosphocreatine (PCr), and the alpha-, beta-, and gamma-phosphorus nuclei of ATP. The frequency axis marked in parts per million (p.p.m.) pertains to both spectra. Electroencephalographic (EEG) tracings with calibration bars labelled in microvolts appear under each spectrum. High-amplitude spike-and-wave discharges in the lower EEG tracing are accompanied by reduced PCr and elevated Pi in the corresponding spectrum, reflecting changes in concentrations of these compounds. (Reprinted with permission from *Proc Natl Acad Sci USA*.)

Novel MRS methods for monitoring flow of ^{13}C from [1-^{13}C-] glucose through pools of cerebral metabolites observable in vivo were under development at this time (Prichard and Shulman 1986), and they seemed to offer a way to investigate the metabolic status of shock-elevated lactate.

Meanwhile, positron emission tomography (PET) supplied a quite interesting finding on brain activation (Fox et al., 1988). Photic stimulation was shown to cause 30–50% increases in blood flow and glucose uptake in human primary visual cortex without a corresponding rise in oxygen extraction. These results suggested that lactate might rise in response to stimulation within the physiological range and could be observed by ^{1}H MRS if the required sensitivity could be achieved.

Still another line of research was developing NMR measurement capabilities that would prove to be quite powerful ways of investigating brain activation non-invasively. Magnetic resonance imaging (MRI) became well established in medical diagnosis in the 1980s. Being based on the very strong signal from water protons, it is free of many of the sensitivity limitations of MRS done on much more dilute compounds. Workers using advanced MRI methods coupled with gadolinium contrast enhancement showed that NMR methods could be used to observe an aspect of the same kind of blood flow change to photic stimulation that had been demonstrated by PET (Belliveau et al., 1991). Other workers building on an observation of deoxyhemoglobin paramagnetic effects on water line width (Thulborn et al., 1982) showed that the effect could be used to image activity related blood volume changes in the brain (Ogawa and Lee 1990; Ogawa et al., 1990).

CURRENT RESEARCH

New ^{13}C labelling methods using combined ^{1}H/^{13}C MRS have recently been used to demonstrate that all of the shock-elevated lactate in rabbit brain is metabolically active (Petroff

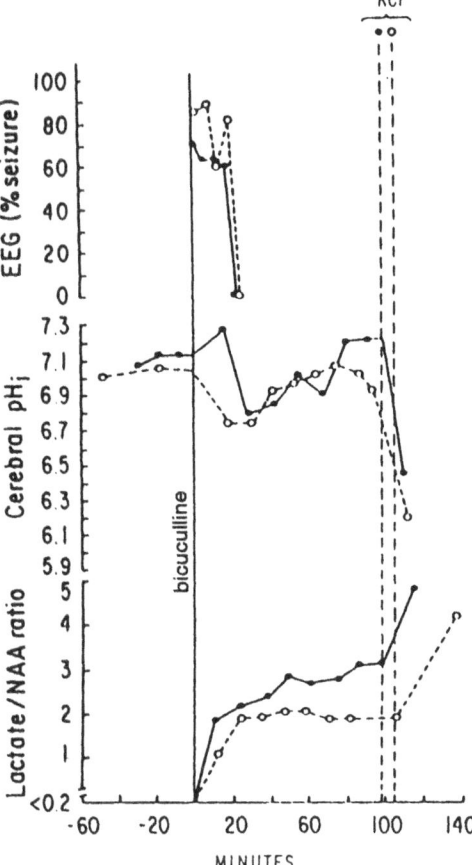

Figure 2. Time course of EEG, intracellular pH (pH), and lactate changes caused by bicuculline-induced status epilepticus in rabbit brain studied in vivo as in the experiment of Figure 1. Intracellular pH was measured in the ^{31}P spectrum and lactate in the proton (^{1}H) spectrum; both spectra were acquired from a double-tuned surface coil. EEG "%seizure" refers to the percentage of 10-second EEG epochs dominated by high-amplitude spike-and-wave discharge. Data from two animals are plotted as filled and open circles. Bicuculline was given at time zero. In both animals, intense seizure discharge persisted for 20 min, during which intracellular pH fell and lactate rose. Over the hour after cessation of seizure discharge, intracellular pH slowly returned to normal, but lactate—plotted as a ratio of its resonance to the unvarying resonance of N-acetyl aspartate (NAA)—remained elevated. Agonal changes in intracellular pH and in lactate followed KCl-induced cardiac arrest. (Reprinted with permission from *Ann Neurol.*)

et al., 1992). No more than 10% can be trapped in dead cells, the extracellular space, or other metabolically inactive compartments. Data illustrating this result are shown in Figure 3. Similar ^{13}C labelling techniques were used to demonstrate turnover of stroke-elevated lactate in a human patient (Rothman et al., 1991) and are, in principle, applicable to studies of brain activation.

Photic stimulation does indeed raise lactate in human visual cortex (Prichard et al., 1991), as predicted by the PET study referred to above. The result is illustrated by the ^{1}H spectra in Figure 4. It reinforces the PET workers' conclusion that the increased energy demand of visual stimulation in the normal range is met by selective activation of glycolysis in the presence of unimpaired respiratory machinery. Conventional biochemical control theory did not predict this result, but it is consistent with other data which suggest that the relationship between biochemistry and function in the nervous system is more complex than had been thought: glycolytic and respiratory enzyme systems appear to be heterogeneously distributed within the brain (Borowsky and Collins, 1989), as they are well known to be in muscle. As in muscle, biochemical heterogeneity in the brain is likely to be related to function, but in ways which are not yet well understood.

Epileptic patients have been studied by several groups using MRS. Elevation of lactate associated with a focus of electrical seizure activity was reported in a patient with Rasumussen's encephalitis (Matthews et al., 1990). A number of other ^{1}H studies have been reported in preliminary form; some of the data are described in other contributions to this symposium. Two groups that have used ^{31}P MRS to study small numbers of patients with complex partial

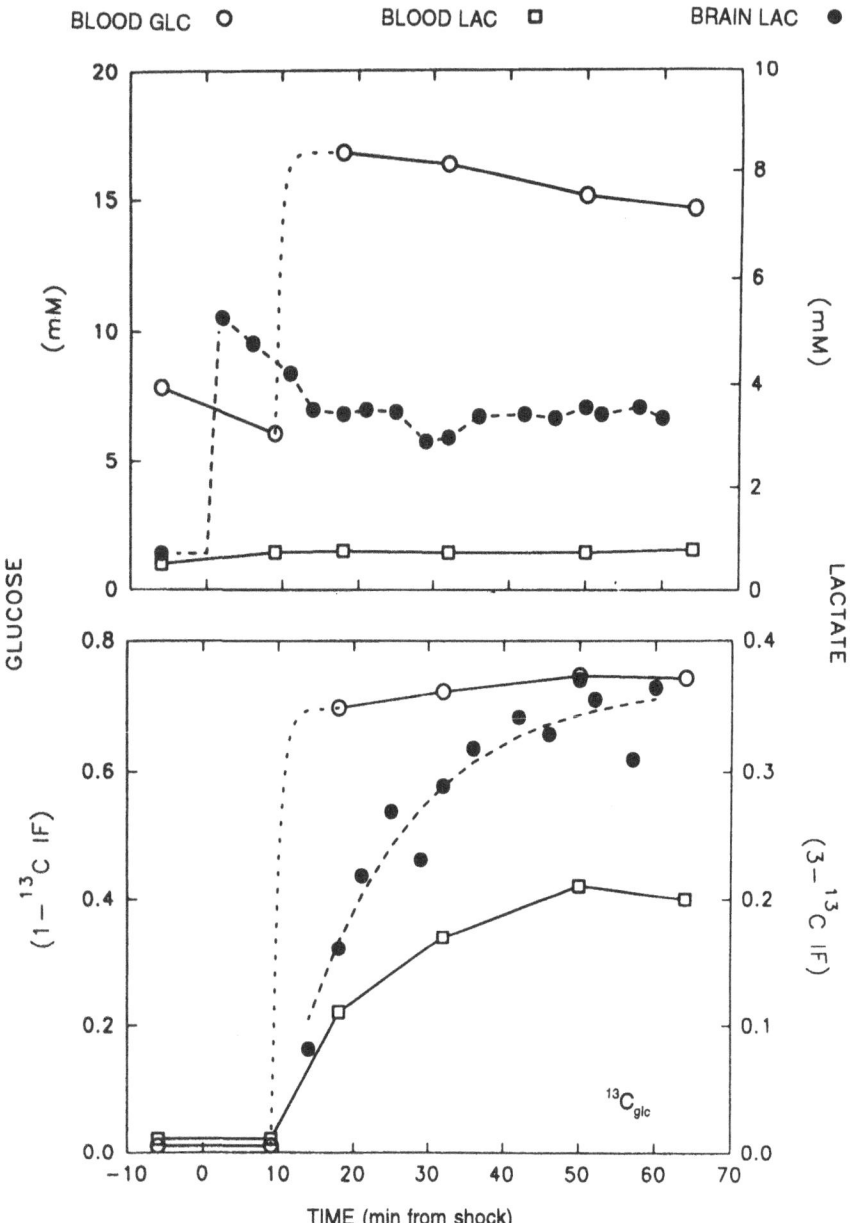

Figure 3. Time course of changes in concentrations (upper graph) and ^{13}C isotopic fractions (lower graph) of blood glucose (squares), blood lactate (open circles) and brain lactate (filled circles) during cortical electroshock followed by labelling of lactate pools with ^{13}C from blood glucose. Data are all from a single rabbit studied in vivo with surface coils by combined $^{1}H/^{13}C$ methods in a 4.7 T Bruker/Oxford Research Systems spectrometer. Following cortical electrical shock at time zero, brain lactate rose to 5 mmol/l (back-calculated from NMR study of an extract of the removed brain), and it remained at 3–4 mmol/l for the remainder of the experiment. In contrast, blood lactate did not change, illustrating the independence of the blood and brain lactate pools. Nine minutes after electroshock, the ^{13}C isotopic fraction (IF) of blood glucose was raised rapidly by computer-controlled intravascular infusion of [1-^{13}C-]glucose. The 3-^{13}C labelled IF of brain lactate gradually rose to the level predicted from steady-state blood glucose IF, showing that the two pools were in full metabolic equilibrium. Blood lactate IF reached an apparent steady state at a lower level, as if blood lactate were exchanging with at least two lactate pools outside the brain, one of which was turning over much faster than the other. (Reprinted with permission from *J Cereb Blood Flow Metab.*

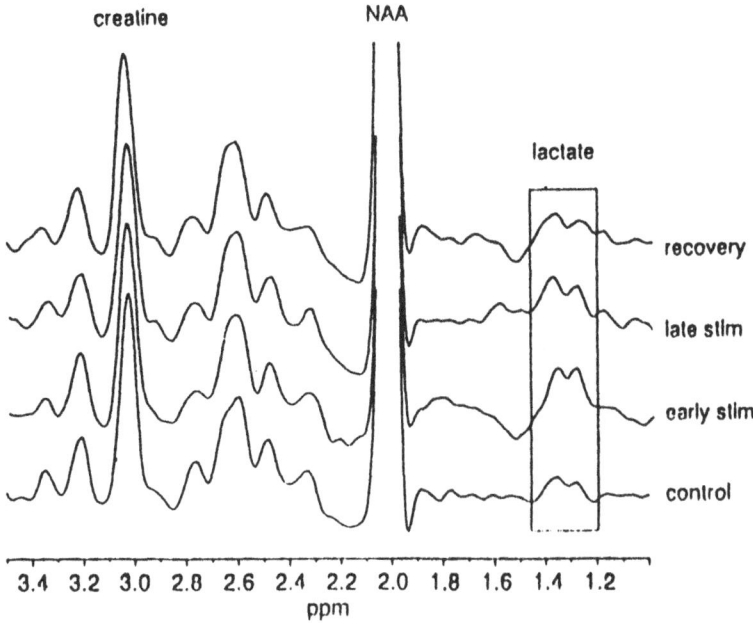

Figure 4. Proton (^{1}H) spectra from calcarine cortex and adjacent brain regions of a normal human subject before, during and after photic stimulation by red LED goggles flashing at 16 Hz. Resonances from creatine, N-acety-laspartate (NAA) and lactate are labelled. The lactate resonance, in which the characteristic two-peaked fine structure can clearly be seen, rose during stimulation and returned to normal afterwards, suggesting that increased energy demand by stimulation within the physiological range was met preferentially by non-oxidative glycolysis. (Reprinted with permission from *Proc Natl Acad Sci USA*.)

epilepsy have obtained different results. One observed decreased phosphocreatine/inorganic phosphate ratio (PCr/Pi) in the temporal lobe containing the primary seizure focus (Kuzniecky et al., 1992). The other observed elevated pH and Pi, and decreased phosphomonoesters in similar regions of the brain (Hugg et al., 1992). Both studies appear to be technically sound. Data from larger groups of patients will be necessary to resolve the differences between them, which may be the result of differences in exact size and placement of the sensitive volumes measured.

Among the most exciting current developments in NMR work on brain activation are measurements of use-related cerebrovascular changes based on the paramagnetic effect of deoxyhaemoglobin, pioneered for this application by Ogawa and his colleagues (Ogawa and Lee 1990; Ogawa et al., 1990). Four groups have shown such changes related to sensory stimulation and motor activity (Bandettini et al., 1992; Frahm et al., 1992; Kwong et al., 1992; Ogawa et al., 1992). One group did the study at 4 T, achieving remarkable anatomical resolution (Ogawa et al., 1992).

Finally, a very recent result pertinent to cerebral excitability has come from an experimental study of diffusion-weighted imaging (DWI) in rats during status epilepticus. Much previous animal work had shown that the average apparent pathlength of water diffusion is substantially decreased in cerebral ischemia (Moseley et al., 1991; LeBihan and Turner, 1992; van Bruggen et al., 1992), and, as was expected, the phenomenon has been observed in human stroke (Warach et al., 1992). A change of the same kind is present during status epilepticus in the rat (Zhong et al., 1993). As cerebral blood flow is greatly increased and ATP is not depleted in status epilepticus, the result poses new questions about the mechanism(s) of DWI changes in both conditions.

PROBABLE DEVELOPMENTS OVER THE NEXT FIVE YEARS

Studies of brain activation by NMR methods are entering a rapid growth phase. A large role for them is already clear, but the limits of it are not. Introduction of the water-based techniques has endowed NMR methods suitable for research on brain activation with sensitivity that had not been anticipated. Benefits of that sensitivity can be realised as anatomical resolution which exceeds that of PET and time resolution unequalled by any technique capable of making in vivo observations related to metabolism.

An important feature of the situation not yet well appreciated outside the NMR community is the inherent mutual compatibility of several different kinds of NMR measurements. In principle, conventional MRI, MRS and all of the new techniques mentioned above, as well as others not mentioned, can be done in the same machine. Arrays of NMR techniques tailored for specific neurobiological and medical purposes will become available in most biomedical research centres in the next few years. They will spread into diagnostic centres as rapidly as they are seen to be cost-effective compared to current techniques; most current state-of-the-art MRI machines used purely for medical diagnosis can be equipped to perform any of the new measurements at relatively small cost.

The role of lactate in the brain may be revealed by the new methods to be more extensive than had been thought. Its long persistence after various perturbations, its dissociation from pH under some circumstances, and its elevation by physiological stimuli raise new questions. The most interesting one is the possibility that lactate may have a signalling function in addition to its metabolic role. At least one piece of experimental evidence can be adduced in support of the idea: lactate suppresses depolarisation-induced release of acetylcholine by Torpedo electroplaques (Gaudry-Talarmain 1986). An effect of this sort in the mammalian nervous system would automatically help retard excessive neuronal discharge, which always seems to cause substantial lactate accumulation in the most active regions. Elevation of lactate by physiological stimulation (Prichard et al., 1991) invites speculation concerning a lactate-signalling role in normal function. A common compound so closely responsive to increased neural activity would be well qualified for integration into adaptive mechanisms of neural control.

The metabolic role of lactate may be specialised in the nervous system. A recent ^{13}C labelling study leaves no doubt that the brain lactate pool is highly sequestered from blood lactate (Petroff et al., 1992). In Chapter 44 Professor H.S. Bachelard reviews data which indicate different patterns of metabolism in neurons and glia when hippocampal slices are stimulated by K-induced depolarisation. Lactate produced in adjacent glia would be a convenient energy reservoir for intensely active synaptic terminals if it could find its way into them. Elevation of glial lactate by selective activation of glycolysis would create a glia-to-neuron lactate gradient favouring the necessary transfer by either facilitated diffusion of lactate anion or passive diffusion of lactic acid.

The new data from NMR studies of brain activation suggest that these novel possibilities should be explored further.

Brain activation studies by NMR methods open vast new possibilities in cognitive neuroscience, the study of motor and sensory processes in humans, and analysis of pathophysiological mechanism in human brain disease. "Revolutionary" is not too strong a word for developments likely to flow from this new NMR methodology as it matures.

REFERENCES

Bandettini, P.A., Wong, E.C., Hinks, R.S., Tikofsky, R.S., and Hyde, J.S., 1992, Time course EPI human brain function during task activation, Magn Reson Med. 25: 390–397.

Belliveau, J.W., Kennedy, D.N., McKinstry, R.C., Buchbinder, B.R., Weisskoff, R.M., Cohen, M.S., Vevea, J.M., Brady, T.J., and Rosen, B.R., 1991, Functional mapping of the human visual cortex by magnetic resonance imaging, Science 254: 716–719.

Borowsky, I.W., and Collins, R.C., 1989, Metabolic anatomy of brain: a comparison of regional capillary density, glucose metabolism, and enzyme activities, J Comp Neurol. 288: 401–413.

Fox, P.T., Raichle, M.E., Mintun, M.A., and Dence, C., 1988, Nonoxidative glucose consumption during focal physiologic neural activity, Science 241: 462–464.

Frahm, J., Bruhn, H., Merboldt, K-D, and Hanicke, W., 1992, Dynamic MRI of human brain oxygenation during rest and photic stimulation, J Magn Reson Imag. in press.

Gaudry-Talarmain, Y.M., 1986, The effect of lactate on acetylcholine release evoked by various stimuli from Torpedo synaptosomes, Eur J Pharmacol. 129: 235–243.

Hida, K., Suzuki, N., Kwee, I.L., and Nakada, T., 1991, pH-lactate dissociation in neonatal anoxia: Proton and 31P NMR spectroscopic studies in rat pups, Magn Reson Med. 22: 128–132.

Hugg, J.W., Laxer, K.D., Matson, G.B., Maudsley, A.A., Husted, C.A., and Weiner, M.W., 1992, Lateralisation of human focal epilepsy by 31P magnetic resonance spectroscopic imaging, Neurology 42: 2011–2018.

Kuzniecky, R., Elgavish, G.A., Hetherington, H.P., Evanochko, W.T., and Pohost, G.M., 1992, In vivo 31P nuclear magnetic resonance spectroscopy of human temporal lobe epilepsy, Neurology 42: 1586–1590.

Kwong, K.K., Belliveau, J.W., Chesler, D.A., Goldberg, I.E., Weisskoff, R.M., Poncelet, B.P., Kennedy, D.N., Hoppel, B.E., Cohen, M.S., Turner, R., Cheng, H-M., Brady, T.J., and Rosen, B.R., 1992, Dynamic magnetic resonance imaging of human brain activity during primary sensory stimulation, Proc Natl Acad Sci USA 89: 5675–5679.

LeBihan, D., and Turner, R., 1992, Diffusion and perfusion, in: "Magnetic Resonance Imaging," 1st edn, D.D. Stark and W.G. Bradley, eds, Mosby Yearbook Inc, St Louis.

Matthews, P.M., Andermann, F., and Arnold, D.L., 1990, A proton magnetic resonance spectroscopy study of focal epilepsy in man, Neurology 40: 985–989.

Moseley, M.E., Wendland, M.F., and Kucharczyk, J., 1991, Magnetic resonance imaging of diffusion and perfusion, Topics in Magnetic Resonance Imaging 3: 50–67.

Ogawa, S., and Lee, T.M., 1990, Magnetic resonance imaging of blood vessels at high fields: In vivo and in vitro measurements and image simulation, Magn Reson Med. 16. 9–18.

Ogawa, S., Lee, T.M., Nayak, A.S., and Glynn, P.,1990, Oxygenation-sensitive contrast in magnetic resonance image of rodent brain at high magnetic fields, Magn Reson Med. 14: 68–78.

Ogawa, S., Tank, D.W., Menon, R., Ellermann, J.M., Kim, S-G., Merkle, H., and Ugurbil, K., 1992, Intrinsic signal changes accompanying sensory stimulation: Functional brain mapping using MRI, Proc Natl Acad Sci USA. 89: 5951–5955.

Paschen, W., Djuricic, B., Mies, G., Schmidt-Kastner, R., and Linn, F., 1987, Lactate and pH in the brain: Association and dissociation in different pathophysiological states, J Neurochem. 48: 154–159.

Petroff, O.A.C., Prichard, J.W., Behar, K.L., Alger, J.R., and Shulman, R.G., 1984, In vivo phosphorus nuclear magnetic resonance spectroscopy in status epilepticus, Ann Neurol. 16: 169–177.

Petroff, O.A.C., Prichard, J.W., Ogino, T., Avison, M.J., Alger, J.R., and Shulman, R.G., 1986, Combined 1H and 31P nuclear magnetic resonance studies of bicuculline-induced seizures in vivo, Ann Neurol. 20: 185–193.

Petroff, O.A.C., Novotny, E.J., Avison, M.J., Rothman, D.L., Alger, J.R., Ogino, T., Shulman, G.I., and Prichard, J.W., 1992, Cerebral lactate turnover after electroshock: in vivo measurements by 1H/13C magnetic resonance spectroscopy, J Cereb Blood Flow Metab. in press.

Prichard, J.W., and Shulman, R.G., 1986, NMR spectroscopy of brain metabolism in vivo, Ann Rev Neurosci. 9: 61–85.

Prichard, J.W., Alger, J.R., Behar, K.L., Petroff, O.A.C., and Shulman, R.G., 1983, Cerebral metabolic studies in vivo by 31P NMR, Proc Natl Acad Sci USA. 80: 2748–2751.

Prichard, J.W., Petroff, O.A., Ogino, T., and Shulman, R.G., 1987, Cerebral lactate elevation by electroshock: a 1H magnetic resonance study, Ann N Y Acad Sci. 508: 54–63.

Rothman, D.L., Howseman, A.M., Graham, G.D., Petroff, O.A.C., Lantos, G., Fayad, P.B., Brass, L.M., Shulman, G.I., Shulman, R.G., and Prichard, J.W., 1991, Localised proton NMR observation of 3-13C-lactate in stroke after 1-13C-glucose infusion, Magn Reson Med. 21: 302–307.

Schnall, M.D., Yoshizaki, K., Chance, B., and Leigh, J.S., 1988, Triple nuclear NMR studies of cerebral metabolism during generalised seizure, Magn Reson Med. 6: 15–23.

Thulborn, K.R., Waterton, J.C., Matthews, P.M., and Radda, G.K., 1982, Oxygenation dependence of the transverse relaxation time of water protons in whole blood at high field, Biochem Biophys Acta 714: 265–270.

van Bruggen, N., Cullen, B.M., King, M.D., Doran, M., Williams, S.R., Gadian, D.G., and Cremer, J.E., 1992, T2- and diffusion-weighted magnetic resonance imaging of a focal ischemic lesion in the rat brain, Stroke 23: 576–582.

Warach, S., Chien, D., Li, W., Ronthal, M.B., and Edelman, R.R., 1992, Fast magnetic resonance diffusion-weighted imaging of acute human stroke, Neurology 42: 1717–1723.

Young, R.S.K., Petroff, O.A.C., Novotny, E.J., and Wong, M., 1990, Neonatal excitoxic brain injury, Dev Neurosci. 12: 210–220.

Younkin, D.P., Delivoria-Papadopoulas, M., Maris, J., Donlon, E., Clancy, R., and Chance, B., 1986, Cerebral metabolic effects of neonatal seizures measured with in vivo 31P NMR spectroscopy, Ann Neurol. 20: 513–519.

Zhong, J., Petroff, O.A.C., Prichard, J.W., and Gore, J.C., 1993, Changes in water diffusion and relaxation properties of rat cerebrum during status epilepticus, Magn Reson Med. 30: 241–246.

53

DIFFERENTIAL DIAGNOSIS OF HUMAN INTRACRANIAL TUMORS IN VIVO USING ^{1}H MR SPECTROSCOPIC IMAGING AND FEATURE SPACE FOR SPECTRAL PATTERN RECOGNITION

Mark C. Preul, D. Louis Collins, and Douglas L. Arnold

MR Spectroscopy Unit
Department of Neurology and Neurosurgery
Montreal Neurological Institute and Hospital
McGill University
Montreal, Quebec
Canada

BACKGROUND

Attaining high specificity in preoperative brain tumor diagnosis is a challenge. Conventional radiological techniques used to diagnose and grade brain tumors such as X-ray CT and MRI not infrequently yield ambiguous results. The gains made by MRI in sensitivity of detection of brain tumors have not been paralleled by improved specificity. (Atlas, 1991; Darwin, 1986; Kazner, 1989)

Although diagnosis and grading of intracranial tumors in non-eloquent areas can be safely established by resection or stereotactic biopsy with accuracy approaching 90%, biopsy of tumors in deep or eloquent brain has serious limitations.(Chandrasoma, 1990; Lunsford, 1990) Needle biopsy in these areas requires image-directed stereotactic techniques, the number of samples obtained is limited, and the risk of neurological deficit is increased. Pathological evaluation of biopsies in such cases may be inconclusive up to 40% of the time.(Chandrasoma, 1990; Lunsford, 1990).

[1]H MR Spectroscopic Imaging

Proton magnetic resonance spectroscopic imaging (^{1}H MRSI) enables noninvasive assay *in vivo* of regional biochemical pathology of brain tumors. Images can be generated that are based on metabolites in the tissue, instead of on water, as is the case in conventional MRI. Spectra are obtained from approximately 1 cm^3 volume elements or voxels within a larger region of interest (ROI). This allows retrospective analysis of chemical spectra for any portion

Magnetic Resonance Scanning and Epilepsy, Edited by S.D. Shorvon et al.,
Plenum Press, New York, 1994

of the ROI and assessment of regional heterogeneity of metabolic changes within tumors and in adjacent and remote brain tissue (Luyten, 1990; Segebarth, 1990). ^{1}H MRSI, thus, has advantages over single-voxel MR spectroscopy techniques (Arnold, 1990; Arnold, 1991; Henriksen, 1991; Kugel, 1991; Luyten, 1991).

Previous Attempts at Analysis of Brain Tumor MR Spectra

Differentiation of intracranial tumors on the basis of individual resonances normally present in the ^{1}H MR spectrum, or even on new resonances that appear in tumors, is difficult. Increases and decreases in individual resonance intensities between different tumor types tends to overlap(Daemerel, 1991; Kugel, 1992; Luyten, 1990; Gill, 1990; Bruhn, 1989). The change in pattern of all the resonances considered together is more likely to be discriminatory. We, therefore, combined ^{1}H MRSI with a statistically-based technique for spectral pattern recognition. This new approach to classification is based on the simultaneous consideration of the 6 main chemical compounds observed in the T2-weighted ^{1}H MR spectrum (NAA, Cho, Cr, LA, lipid [Lip], alanine [Ala]) and analysis of the minimum distance to group mean in six-dimensional metabolite feature space. We have begun to assess the ability of this approach to classify different brain tumors.

PATIENTS AND METHODS

^{1}H MRSIs were obtained using a 1.5 T imaging/spectroscopy system (Philips, The Netherlands). Changes in MR signals from choline-containing phospholipids (Cho—3.2 ppm), phosphocreatine + creatine (Cr—3.0 ppm), N-acetylaspartate (NAA—2.0 ppm), alanine (Ala—1.4 ppm), lactate-lipid (LA—1.3 ppm), and lipid (Lip—0.9 ppm) were measured in 60 untreated (except for corticosteroids) patients with histology-proven brain tumors (glioblastoma multiforme, n = 14; intermediate-grade astrocytoma, n = 14; low-grade astrocytoma, n = 15; metastasis, n = 12; meningioma, n = 5) and 10 normal control subjects. Biochemical characteristics in vivo were compared with histology of the tumor.

^{1}H MRSIs were acquired from a large ROI, including the tumor and contralateral or remote brain that appeared normal on MRI. Water-suppressed ^{1}H MRSI were acquired using inversion-suppression of the water signal and a 90°–180°–180° pulse sequence (TR 2 s, TE 272 ms, 250 × 250 FOV, 32 × 32 phase-encoding profiles, 1 signal average per profile). A second MRSI was also obtained without water suppression (TR 850 ms, TE 272 ms, 250 × 250 FOV, 16 × 16 phase-encoding profiles, 1 signal average per profile). After zero-filling the latter to 32 × 32 profiles, the water suppressed 1H MRSI was divided by the non-water suppressed ^{1}H MRSI to correct for artifacts from magnetic field inhomogeneity (den Hollander, 1991; Traber, 1992).

Metabolite resonances intensities were normalized to the contralateral Cr resonance intensity. Control values came from homologous contralateral or remote voxels and from normal subjects. Post-processing of data was peformed with SUNSPEC1 software (Philips Medical Systems, The Netherlands).

All patients had either craniotomy or at least three stereotactic biopsies from different areas of the tumor. Histology was evaluated by a neuropathologist using Reinertz grading for astrocytomas. All tumors were supratentorial and ≥ 2 cm in the cranio-caudal diameter. The ROI was positioned so that the cranio-caudal dimension of the ROI was completely filled by tumor, thus eliminating partial volume effects from surrounding non-tumorous brain tissue.

OBSERVATIONS

Maximal abnormalities in metabolites occurred in voxels at the center of the tumor. Voxels at the tumor periphery were also abnormal, but less so than central voxels. Chemical abnormalities extended outside the tumor boundaries on MRI. Relative resonance intensity ratios for individual metabolites according to tumor type are shown in Figure 1.

Meningiomas showed prominent Cho, low Cr, and a characteristic Ala peak in the absence of LA (Figure 2).

Low-grade astrocytomas showed relatively normal Cr, the highest Cho and NAA peaks of the all tumors, and low LA peaks (Figure 3).

The histologically malignant tumors showed the highest LA and/or Lip. Metastases had very low Cr and NAA. Glioblastomas showed high Cho, low Cr, the lowest NAA of the glial tumors, and a relatively smaller Lip peak than the metastases. Intermediate grade astrocytomas often showed slightly higher Cho than glioblastomas, near normal Cr, and LA which was increased, but to a lesser extent than in glioblastomas (Figures 4, 5, 6).

Lip was higher in metastases than in glioblastomas. Intermediate and low grade astrocytomas did not show Lip. Metastases and glioblastomas had much higher LA than intermediate or low grade astrocytomas. LA was higher in intermediate than in low grade astrocytomas. Cr and NAA were lower in mets than in glioblastomas. No differentiation could be made between the metastatic tissue types on the basis of the 1H MR spectra.

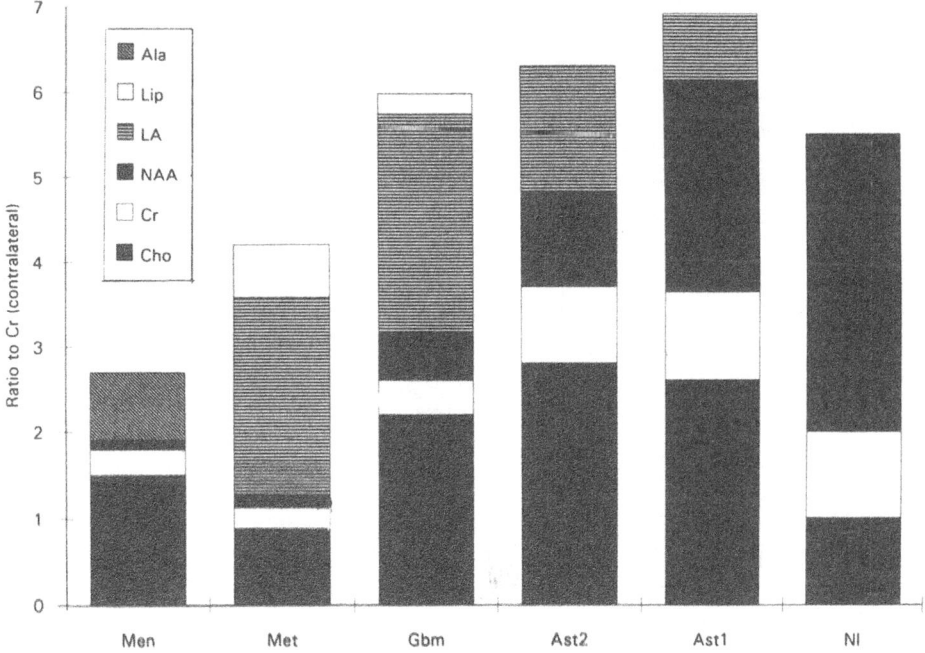

Figure 1. Average metabolite values from central tumor voxels. The five major classes of intracranial tumors and the normal subjects are separable by their "typical" 1H spectral patterns. (Men = meningioma; Met = metastasis; Gbm = glioblastoma; Ast2 = intermediate grade astrocytoma; Ast1 = low grade astrocytoma; Nl = normal subject; Cho = choline; Cr = creatine; NAA = N-acetylaspartate; LA = lactate; Lip = lipid; Ala = alanine).

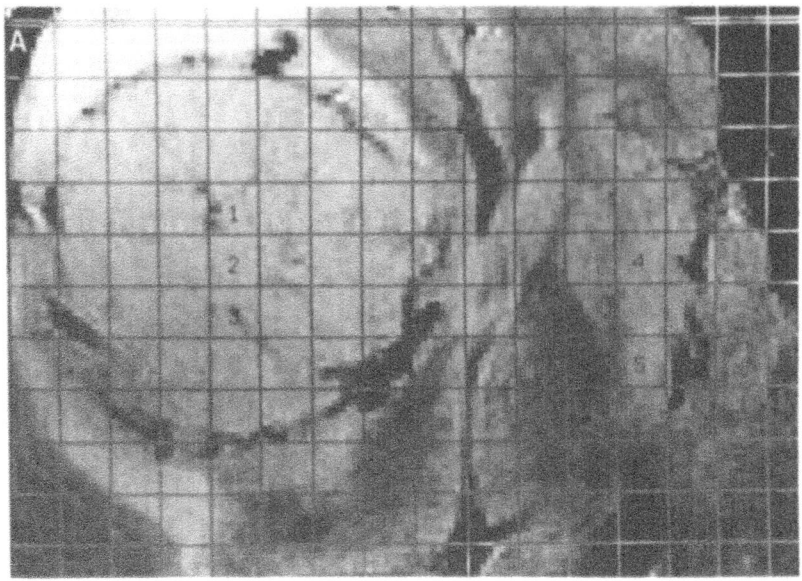

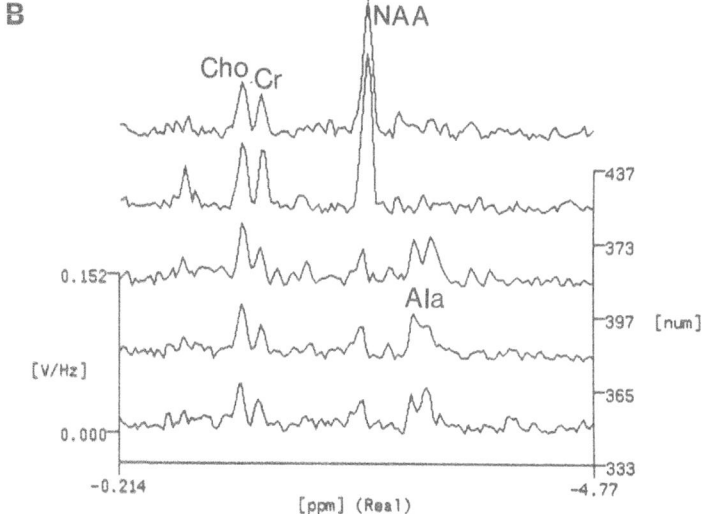

Figure 2. A & B ^{1}H MR spectra from a 32-year-old woman with a large right sphenoid meningioma. The spectra numbers 333, 365, 397 originate from voxels 1, 2, 3, respectively. Spectra 373 and 437 originate from voxels 4 and 5 that appear normal on MRI. Note the mildly increased Cho, decreased Cr and NAA, and the characteristic resonance from Ala at 1.4 ppm. The latter must not be confused with LA which is a doublet at 1.3 ppm. The residual NAA may reflect contributions from other N-acetyl groups.

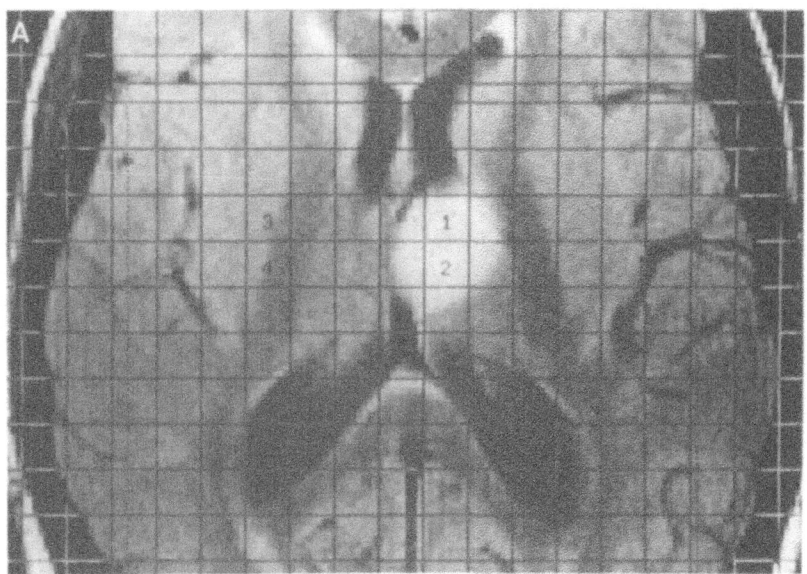

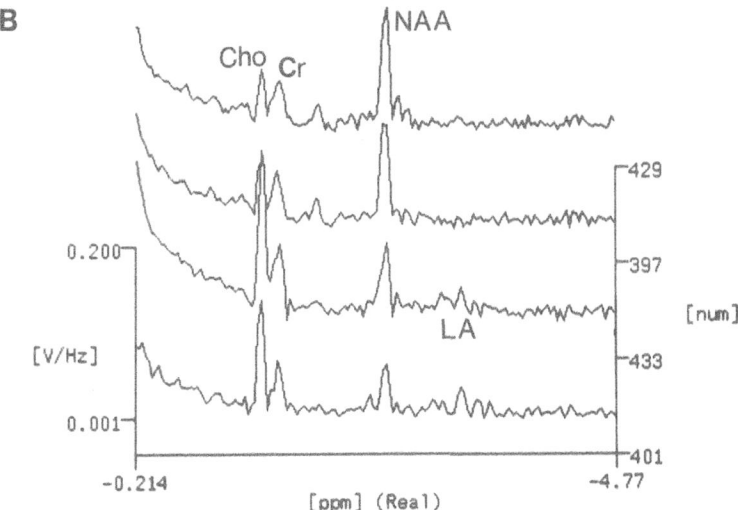

Figure 3. A & B ^{1}H MR spectra from a 28-year-old female with a low grade astrocytoma in the left thalamus and involving the optic tract. Spectra 401 and 433 originate from the tumor and correspond to voxels 1 and 2, while spectra 397 and 429 originate from voxels 4 and 5 which are in contralateral brain that appears normal on MRI. Note the very high signal intensity from Cho, near normal Cr, moderately decreased NAA and a very low signal from LA.

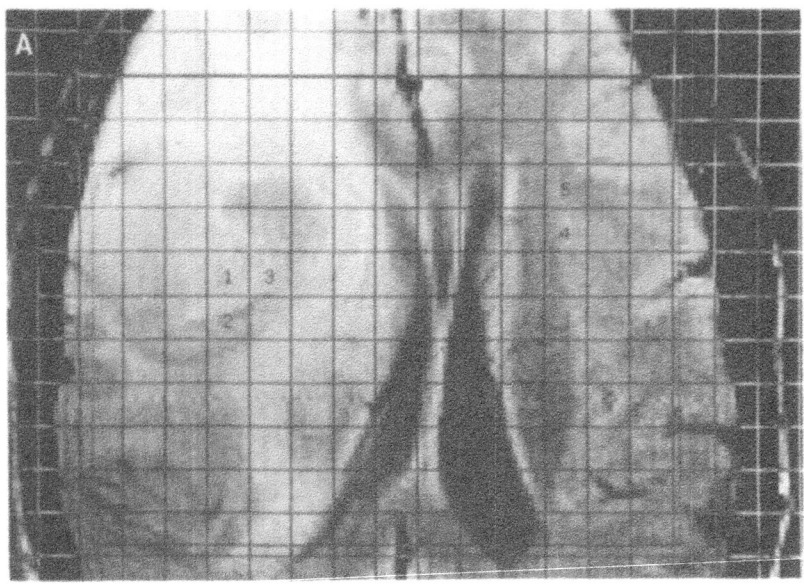

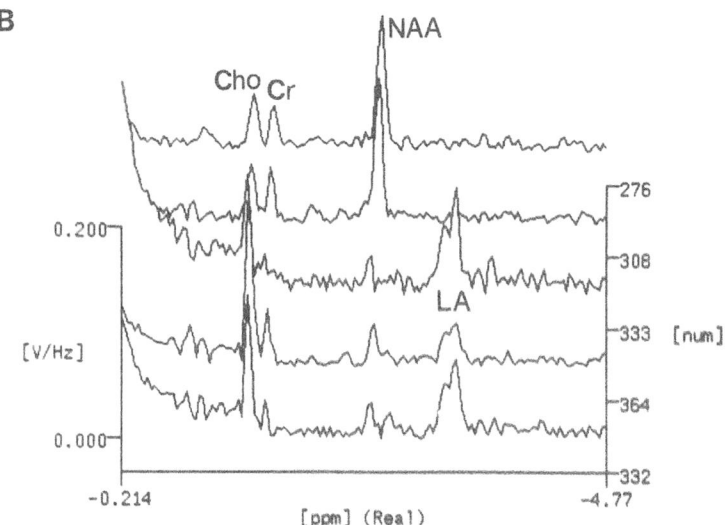

Figure 4. A & B ^{1}H MR spectra from a 43 year old man with a right frontal intermediate grade astrocytoma. Spectra 332, 364, 333 are from voxels 1, 2, and 3, respectively, and spectra 308 and 276 are from contralateral MRI normal-appearing brain. Note the high Cho signal, lower Cr and NAA compared to the low-grade astrocytoma, and moderately high LA peak.

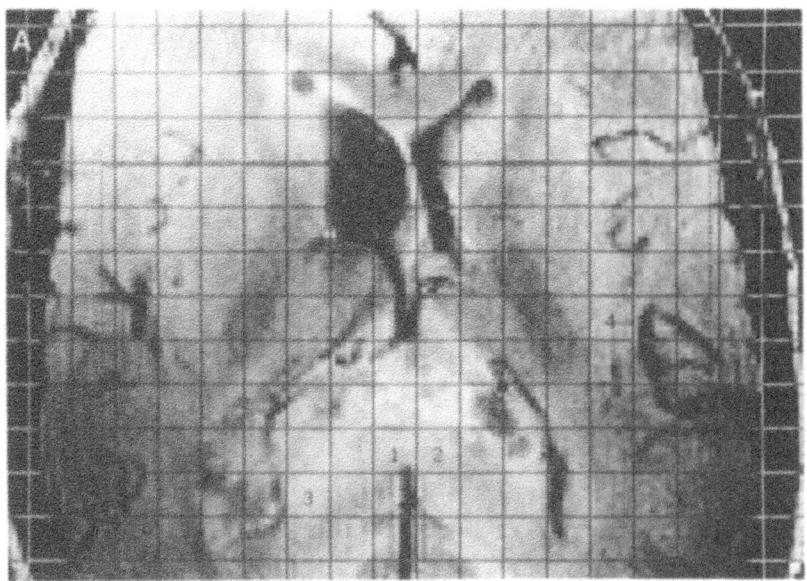

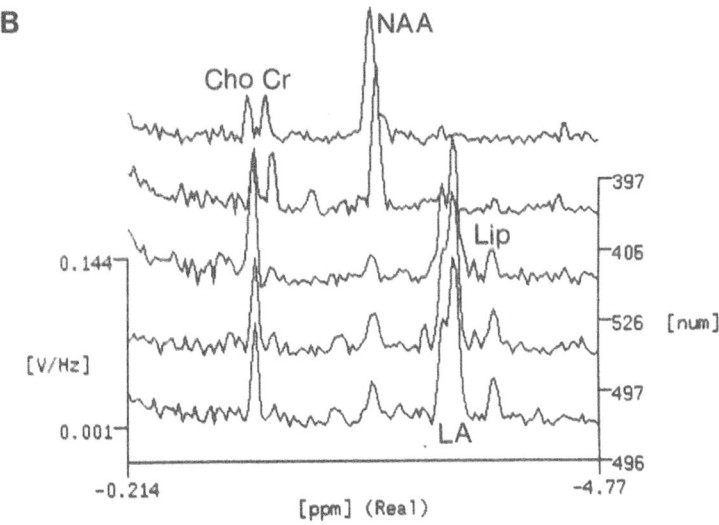

Figure 5. A & B ^{1}H MR spectra from a 55-year-old man with a glioblastoma of the splenium of the corpus callosum. Spectra 496, 497, 526 are from voxels 1, 2, 3, respectively and spectra 405 and 397 are from voxels 4 and 5, respectively. Note the very high LA and prominent Lip peak at 0.9 ppm. Cho is high, Cr and NAA are low.

Compared to normals, NAA was decreased in MRI normal-appearing contralateral brain tissue in all patients with glioblastomas, intermediate grade astrocytomas, metastases, and in 8 patients with low-grade astrocytomas. In the same region LA was increased in all patients with glioblastomas and metastases, in 9 patients with intermediate grade astrocytomas and in 3 meningiomas. Spectra from normal subjects did not show resonance from LA, Lip, or Ala, but had well defined Cho, Cr, and the highest NAA peaks (Figure 7).

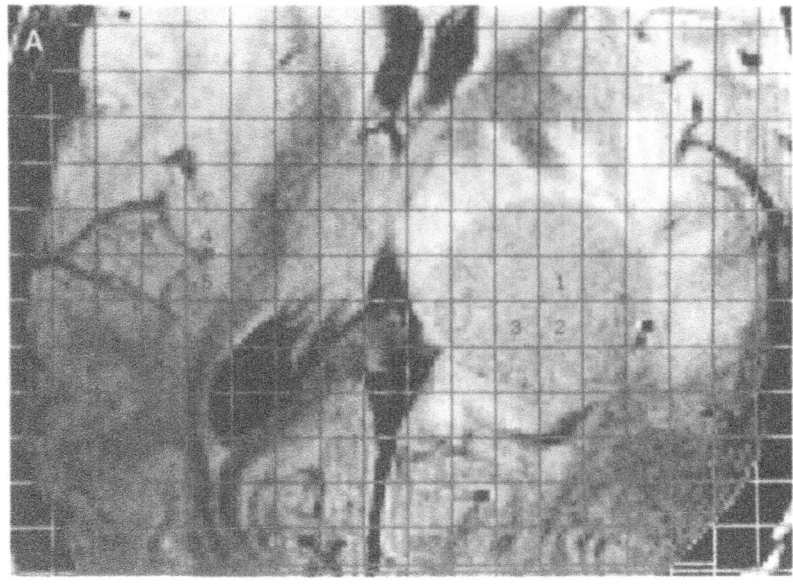

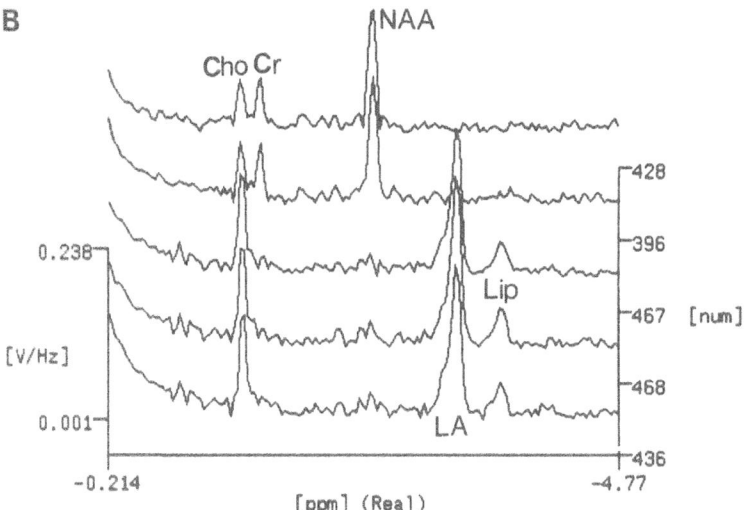

Figure 6. A & B ^{1}H MR spectra from a large, deep temporal-parietal adenocarcinoma of the lung in a 38-year-old man. Voxels 1, 2, 3 correspond to spectra 436, 468, 467, respectively, which show very high Cho, very low Cr and NAA, very high LA with a prominent Lip peak at 0.9 ppm. Compared to the spectra from the glioblastoma, the metastases have very low or absent NAA.

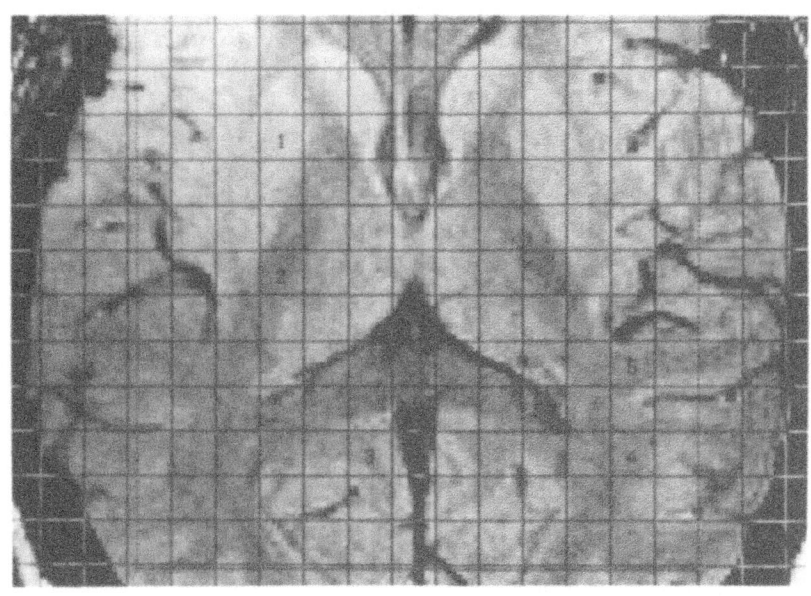

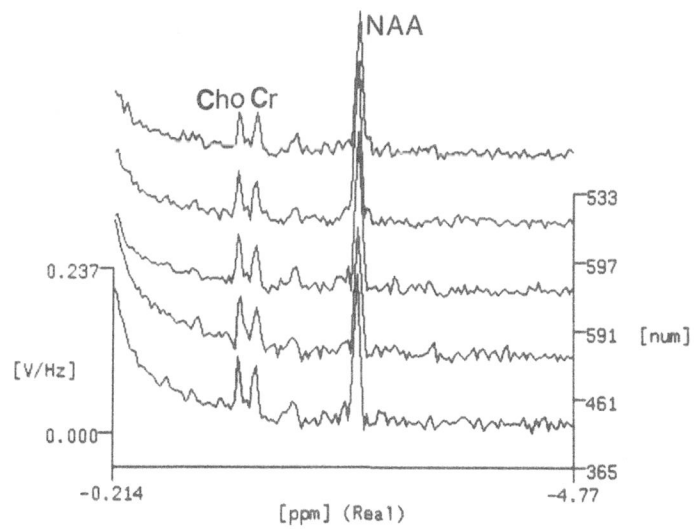

Figure 7. A & B ^{1}H MR spectra from a normal 42-year-old man. Spectra 365, 461, 591, 597, 533 correspond to voxels 1–5, respectively. Note the well defined Cho and Cr peaks, the high signal from NAA and no detectable signal from LA, Ala, or Lip.

DISCUSSION

Interpretation of Chemical Changes

NAA is found exclusively in neurons and their processes, and can be used as a neuronal marker (Nadler, 1972; Coyle, 1989; Gill, 1989; Gill, 1990). NAA has been shown to be generally decreased in tumor spectra (Arnold, 1990; Bruhn, 1989; Alger, 1990; Segebarth, 1990). Several factors may be responsible for the low NAA. Tumors may not contain neurons, there may be neuronal damage from tumor infiltration or compression of normal brain tissue, or there may be metabolic differences in those neurons that are surrounded by astrocytes or are non-functional in the tumor. More NAA is present in glial tumors than metastases or meningiomas, presumably because the latter do not contain neurons. NAA tends to be higher in low grade astrocytomas and intermediate astrocytomas compared to glioblastomas, likely reflecting the greater neuronal loss or damage in the more malignant tumors. Decreased NAA is not a specific feature of neoplasia, however, since any pathologic condition that causes neuronal loss will cause this same spectroscopic finding (Arnold, 1990; Arnold, 1992; Gill, 1989; van der Knaap, 1992; Duijn, 1992; Graham, 1992).

Although no abnormality was apparent on MRI of the contralateral hemisphere of our patients with tumors, NAA was significantly decreased in brain contralateral to the tumors of all our patients. LA was slightly increased in the contralateral hemisphere of all patients except those with low grade astrocytomas compared to the normal subjects. Abnormal metabolite and pH distributions have been demonstrated in the contralateral hemisphere that appeared normal on MRI in two patients with tumors using ^{31}P MRSI and in one studied with ^{1}H MRS (Segebarth, 1990; Hugg, 1992). The decrease of NAA and increase in LA probably results from damage to axonal projections and mass effect.

LA signals have been demonstrated in most malignant tumors and in some benign neoplasms. Increased LA on ^{1}H MRS has been topographically correlated with increased glucose metabolism on PET scans (Alger, 1990; Luyten, 1990). LA may be increased in and around more malignant tumors because they have outgrown or compromised their blood/nutritional supply, or because they are intrinsically glycolytic (Warburg, 1930). LA may also be increased in tumors with large cystic components as these cysts appear to be composed of fluid in which LA accumulates.

Some studies with ^{1}H or ^{31}P MRS or ^{1}H MRSI have failed to show a correlation between LA and histologic grade (Kugel, 1992; Sutton, 1992) although others have (Segebarth, 1990; Luyten, 1990; Arnold, 1990). We observed higher LA signals in all glioblastomas and metastases than low or intermediate-grade astrocytomas. Although it has been suggested that lower-grade astrocytomas, lacking evidence of necrosis, are not hypoxic and therefore do not use anaerobic metabolism, in our experience they appear to generate significant amounts of LA compared to normal brain (Sutton, 1992). Aerobic glycolysis has been known to be a feature of brain tumors for many years.

In our study, very large Lip peaks appear to be characteristic of malignant tumors, especially metastases and glioblastomas. We have not examined other tumors such as dermoids, but Lip was not present in two large epidermoids that we have studied. Two recent examinations of primary intracranial lymphoma (not included in this study) have also shown high LA and Lip peaks. Glioblastomas often show prominent signals from Lip, but these are usually smaller than those of metastases in our untreated patients. Experimental C6 glioma growth in rat brain has shown that Lip increases more than LA with increasing size and grade of the tumor (Remy, 1989). Several explanations are possible for the association of a high Lip signal and malignancy. The Lip may be seen because of release of Lip from membranes or changes in Lip mobility in membranes as the cells become more malignant. High Lip signals probably largely reflect myelin breakdown and the destructive nature of these tumors. In our experience, the highest Lip peaks are detectable in areas of necrosis (very low signal from Cho, Cr, and NAA) (Gill, 1990). Thus, Lip and LA when present may serve as markers for malignant tumors. Characterization of various portions of the tumor differing in malignancy may be possible using LA and Lip values from ^{1}H MRSI. This may be helpful in directing stereotactic biopsy to areas of the tumor which may show the highest degree of malignancy, or away from areas which are only necrotic (Figure 8).

Meningiomas show a characteristic spectral pattern with a resonance from Ala not normally observed in brain (Gill, 1990; Henriksen, 1991; Kugel, 1991; Demaerel, 1991). Ala may be present in other tumors such as glioblastomas, but it is not usually observed in vivo because of the LA resonance (Peeling, 1992; Gill, 1990; Bruhn, 1989).

Cho signals have been noted to be increased in tumor spectra (Arnold, 1990; Gill, 1989; Gill, 1990; Bruhn, 1989; Sutton, 1992). The significance of an increased Cho peak must be assessed in the context of the tumor. In gliomas or metastases, it may reflect cell membrane breakdown. In meningiomas high Cho probably does not reflect cell membrane degradation, but rather higher steady state levels or a change in mobility.

Total Cr concentration is relatively constant throughout normal brain thus, Cr has been used as an internal standard for other resonances that change such as NAA, Cho, and LA. ^{1}H MRSI clearly shows that Cr changes in tumors. Hence we used contralateral or remote areas where Cr appeared unchanged to normalize our spectra.

Analyses for Classification of Tumor Spectra: Making the Spectra Useful

In most reports of tumor spectroscopy, statistical analysis of diagnostic value has been relatively simplistic, usually considering changes in individual resonances one at a time. This ignores information present in the pattern of changes in all the peaks considered together. We utilized a computer-based pattern recognition technique to classify tumor spectra and compared this with histological diagnosis.

Pattern recognition analyses of in vitro spectra has been reported by Howells et al., who developed a scheme employing principal component analysis to classify of ^{1}H MR spectra from normal and malignant rat tissue biopsies, and from other types of cancer using a final cluster analysis (Howells, 1992). Reininghaus et al., were able to perform similar successful analyses on the ^{1}H MR spectra of urine from cancer patients (Reininghaus, 1992). These methods avoid assigning any one chemical peak excessive importance and thus making assumptions regarding the metabolites that are chosen for study. The objective of such pattern recognition is to predict an otherwise obscure property, such as tumor grade or type, of a sample on the basis of indirect measurements.

In the basic classification model which we have utilized (Duda, 1973), input features (e.g. six peak intensities) are passed through a classifier process that assigns a label to the object. The limited size of the initial data sample does not justify the estimation of the underlying probability distribution for the features of the different types of tumors in question, thus eliminating the use of parametric methods such as bayesian classifiers. Therefore, we used a simple non-parametric classification scheme known as the "nearest distance to the mean classifier." Classification was done in six-dimensional metabolite feature space according to which class mean was nearest. The process employed two steps:

(1) In the training step, the mean feature vector for each class of tumor was determined by averaging the feature vectors for each patient for each voxel in the class. certain features such as Ala resonance intensity have high specificity and were consequently weighted.

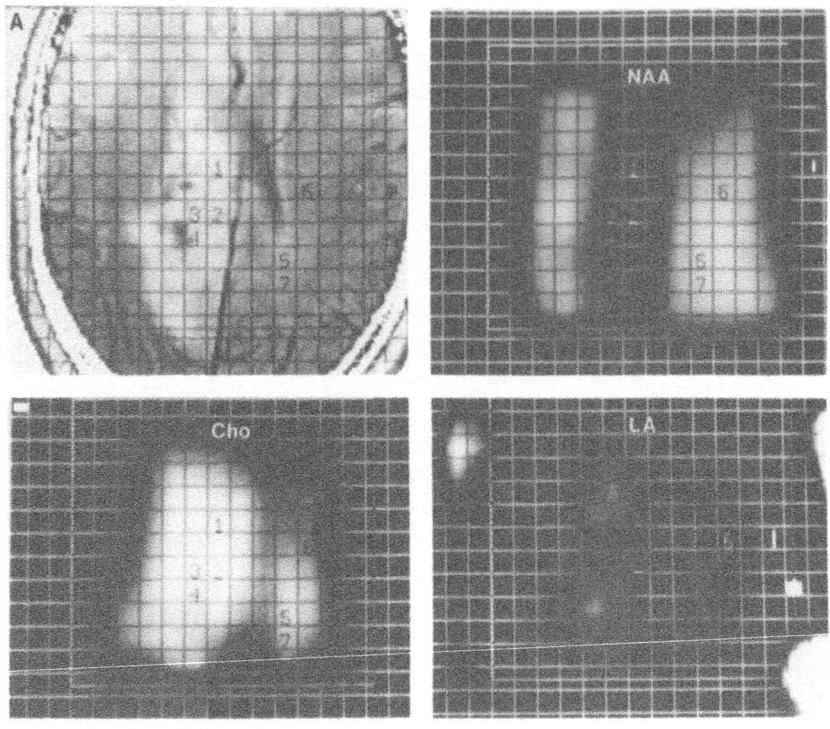

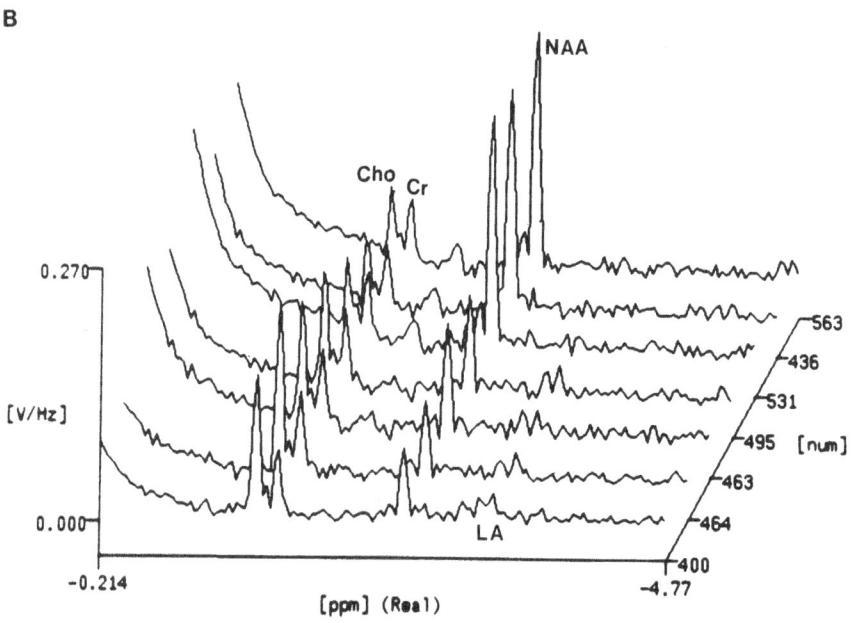

Table 1.

Misclassification Results	Tumor CT/MRI[a] ± Angiography	^{1}H MRSI & Feature Space Classification[a]
Glioblastoma	4/14	0/14
Astrocytoma II[b]	5/14	0/14
Astrocytoma I[c]	3/15	0/15
Metastasis	3/11	0/11
Meningioma	1/5	0/5
Overall Error	16/60 (26%)	0/60 (0%)[d] (6%)[e] (11%)[f]

[a]Number misinterpreted/number total.
[b]Intermediate grade astrocytoma.
[c]Low-grade astrocytoma.
[d]Using averaged central tumor voxels.
[e]Using individual voxels from the center of the tumor.
[f]Using classification of all central and peripheral tumor voxels.

(2) In the classification step, each voxel was assigned the label of the class with the nearest distance to the mean in feature space. In this manner, voxels were labeled with the class that had the most similar features.

The results obtained from the classification based on the average of central voxels were more accurate than classification based on individual central voxels or central and peripheral voxels. Error associated with individual central voxels is "averaged out" by this method allowing the common, unique tumor characteristics to be more obvious, thus allowing for improved tumor discrimination. Because of the error from artifacts due to partial volume effects in peripheral compared to central voxels, diagnostic accuracy was lower using peripheral voxels, although this did not prevent accurate measurements of metabolites in the periphery.

Average central voxel spectra from the 60 tumors and miscellaneous spectra from 10 normals from the training set were correctly classified on retesting. Primary differential diagnosis suggested by neuroradiologists for the same group of tumors using X-ray CT, MRI, with or without angiography was incorrect in 26% of patients (Table 1).

Figure 8. A & B 1H MRSI of a 52-year-old woman admitted for increasing seizure frequency with a known right hemisphere mass for 10 years. One 8 mm proton density-weighted MR image through the 22 mm (cranio-caudal dimension) thick ROI is shown (upper left). Images are labelled according to metabolite. The outline of the ROI is seen as a dotted (vertical) and a continuous (horizontal) line in all images of A. Spectra (nos. 400–563) in B correspond to voxels 1–7, respectively, in A. The mass extended from the right centrum semi-ovale, through the right parietal occipital cortex and into the mesial right temporal structures. Upper right image in A is based on the signal from NAA and shows decreased NAA in the area of the mass. It was believed from conventional MR images that the lesion did not cross the right half of the splenium of the corpus callosum. However, based on information provided by the images based on Cho (lower left) and LA (lower right), a large area of increased Cho signal extends beyond the borders of the mass and even across the splenium into the left hemisphere. The LA image shows two separate areas of slightly increased LA signal in the mass in the right hemisphere and an area of subtly increased LA signal in the area of voxels 5 & 7 which corresponds to an area of slightly increased intensity on the conventional MR image. The latter was thought to be chemical imaging evidence of spread of the tumor across the splenium of the corpus callosum. Histology from image-guided stereotactic biopsies demonstrated that there was increased cellular pleomorphism of the tumor in the area of voxels 3 and 4 and confirmed that there was tumor in the area of voxels 5 and 7.

CONCLUSIONS

Proton MRSI provides non-invasive chemical characterization of brain neoplasia not possible from X-ray CT and MRI. A large training set in six-dimensional feature space modeling the typical biochemical profiles of 60 tumors of the 5 most common human intracranial supratentorial tumor types has been created. This training set is now of adequate size to begin application of automatic classification techniques. By combining ^{1}H MRSI with a computer-based pattern recognition scheme, these data suggest that it may be possible to assign lesions in vivo to diagnostic categories (e.g. tumor or non-tumor, malignant or benign) with known degrees of certainty on the basis of their biochemical nature. These techniques may reduce the need for surgical biopsy, thereby decreasing patient morbidity.

REFERENCES

Alger J.R., Frank J.A., Bizzi A., Fulham M.J., DeSouza B.X., Duhaney M.O., Inscoe S.W., Black J.L., van Zijl P.C.M., Moonen C.T.W., DiChiro G: Metabolism of human gliomas: assessment with H-1 spectroscopy and F-18 fluorodeoxyglucose PET. Radiology 177: 633–641, 1990.

Arnold DL, Shoubridge EA, Villemure JG, Feindel W: Proton and phosphorus magnetic resonance spectroscopy of human astrocytomas in vivo. Preliminary observations on tumor grading. NMR in Biomed 1990; 3: 184–189.

Arnold DL, Emrich JF, Shoubridge EA, Villemure JG, Feindel W: Characterization of astrocytomas, meningiomas, and pituitary adenomas by phosphorus magnetic resonance spectroscopy. J Neurosurg 1991; 74: 447–453.

Arnold DL, Matthews PM, Francis GS, O'Connor J, Antel J: Proton magnetic resonance spectroscopic imaging for metabolic characterization of demyelinating plaques. Ann Neurol 1992; 31: 235–241.

Atlas SW: Intraaxial brain tumors. In: Magnetic Resonance Imaging of the Brain and Spine. SW Atlas (ed). New York: Raven Press, 1991, pp. 223–326.

Bruhn H, Frahm J, Gyngell ML, Merboldt KD, Hanicke W, Sauter R, Hamburger C: Noninvasive differentiation of tumors with use of localized H-1 MR spectroscopy in vivo: initial experience in patients with cerebral tumors. Radiology 172: 541–548, 1989.

Chandrasoma PT: Pathologic evaluation of imaging directed stereotactic biopsy materials. In: Apuzzo MLJ (ed): Malignant Cerebral Glioma. Park Ridge, IL: American Association of Neurological Surgeons, 1990, pp 129–140.

Coyle JT, Robinson MB, Blakely RD, Forloni G-L. The neurobiology of N-acetyl-aspartyl-glutamate. In: Barnard EA, Costa E (eds). Allosteric modulation of amino acid receptors: Therapeutic implications. New York: Raven Press 1989: 319–333.

Darwin RH, Drayer BP, Riederer SJ, Wang HZ, MacFall JR: T2 estimates in healthy and diseased brain tissue: a comparison using various MR pulse sequences. Radiology 1986; 160: 375–381.

Demaerel P, Johannik K, Van Hecke P, Van Ongeval, Verellen S, Marchal G, Wilms G, Plets C, Goffin J, Van Calenbergh F, Lammens M, Baert AL: Localized ^{1}H NMR spectroscopy in fifty cases of newly diagnosed intracranial tumors. J Comput Assist Tomogr 15: 67–76, 1991.

den Hollander JA, Oosterwaal B, van Vroonhoven H, Luyten PR: Elimination of magnetic field distortion in 1H NMR spectroscopic imaging. Society of Magnetic Resonance in Medicine 10th Annual Meeting, 1991; 1: 472 (Abstracts).

Duda RO, Hart PE: Pattern classification and scene analysis. New York: Wiley and Sons, 1973.

Duijn JH, Matson GB, Maudsley AA, Hugg JW, Weiner MW: Human brain infarction: proton MR spectroscopy. Radiology 1992; 183: 711–718.

Gill SS, Small RK, Thomas DGT, Patel P, Porteus R, Van Bruggen, Gadian DG, Kauppinen RA, Williams SR: Brain metabolites as 1H NMR markers of neuronal and glial disorders. NMR in Biomed 2: 196–200, 1989.

Gill SS, Thomas DGT, Van Bruggen N, Gadian DG, Peden CJ, Bell JD, Cox IJ, Menon DK, Iles RA, Bryant DJ, Coutts GA: Proton MR spectroscopy of intracranial tumors: in vivo and in vitro studies. J Comput Assist Tomogr 14: 497–504, 1990

Graham GD, Blamire AM, Howseman, AM, et al.: Proton magnetic resonance spectroscopy of cerebral lactate and other metabolites in stroke patients. Stroke 1992; 23: 333–340.

Henriksen O, Wieslander S, Gjerris F, Jensen KM: In vivo 1H-spectroscopy of human intracranial tumors at 1.5 Tesla. Preliminary experience at a clinical installation. Acta Radiol 1991; 32: 95–99.

Howells SL, Maxwell RJ, Griffiths JR: Classification of tumor 1H NMR spectra by pattern recognition. NMR Biomed 1992; 5: 59–64.

Hugg JW, Matson GB, Twieg DB, Maudsley AA, Sappey-Marinier D, Weiner MW: Phosphorus-31 MR spectroscopic imaging of normal and pathological human brains. Magnetic Reson Imaging 1992; 10: 227–243.

Kazner E, Wende S, Grumme T, Stochdorph O, Felix R, Claussen C: Computed tomography and magnetic resonance tomography of intracranial tumors. Berlin: Spinger-Verlag, 1989.

Kugel H, Heindel W, Ernestus RI, Bunke J, du Mesnil R, Friedmann G: Human brain tumors: spectral patterns detected with localized H-1 MR spectroscopy. Radiology 1992; 183: 701–709.

Lundsford LD, Coffey RJ: Stereotactic surgery in the diagnosis and therapy of malignant intracranial gliomas. In: Apuzzo MLJ (ed): Malignant Cerebral Glioma. Park Ridge, IL: American Association of Neurological Surgeons, 1990, pp 115–128.

Luyten PR, Marien JH, Heindel W, van Gerwen PH, Herholz K, den Hollander JA, Friedmann G, Heiss WD: Metabolic imaging of patients with intracranial tumors: H1 MR spectroscopic imaging and PET. Radiol 1990; 176: 791–799.

Luyten PR, Marien AJ, den Hollander JA: Acquisition and quantitation in proton spectroscopy. NMR Biomed 1991; 4: 64–69.

Nadler JV, Cooper JR: N-Acetyl-L-aspartic acid content of human neural tumors and bovine peripheral nervous tissues. J Neurochem 1972; 19: 313–319

Peeling J, Sutherland G: High-resolution ^{1}H NMR spectroscopy studies of extracts of human cerebral neoplasms. Mag Res Med 24: 123–136, 1992.

Reininghaus FE, Maxwell RJ, Howells SL, Zanker KS, Griffiths JR: Analysis of 1H NMR spectra of urine from cancer patients using pattern recognition technique. 11th Annual Meeting Society of Magnetic Resonance in Medicine, 1992; Works in Progress: 3423 (Abstracts).

Remy C, Von Kienlin M, Lotito S, Francois A, Benabid AL, Decorps M: In vivo 1H NMR spectroscopy of an intracerebral glioma in the rat. Magn Reson Med 1989; 9: 395–401.

Segebarth CM, Baleriaux DF, Luyten PR, den Hollander JA: Detection of metabolic heterogeneity of human intracranial tumors in vivo by 1H NMR spectroscopic imaging. Magn Reson Med 1990; 13: 62–76.

Sutton LN, Wang Z, Gusnard D, Lange B, Perilongo G, Bogdan AR, Detre JA, Rorke L, Zimmerman RA: Proton magnetic resonance spectroscopy of pediatric brain tumors. Neurosurgery 1992; 31: 195–202.

Traber F, Bunke J, Kaiser WA, Layer G, Muller-Lisse U, Reiser M: 1H-MR spectroscopic imaging (MRSI) of brain lesions using improved techniques for water suppression and correction of magnetic field distortions. Society of Magnetic Resonance in Medicine 11th Annual Meeting, 1992; Works in Progress: 1947 (Abstracts).

van der Knaap MS, van der Grond J, Luyten PR, den Hollander JA, Nauta JJP, Valk J: ^{1}H and ^{31}P magnetic resonance spectroscopy of the brain in degenerative cerebral disorders. Ann Neurol 1992; 31: 202–211.

Warburg O: The Metabolism of Tumors. London: Arnold Constable, 1930: 75–325.

INDEX

The manufacturer's authorised representative in the EU is Springer
Nature Customer Service Centre GmbH, Europaplatz 3, 69115 Heidelberg,
Germany. If you have any concerns regarding our products, please
contact ProductSafety@springernature.com

Printed and bound by CPI Group (UK) Ltd, Croydon, CR0 4YY
23/04/2026
02095628-0012